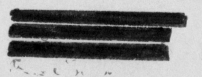

15-21

Second Edition

teaching
elementary
health
science

walter d.
sorochan

stephen j.
bender

san diego
state university

ADDISON-WESLEY PUBLISHING COMPANY

reading, massachusetts • menlo park, california
london • amsterdam • don mills, ontario • sydney

This book is in the
ADDISON-WESLEY SERIES IN HEALTH EDUCATION

Photograph credits:

David Austin/Stock, Boston: p. 1
George Bellerose/Stock, Boston: p. 21
Jean Boughton/Stock, Boston: p. 300
D. Dietz/Stock, Boston: p. 239
Owen Franken/Stock, Boston: p. 318
Rosemary Good: pp. 2, 22, 60, 174, 182, 264, 378, 398
Patricia Hollander Gross/Stock, Boston: p. 240
Marshall Henrichs: pp. i, 208
Ellis Herwig/Stock, Boston: pp. 98, 132,
Ken Heyman: pp. 44, 72, 163, 164, 230, 288, 420
Wally Huntington Photo: p. 118
Anna Kaufman Moon/Stock, Boston: pp. 354, 440
Florence Sharp: pp. 32, 328
Peter Vandermark/Stock, Boston: p. 117

Portions of this text are adapted from Walter D. Sorochan and
Stephen J. Bender, *Teaching Secondary Health Science*, New
York: Wiley, 1978.

Library of Congress Cataloging in Publication Data

Sorochan, Walter D
   Teaching elementary health science.

   (Addison-Wesley series in health education)
   Includes bibliographies and index.
   1. Health education (Elementary) I. Bender,
Stephen J., joint author. II. Title.
LB1587.A3S67 1979   372.3'7   78-62551
ISBN 0-201-07492-3

ISBN 0-201-07492-3
ABCDEFGHIJ-MA-79

To all those prospective elementary teachers who will, we hope, benefit from this book.

preface

This second edition of *Teaching Elementary Health Science* places new emphasis on the specific areas of preparation deemed essential in the development of a competent elementary health educator. A logical approach to teacher preparation has been developed by first introducing the reader to the concept of health. Following is an in-depth study of the child. Additional information focuses on health as a part of the elementary school curriculum, and then a lengthy discussion of process as it relates to elementary health instruction is presented. The concluding material is devoted to exemplary concept lesson plans.

The overall purpose of the text is simple. We have carefully structured the textual material so that even the most uninformed will be aware that a great deal can be done to assist children in attaining optimal well-being. Health, as a quality of life, is a complex concept. Further, it can be defined as a dynamic and evolving process affected by many factors. One of the more influential of these factors is the direction and guidance of a health nature that the child receives in his or her early years. It follows that the elementary teacher can be a strong force in the shaping of a child's health knowledge, attitudes, and habits.

In an effort to assist the elementary teacher in accomplishing such a goal, the second edition of *Teaching Elementary Health Science* is divided into five parts. The first part examines the many meanings of health and suggests a two-dimensional model of well-being. No doubt the reader will have a much better understanding of just what optimal well-being is after reading Chapter 1.

Part II is devoted to an in-depth discussion of how children grow and attain health. Attention is focused on the typical developmental tasks and physical problems experienced by elementary children. Emphasis is also placed on potential emotional and behavioral problems of elementary school youngsters. This information is supplemented by a chapter new to this edition, dealing with values development. Concluding Part II is a chapter concerning the general guidelines for emergency care. Part II is truly unique in that it focuses exclusively on the child.

Part III focuses on the relationship of health education to the elementary school curriculum. Emphasis is placed on the role of the elementary teacher in the school health program. In addition, the elementary health education curriculum is discussed, and the *California Framework for Health Instruction* is provided as an exemplary model.

Part IV deals solely with elementary health instruction. It is in this section that the reader is provided with detailed chapters concerning the conceptual approach, behavioral objectives, learning experiences, evaluation, and finally, concept lesson planning, all of which provide for a sound basis for Part V of the text.

Part V of the text should prove most helpful for all elementary school teachers. Eleven chapters are devoted to exemplary concept lesson plans dealing with most of the health-topic areas relevant to elementary school children. Topical areas covered include the human body, emotional-social health, drugs, tobacco, alcohol, environmental conservation, nutrition, dental health, safety, disease, and family living. Although the complement of lesson plans in each of these areas is not comprehensive, they should provide an excellent basis from which to develop a functional teaching unit.

Last, but certainly not least, we wish to express our sincere appreciation to all those who helped make this book a reality. It is our profound hope that many will benefit from its contents.

San Diego, California   W.D.S.
February 1979   S.J.B.

contents

About the Authors

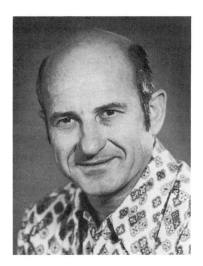

Walter D. Sorochan, H.S.D.
Professor of Health Science
San Diego State University

Walter D. Sorochan was born in Lamont, Alberta, Canada, and reared in a farming community near Vancouver, British Columbia. He received his undergraduate degree in biology and physical education from the University of British Columbia in 1952. Upon receiving his Teacher Training Diploma in 1953, he taught for a year in Kamloops, British Columbia.

After receiving his Master of Science degree from the University of Oregon, Dr. Sorochan taught and coached for six years at the junior and senior high school levels in Vancouver.

He taught health education at Bemidji State College in 1962, thereafter accepting an appointment at Eastern Kentucky University, where he taught health education from 1963 to 1968. During this time, he worked on his terminal degree at Indiana University, receiving his Doctor of Health Science degree in 1969. Since then he has been teaching at San Diego State University, where he is now Professor of Health Science.

His lifestyle reflects his interests: He enjoys music of all kinds, as well as dancing, concerts, and plays; is an avid sports fan; plays sand volleyball on the beach; and often jogs on the beach. Besides fostering health research, he is keenly interested in orthobiosis, self-actualization, and prospective medicine. Professor Sorochan is the author of two other health education texts and numerous articles.

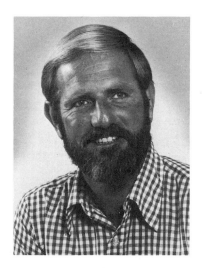

Stephen J. Bender, H.S.D.
Professor of Health Science
San Diego State University

Stephen J. Bender was born and reared in the upstate New York community of Rochester. He received his Bachelor of Science degree in health science from the State University of New York, Brockport, in 1966. He then did graduate study at Indiana University, receiving his Master of Science and Doctor of Health Science degrees in 1968.

Dr. Bender then accepted an appointment as Assistant Professor of Health Science at Memphis State University, Memphis, Tennessee. In 1970 he accepted an appointment in the Department of Health Science at San Diego State University, where he is now Professor of Health Science.

An avid sportsman, Professor Bender's interests include jogging, racquetball, and sports cars, as well as real estate and plants. He is the author of four other health science texts and numerous periodical articles.

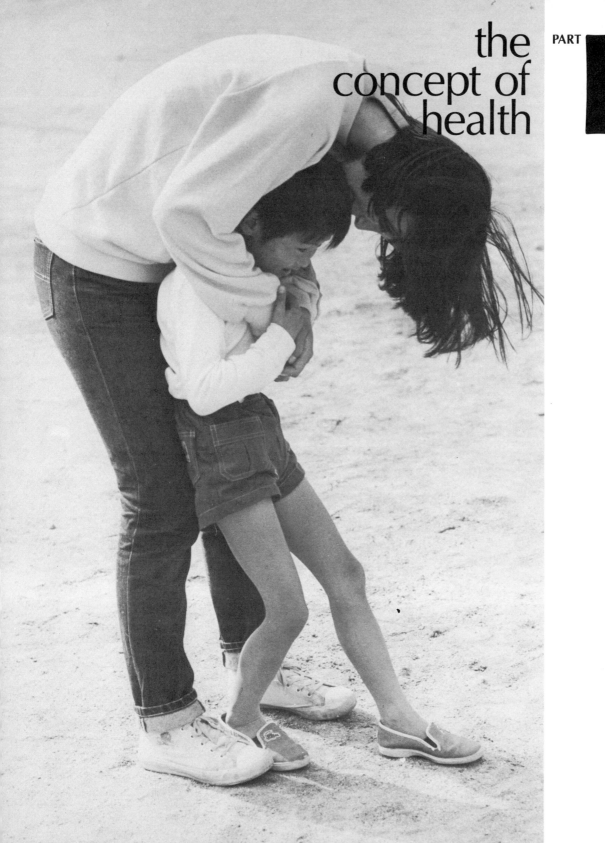

the concept of health

1

CHAPTER 1

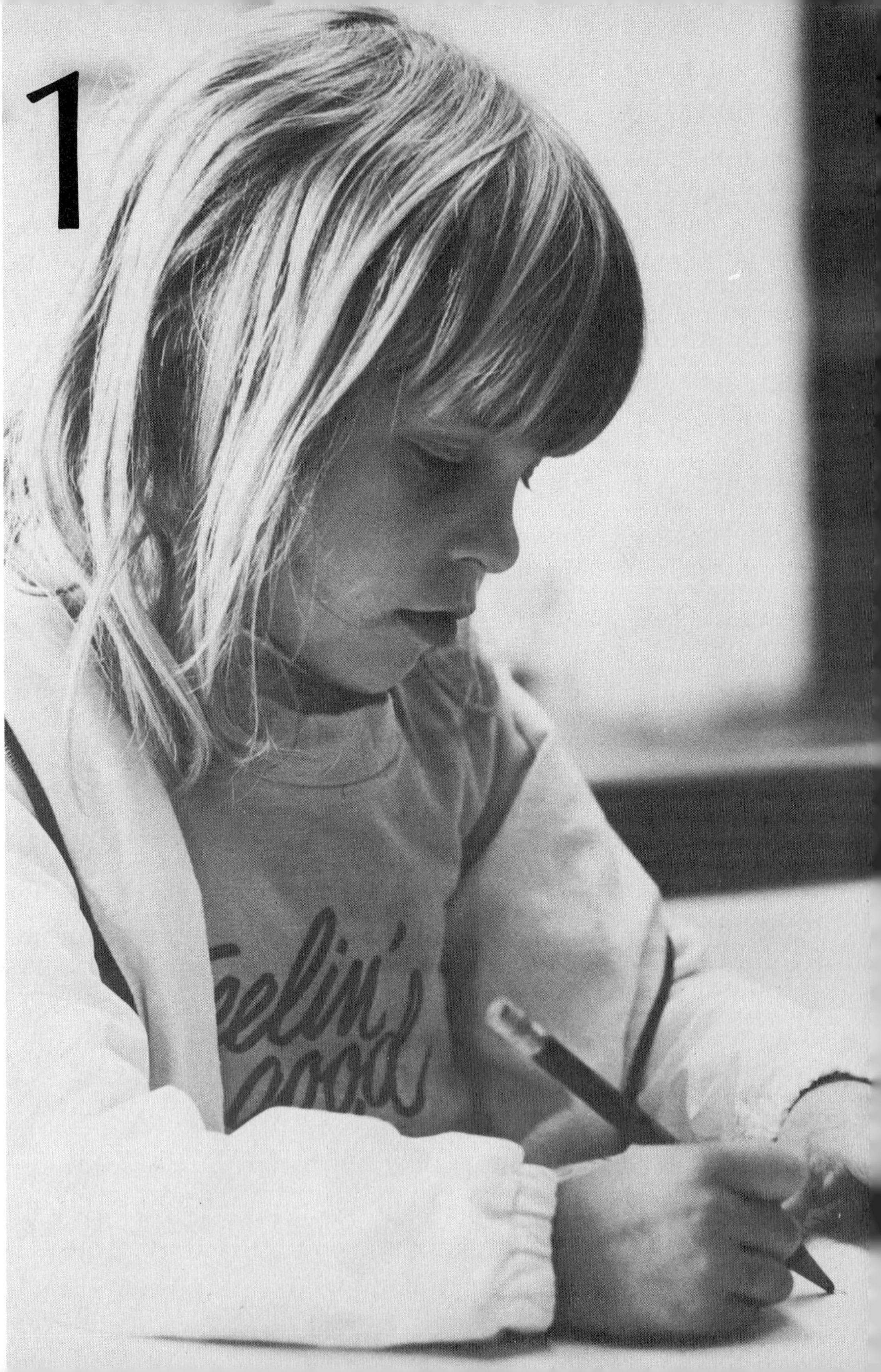

the meaning of health

INTRODUCTION

We spend half our lives getting and keeping health—the other half using health to do those things we want to do. Health is the most precious of gifts!

Americans are becoming more and more concerned about the quality of their lives, and their concern takes many forms. Environmentalists are pointing out how industry and the person on the street are degrading our environment. Ralph Nader and his raiders are focusing attention on the need for more constructive consumerism. Various federal departments and agencies are trying to safeguard the American public from dangerous and new drugs, false advertising, and pollutants and other health hazards. These and many other efforts by voluntary groups, public agencies, and private individuals reflect a genuine concern about the quality of life. Health is to quality of life as foundation is to a house. A sound house is built on a sound foundation. And so it is with life. To fulfill the aspirations of life, we need good health. Unfortunately, such a state is difficult for many Americans to attain.

The health dilemmas for most of us, including elementary teachers, may arise when: (1) our pres-

ent health values are in conflict with one another; (2) our current values are not strong enough as health-mediating variables; (3) our traditional values, in many cases, are in conflict with the values of today; and (4) our present lifestyle is not a strong reinforcer of optimal well-being (or of a high quality of health). Those individuals who have only a shallow and confusing concept of health are most likely to be preyed on by such dilemmas. Furthermore, an inadequate understanding of health creates apathy toward concern for individual, family, and community health. Teachers lacking an adequate concept of health may not be too concerned about the health of the children in their classrooms. They may even be unaware of and unconcerned about their own health status. This is indeed unfortunate, because the elementary teacher can have tremendous influence on the child's evolving constructive hygienic attitudes and habits.

In an effort to orient the prospective elementary teacher to the meaning of the concept "health," this chapter deals with: (1) the contrast between the old and the new concepts of health; (2) the interpretation of health as a concept of well-being; (3) the

3

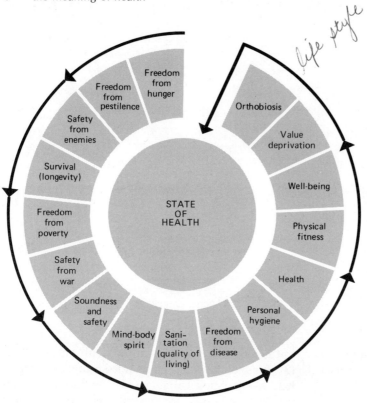

life style

What was your experience
How has it changed?

Fig. 1.1 A historical summary of the meanings that have been given to health.

factors determining well-being; and (4) the relationship of well-being to lifestyle.

OLD CONCEPTS OF HEALTH CONTRASTED WITH NEW CONCEPTS

The meaning of health changes with the times and human social conditions. A historical review of the numerous meanings people have attached to health should be helpful in interpreting the concept of health. Such a review should also help to set the stage for conceptualizing about the modern meaning of health.

Health, in the hygienic sense, evolved over thousands of years as an approach to survival and longevity. Like medicine, health had its beginnings in mystery and superstition in the dark, backward abysm of time. The three Ms—mystery, magic, and medicine—were one and the same. More often than not, they were fixed in the religion of primitive cultures. Life and health were indistinguishable from the three Ms, for all were intertwined in the process of living. Such a concept of living is understandable when we recall that primitive peoples were terrified by the world around them and ascribed disease, as well as other misfortunes, to supernatural and malevolent forces and to the influence of spirits to be placated by sacrifice. Death was, and still is in some cultures, considered a punishment for disobedience. Thus style of life evolved as a struggle to be healthy enough to survive the forces of nature and the environment. The myths and religions of the past reflect the riskiness and complexity of life in ancient and medieval times.

One cannot contemplate the concept of health without considering life, religion, and medicine as integral parts of the whole process. Indeed, the history of either of these would be incomplete and incoherent without some cross-fertilization. And so it is with trying to understand how health has changed with human history.

As has already been pointed out, health evolved as a prerequisite to *survival* and *longevity*. This dual approach was accompanied by the *aspiration for happiness*. Social and hygienic problems evolved the meanings ascribed to health by various cultures. As the problems changed in each culture over the centuries, so too did the concept of health. People's major concern during those adverse times was survival from wars, poverty, hunger, and communicable diseases. Indeed, this ability to survive became a part of the concept of health. Concern over the origin of diseases from the sixteenth to the eighteenth centuries reflects the great adversity of those times—pestilence, illnesses, famine, poverty, and ignorance. The dilemma posed was how to survive against nature—to survive not only wars, but also communicable diseases spread by contaminated water supplies and overcrowding— and it formed a great part of the concept of health.

Eventually, from the threats of suffering or dying from pestilence, starvation, and war, there evolved the health concept of being *sound* and *safe*. With the advent of the Industrial Revolution (1800) and the escalation of trade with the New World, the old problems of living were compounded. Overcrowding, poor sanitation, and adverse living conditions focused attention on health as a *quality of living*. To the Englishman Southwood Smith and to the engineer Edwin Chadwick, it appeared in the 1830s that since disease always accompanied want, dirt, and pollution, health could be restored only by bringing back to the multitudes pure air, pure water, pure food, and pleasant, aesthetic surroundings (a common cry of 1969 and 1970).

The initial sanitary movement in England spread to Boston in the 1840s. Now health became symbolic of *sanitation* and justly so, for poor health was essentially caused by the diseases of insanitation. Health became symbolic of *freedom from disease*. Concern about health was transferred from the individual to the social level. Out of this approach arose social reforms that contributed to the partial solution of the problems in nineteenth-century Europe and America. Awareness of crowd diseases also stimulated a strong humanitarian feeling that the state should become responsible for the people's health.

It took almost 50 years of sanitary and social engineering to bring environmental health of industrial America under control. The problems presented by communicable diseases and insanitation were considerably reduced by 1900. With sanitation no longer a major social problem, attention once again shifted from the public in general to the individual. Personal problems, such as nutrition, personal cleanliness, and health care, focused attention on personal hygiene. Conceptualizing health as *personal hygiene* was in vogue until about 1920, when the term *health* was reintroduced and applied in public and private spheres of life. This concept of health persisted until about 1955, when the national emphasis turned to *physical fitness* as a health concept for many.

As technology flowered into full bloom in the early 1960s, bringing with it new understandings, new lifestyles, and rapid social changes, another major shift of emphasis in conceptualizing health occurred. *Well-being* began to compete with health for recognition and acceptability. Dunn (1961, p. 159) defines well-being as follows:

. . . *high level wellness for the individual is an integrated method of functioning which is oriented toward maximizing the potential of which the individual is capable. It requires that the individual maintain a continuum of balance and purposeful direction within the environment where he is functioning.*

Well-being is based on the concept that our level of well-being is a process that fluctuates from time to time. This semantic-concept struggle is still going on, and most laypeople are unaware of it.

Well-being has now been jolted by another new concept of health: *"valueness* or *value wellness."* Valuelessness is simply a state of apathy or indecision about life in general. Such a state may result from either a conflict of old and new values or a deprivation or lack of values by which to conduct one's life. Persons living with value conflicts have difficulty adjusting to life in the United States today. People feeling a deprivation of values tend to withdraw from society or to reject the establishment programs and consequently feel thwarted in living up to their optimal potentials. We need more background on the evolution of valuelessness to be able to interpret health as value wellness.

Value wellness reflects another major shift of emphasis about health since 1960. It reflects a reaction to an emerging health problem in our society—a problem originating in technology and the new sociohygienic needs of our ever-changing society. Technology has rocketed us into a new epoch, one characterized by new values toward health, education, industry, war, politics, religion, and life. This new epoch began about 1950 and resulted from the sudden transition from mechanical to electronic technology. Machines have provided us with an abundance of the commodities and services that are essential for providing the biological necessities of life. Electricity has simply accelerated the availability of the products and services of the machine age and more or less assured us of survival.

People who have sufficiently fulfilled all of their basic biological needs are no longer motivated by them primarily. Instead, they are turned on by higher needs, or metavalues. People feeling such higher needs are capable of becoming self-actualizing persons. Although such persons are sufficiently free of illness and sufficiently gratified in their biological needs, they are motivated by altruistic and self-realization values. When such persons are deprived of or are culturally stifled in attaining their metavalues, they evolve valuelessness feelings, such as alienation, loss of identity, extrapunitiveness, whining, emptiness, rootlessness, the feeling of helplessness, and other psychosocial frustrations. Such persons have a conflict of values, for they have difficulty in placing a priority on *metaneed* over biological needs. In addition, the old values that had directed human behavior since the dawn of civilization have now come into conflict with the new values of the electromagnetic era. Technology has brought destruction of the ethical values to the Western world just as the Industrial Revolution brought vast destruction of human values. Maslow (1964, p. 82) perceives the destruction, the stifling, and the conflict of human values as the ultimate social disease of our time.

Reinforcing Maslow's recognition of valuelessness as the ultimate social disease of our time is the concept of *"future shock"* described by Alvin Toffler (1970). Future shock occurs when people cannot adjust quickly enough to changes. People become bewildered by the razzle-dazzle of change, frustrated in not being able to understand it, and psychologically disoriented and emotionally distressed by not being able to cope successfully or quickly enough to keep pace. Accelerated change appears to disturb our inner equilibrium, cause a misreading of reality and a breakdown in communication, and paralyze our ability to make decisions. We experience feelings of transience, or temporariness and rootlessness, in everyday life. Such feelings carry over to our relationships with people, things, places, ideas, and time. The duration of relationships is cut short, and we experience a rapid turnover of them. As a consequence, we have become a *"throwaway"* society and have adapted this mentality to most aspects of our lives. We rent instead of buying a house; we buy a new car instead of repairing an old one; we use disposable paper towels, plates, and cups; we have shorter-lasting friendships and marriages; we eat out more often; we buy fashionable clothes more often; and so on. Thus the more rapidly changing our society, the more temporarily our needs are fulfilled.

Such changes, a consequence of uncontrolled consumerism technology, result in psychological injury or future shock. The initial symptoms of such shock have already been identified under value deprivation. Many of these initial feelings of discontent and frustration become transformed into secondary behavioral aberrations and are expressed overtly as bizarre dress, drug abuse, alcoholism, withdrawal from society, belligerence, vulgarity, lawlessness, and other psychopathologies. Collectively, these form a syndrome of value deprivation, or valuelessness. Thus value wellness needs to be included in the concept of well-being (or health). Although this approach may be startling, it is an essential one if teachers in this country are going to be effective in preventing millions of children from developing emotional problems and disorders and psychological aberrations.

Finally, health has recently been conceived as a style of living (Sorochan, 1968, pp. 673-686). The term "orthobiosis" was originally coined by the Russian microbiologist Metchnikoff to mean "right or proper style of living." The definition implies behavioral and ecological interaction of human beings with their physical and social environments. It reflects how we conduct our lives each day. Right style of living engenders all factors that may affect longevity, quality of well-being, and a more abundant life. It should be considered as conceptualizing health, for many sociohygienic problems stem from the consequences of our misbehaviors and maladaptations.

It should be obvious by now that the meaning people give to health changes with the times and social conditions, Health has been conceptualized as survival and longevity, soundness and safety,

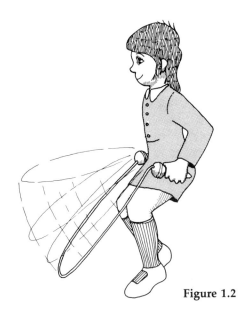

Figure 1.2

quality of living, freedom from disease, personal hygiene, physical fitness, well-being, value wellness, and orthobiosis (style of living).

Teachers should be aware that the meaning they give to health reflects the quality and quantity of health that they themselves possess. Their interpretation of health probably evolved in a number of ways from: the sociocultural climate that was created at the time of child rearing and schooling, experiences of suffering from diseases, and experiencing good and positive feelings about health and living in general. The meaning a teacher gives to health becomes a mediating behavioral force in his or her personal life and in the emphasis he or she places on teaching for health.

LEVELS OF WELL-BEING

Exploring further the concept of health from a contemporary point of view, we find that it can be more precisely conceptualized as levels of well-being. The interpretation by the President's Commission on the Health Needs of the Nation of health as

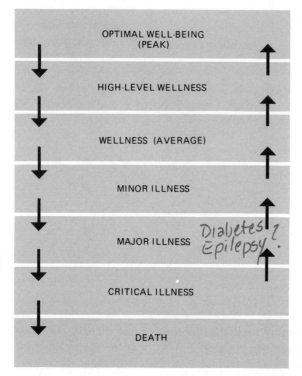

OPTIMAL WELL-BEING
(PEAK)

HIGH-LEVEL WELLNESS

WELLNESS (AVERAGE)

MINOR ILLNESS

MAJOR ILLNESS   *Diabetes?*
                     Epilepsy.

CRITICAL ILLNESS

DEATH

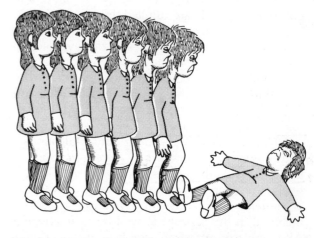

Fig. 1.3 Levels of wellness. The levels of well-being extend from zero wellness (death) at one end of a continuum to optimal well-being at the other end.

levels of well-being (Dunn, 1957, 1961; Hoyman, 1962), and as gradations of health (Rogers, 1960) reinforce such conceptualization. Well-being may be interpreted as a stepladder, with optimal well-being at the top and death at the bottom of the continuum (see Fig. 1.3). In between are gradations, or levels, of wellness.

Health is not a state, but a process. The word "state" implies a static and stable condition, whereas process implies continual adaption or adjustment. Hence wellness, when symbolized by the stepladder idea, implies that one's level of well-being may fluctuate from time to time. As a process, it is dynamic and ever-changing. For example, while reading this paragraph, you may categorize your level of well-being as near the upper third of the stepladder in Fig. 1.3. But suppose that in a few minutes, you decide to cross the street. While cross-

ing the street, you are struck by an automobile. Bleeding profusely from a severed artery, you are faint, in shock, and in a critical-illness level, approaching death. Your level of well-being dropped from a high level to a low level in a matter of a few minutes. But this example highlights the fact that wellness is a dynamic process; the level of well-being can change very suddenly. It also points out that a person's well-being is the integrated result of continuous body changes and the ongoing adaptation to one's physical and social environments. Well-being obviously is a nebulous and abstract concept. It is one that is impossible to measure precisely or to define lucidly.

Although well-being cannot be measured at the present time, it may be theoretically identified by five fitness components: physical, emotional, social, spiritual, and cultural fitness (see Fig. 1.4).

Each type of fitness identifies a different dimension of wellness. The fitness components may be characterized by the following salient features:

1. Physical fitness (maintenance of body processes):
   a) efficient functioning of body systems and organs
   b) ability to resist infections and communicable diseases
   c) freedom from disease, infirmity, or physical disorder
   d) avoiding substances and experiences hazardous to optimal physical fitness
   e) eating a variety and a balance of foods regularly
   f) overall minimum muscular strength
   g) minimum cardiovascular-respiratory-muscular endurance
   h) neuromuscular coordination, flexibility, and balance
   i) weight normal for body height, age, sex, and body density

2. Emotional (mental) fitness (feelings, thoughts, and self-identity):
   a) coping successfully with the stresses of daily living
   b) being flexible in all social situations
   c) feeling worthwhile and adequate as a person
   d) feeling content and happy
   e) feeling a sense of accomplishment and self-realization
   f) facing up to and accepting reality
   g) feeling worthwhile as a member of society by meeting the demands of life
   h) having emotional stability

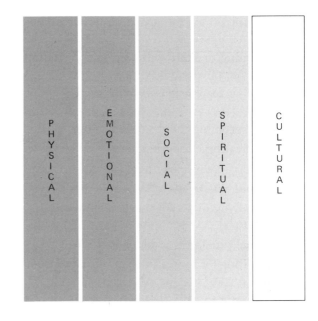

Fig. 1.4 Five fitness components of well-being are interrelated and interdependent.

   i) exercising self-discipline and self-confidence
   j) accepting responsibility for one's behavior and social roles
   k) feeling good about self and others
   l) having worthwhile hobbies and recreational interests
   m) being able to give, express, and accept love
   n) having an adequate self-image

3. Social fitness (relating to others):
   a) having a human approach to living and to dealing with others
   b) setting up own minimum moral standards of conduct (rectitude)

c) having ethical integrity in interpersonal relationships

d) wanting to share with and to contribute to the happiness and welfare of others

e) feeling responsible for others

f) socializing by doing things with others and by becoming involved with others

g) cultivating close friends

h) being able to make new friends

i) being able to relate to people of all ages

j) behaving in socially acceptable ways (morals)

4. Spiritual fitness (aspirations and ideals):

a) aspiring for a safer and a more abundant life for oneself and for one's society

b) aspiring toward "the better things in life"

c) feeling an awareness of a purpose in life and that living, and life itself, are worthwhile

d) being able to appreciate aesthetics

e) having ambition to achieve and to accomplish

f) being able to give way to creative imagination as well as aptness to express creativity

g) being able to set attainable goals and to experience success and self-fulfillment of these

h) having courage to face the unknown

i) willing to take calculated risks

j) feeling that what you do is worthwhile and appreciated by others

5. Cultural fitness (identity with community):

a) responsible involvement in community affairs

b) serving others as a public servant

c) being a contributing member of society

d) attending and/or participating in cultural festivities and social functions, e.g., concerts, plays, and museums. Cultural involvement would include music, art, dance, drama, and other aesthetic aspects of living wherein the talents and creativities of self and/or others may be publicly appreciated.

Although these fitnesses have been exemplified as separate entities, they are normally undetectable, are a part of the whole, and are interdependent. For example, physical fitness is conceived as the prerequisite for all the remaining fitnesses and is the easiest of the fitnesses to identify. It is not possible for a person with a high degree of physical fitness but a low social or a low spiritual fitness to have optimal well-being. Collectively, all five fitnesses complement one another additively and are responsible for contributing to a qualitative lifestyle. Each expresses a different and distinct dimension of wellness.

The characteristics of each of the components of wellness reflect American values. Cultural and subcultural value differences would modify some of the characteristics in each of the components.

When we superimpose the concept of fitness in Fig. 1.4 over the concept of levels of wellness in Fig. 1.3, we can visualize health. It becomes a dynamic, ever-changing concept. In addition, we provide a certain degree of accountability to the concept of wellness. The superimposed model is illustrated by Fig. 1.5. Consider the vertical stepladder symbolizing wellness as having horizontal gradations. Also consider the possibility of physical, emotional, social, spiritual, and cultural fitnesses functioning as separate dimensions that would run up and down the stepladder of wellness. If each fitness could independently fluctuate up and down, each fitness by itself could drop one's level of wellness. This could also happen if two or more fitnesses collectively dropped into the middle or lower third of the wellness stepladder. Each fitness could be conceived as a two-directional conveyor belt, capable of moving up and down. With such mobility, it would have the ability to somehow influence the remain-

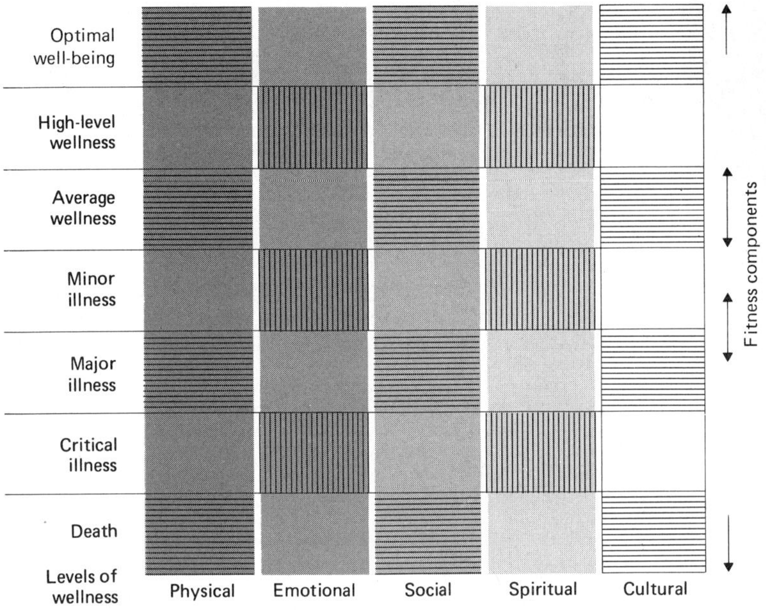

Fig. 1.5 Fitness components superimposed over levels of wellness. Each fitness fluctuates interdependently, modifying the levels of other fitnesses, thereby raising or lowering the whole level of well-being.

ing fitnesses, thereby lowering one's former level of total well-being and consequently one's potentials for self-actualization. The reverse would also be true.

The potentials for optimal well-being for persons with various disorders and disabilities are graphically illustrated in Fig. 1.6. Each example is a projected estimate of the effect that the disorder or disability may have in enhancing the person's potential for optimal well-being. Although each of the fitnesses appears to be unidimensional and to exclude the others, the opposite is probably true in everyday living. Fitnesses may either complement or diminish one another. Often, a person will have a diminished fitness as the result of alcoholism, a cardiovascular disorder (heart disease), or emphysema. Such conditions physiologically incapacitate a person, although he or she may appear and function as though having optimal well-being. In all probability, the other fitnesses compensate for the diminished fitness, thereby masking out and

balancing the alcoholic's disability or disorder. But the optimal potential for physical fitness has been somewhat diminished and may thereby lower the person's potentials for maximizing the other fitnesses. In this case, the cumulative effect of all five fitnesses is such that peak optimal well-being is reduced, and consequently the disabled would experience a lowered level of well-being.

There is no doubt that disability interferes with the realization of one's full genetic potential as a human being. Although one can fulfill one's basic life-maintenance needs, one may often have difficulty in obtaining complete and ultimate satisfaction and happiness from life. Futhermore, the person with diminished health may have difficulty becoming a self-actualizing person in the ultimate sense, for she or he cannot function at top level. However, the degree to which a disability imposes limitations varies greatly. The well-adjusted and controlled diabetic whose morale is high, who is confident and secure in the face of his or her limita-

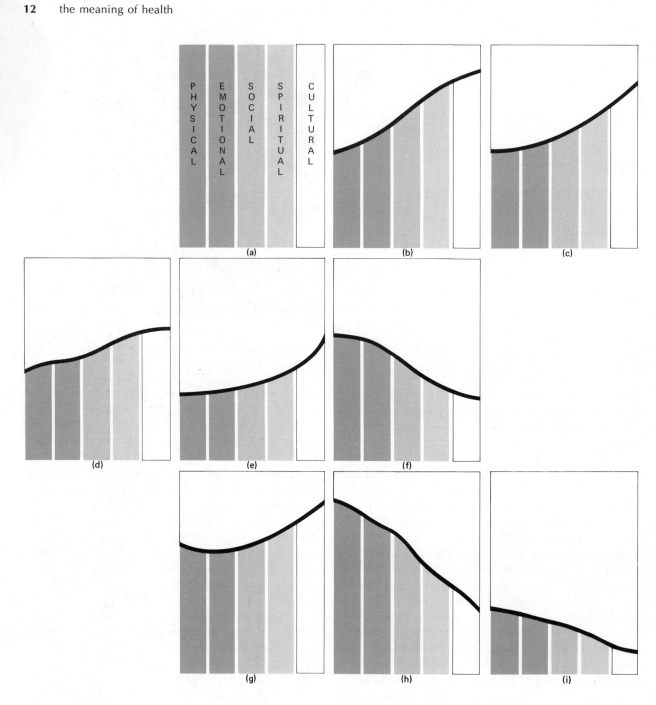

tions, and who accepts the obstacles presented by the condition as a challenge to be responded to positively and successfully may well feel self-actualized. Despite a less than optimal well-being, the person with a disability may achieve a high level of satisfaction in knowing that he or she has fulfilled his or her ultimate personal potential.

Elementary teachers in particular need a positive concept of well-being—one that enhances their personal lives and is relevant to fulfilling their responsibilities as health educators. Elementary school teachers serve as exemplary models of optimal well-being to their children and directly and indirectly influence their sociohygienic behaviors. When a teacher symbolizes a level of optimal well-being, pupils tend to respect him or her more as a person. By respecting the teacher and his or her wellness status, children are more willing to accept that teacher as a source of health information or as one whose sociohygienic habits they can emulate. For example, it is difficult for an obese teacher to teach effectively about nutrition and dieting, for the obesity makes the children perceive the teacher as an obvious hypocrite. Likewise, the teacher who is a chronic cigarette smoker and who points out the hazards of smoking is both a poor exemplary model

◀ **Fig. 1.6** A comparison estimate of the potentials for optimal well-being for persons with various disorders and disabilities: (a) normal, healthy person; (b) diabetic; (c) lack of excersise; (d) cardiovascular disorder; (e) emphysema; (f) chronic alcoholic; (g) overweight; (h) value deprivation; (i) cumulative effect of (c) and (f). The height of each fitness column is a projected estimate of the effect that the disorder or disability may have on the person's realizing his or her potential for optimal well-being.

and a very weak source of information about cigarette smoking.

On the other hand, teachers who practice the mediating concepts of well-being in their everyday lives evolve credibility for wellness in the eyes of their pupils. The importance of teachers' exemplifying a style of life that reinforces optimal well-being cannot be overemphasized. An understanding of the concept of well-being will help you as a prospective teacher to clarify your own concepts of wellness. A teacher with a meaningful and relevant concept of well-being will undoubtedly be more effective in helping children evolve sound sociohygienic habits than will a teacher lacking such a concept.

FACTORS DETERMINING WELL-BEING

Well-being is determined by three things: (1) heredity; (2) environment; and (3) ecological interactions or behaviors. These three factors influence the quality and quantity of optimal well-being as well as lifestyle. All phenomena of well-being and life are conditioned by the interplay of these three determinants.

The potentials for optimal well-being are genetically determined at birth. This endowment includes potentialities for behavior and development throughout one's lifetime. Ability to resist diseases, to fight infections, and to withstand stresses is largely due to genotypic makeup. Medical research points out that people inherit disorders such as diabetes, poor vision, poor muscle tone, and susceptibilities to epilepsy, obesity, various allergies, dental caries, cancer, heart disease, and respiratory infections. Likewise, cognitive, or intellectual, creative, musical, artistic, athletic, and other talents and abilities are inherited. Within these inherited traits are potentialities for behavior and growth. Although a person may have a predisposition to an ability, it is usually latent and needs to be developed. Often an ability evolves in a natural manner when conditions in the environment foster its growth. Basically, the raw material structuring what one is or can be and the kind of well-being that person can enjoy are limited by inheritance.

No genetic trait is so dependent on heredity as not to require certain minimal environmental conditions for its development. This is true even of physical traits and certainly more so of intellectual and emotional ones. At any given moment an individual is the product of countless interactions between his or her genetic endowment and the physical and sociocultural environments.

The physical environment is more stable than social and cultural environments. Making up the physical, or natural, environment are water, air, soil, food, and the numerous plants, animals, and microorganisms. It also includes the by-products of human activities, such as industrial wastes, garbage and sewage, housing, automobiles and their exhausts, pesticides and other drugs and chemicals, empty bottles and cans, and even heat and noise. All of these things are capable of enhancing or undermining one's physical, emotional, social, spiritual, and cultural well-being.

In much the same way that we receive a genetic heritage, we also receive a sociocultural heritage. Every culture and group has its language, family and social structure, customs, values, and aesthetic arts. Life in the human environment is mediated by cultural values. Values, in turn, direct our behaviors and social and ecological interactions. Our social environment molds our status and role in the group, as well as the quality of interpersonal relationships within the group. Under ordinary conditions the sociocultural environment plays a far more crucial role than the physical surroundings in shaping our personalities and in fostering the realizations of our skills, abilities, and potentialities.

The individual has the ability to thrive in his or her environments. A person is continuously interacting with everything in the surroundings. The thrust of these interactions may be thought of as

being directed toward the establishment of a harmonious balance between the forces in the environment and the individual. Such a person-environment relationship is referred to as ecological interaction. Through these interactions an individual is expressing the particular ways in which she or he chooses to adapt and adjust to the stresses presented by the environments. Behavioral scientists would probably refer to ecological interactions as simply adaptive behavior. The point to be made here is that ecological interactions or behaviors are strong determiners of one's well-being.

For example, the polluted air in Los Angeles predisposes many children to respiratory irritations, and some children already have premature initial symptoms of emphysema. Other children in the area suffer from many recurring respiratory infections. The air they breathe has been polluted because of the widespread use of the car as a means of transportation. Such adaptation has been conditioned by people's cultural expectations and needs for locomotion. In response to social and cultural pressures, people's behavior has resulted in polluting the very atmosphere that they and their children breathe. On the other hand, social interactions also determine our well-being. A child who does not play by the rules may not be accepted by his or her playmates. Such a child will feel rejected and emotionally distressed. Both of these examples illustrate the concept of adaptive behavior influencing well-being.

Adaptive behavior is most difficult to understand. One's well-being may be an indirect outcome of two, three, or more factors or circumstances in the environment working together to initiate a disorder or disease on the one hand or to foster well-being on the other. Dubos (1968) suggests that one's well-being and lifestyle are an indirect outcome of a constellation of circumstances rather than the direct result of a single determined factor. Hence the prevailing factors or circumstances do not cause a disease state individually, but only through their collective interplay. For example, heart disease may be the consequence of eating too many rich foods, lack of regular exercise, cigarette smoking, and the emotional stress of living. A cold may eventuate when the cold virus becomes virulent in a child who has not been eating properly, who feels depressed, who is fatigued, and whose viral immunity is low. People who retire from work, have no job to go to, are depressed, have few friends, live alone, and have no outside social interests become tired of living and tend to die early. In all of these examples, the disease or death state may be initiated through a collective interplay of physical and social forces acting together as a syndrome in the environment. Such interplay is the basis for suggesting the *multicausation* theory of not only disease and illness, but also optimal well-being. The multicausation syndrome for optimal well-being would be the collective interplay of the physical, emotional, social, spiritual, and cultural fitnesses. Whether these fitnesses are maximized in the person depends on how he or she interacts with the environments.

Many of our adaptive behaviors are destructive and do not maximize the potentialities for optimal well-being. For example, in the process of adjusting to the fast pace of life in the United States and trying to cope with the problems of life in general, Americans often adapt to emotional stress by trying to find immediate gratification instead of relief for their tensions and anxieties. They may not fulfill their real need in satisfying ways. Smoking cigarettes, having several cups of coffee during work, or having a cocktail or two after work seems to relieve tension. However, such behaviors may become maladaptive in that they may eventually, if repeated long enough, become destructive to the individual. Behavior may also be perceived as destructive in that it may not be the best alternative for coping with the stress of living. Such behaviors can often become misbehaviors, as when a person becomes a chronic cigarette smoker, consequently in-

creasing not only his or her susceptibility to respiratory infections, but also the chances of possibly contracting emphysema and/or lung cancer. Likewise, having a cocktail may become self-defeating if the intoxicated person has a serious car accident, fails to be responsible for his or her actions, or neglects to eat a balanced diet regularly.

In similar fashion, children's coping behaviors can become either destructive or constructive habits. Ideally, elementary children, in their formative years, will be exposed to teachers and parents who can and will help them to adapt positively by providing healthy sociocultural reinforcers for optimal well-being.

In summary, level of well-being is the resultant of the entire complex of a person's interactions with his or her environments. Wellness may also be interpreted as a sense of balance or equilibrium resulting from adaptation between people and their environments. Although heredity, environment, and behavior all play a hand in determining one's well-being, today that being is conditioned largely by cultural behaviors. Teachers should be aware that the school needs to be a cultural environment that reinforces opportunities for optimal well-being.

LIFESTYLE INFLUENCES WELL-BEING

The process of living is made up of fulfilling basic health needs. The model of well-being suggests this idea. One's style of living is reflected by how one performs daily household chores, daily tasks, and how one assumes responsibility for self, family, and society. The "rules of good living" include how and when one brushes one's teeth, washes and dries dishes, relaxes and rests, uses drugs—including cigarettes, coffee, soft drinks, and alcoholic beverages—uses seat belts, and exercises; how, when, and what one eats; toilet habits; how one disposes of garbage, does things or plays with friends, and gets to and from work; how often and when one watches television; how, when, and whether one gives and receives love; whether one is prompt for work; how one aspires for safety and security, copes with the problems of living, relates to people of all ages; the degree of involvement in community affairs; and so on. Maslow refers to these examples in his hierarchy of human needs as basic, or low-level, needs. These are the life-support activities that keep us alive (see Fig. 1.7).

A style of living may either stifle or enhance well-being. Awareness of this possibility prompted Russian microbiologist Metchnikoff (Dubos, 1961, p. 141) to suggest that there is a right, or proper, style of living that allows one to have optimal health, thereby extending one's longevity. He referred to this mode of living as "orthobiosis." It reflects how we conduct our lives each day, including how we carry out the daily chores so essential to maintain and keep us alive. Orthobiosis implies responsible, abundant, fulfilling, purposeful, and prudent daily living for both individuals and society.

Orthobiosis is more important than health, because health is a by-product of how we live. A right style of living is one that is constructive instead of destructive, salubrious instead of deleterious, enhancing instead of diminishing, healthful instead of illness-inducing, adaptive instead of maladaptive, fulfilling and gratifying instead of frustrating, socially acceptable instead of socially rejectable, and so on. Obviously, one's lifestyle needs a sense of balance and correctness to it for one to be an "orthobiot."

One's lifestyle evolves in an effort to fulfill one's needs (see Fig. 1.8). Note that a person will be healthy if he or she is able to fulfill most of his or her needs. On the other hand, a person's lifestyle may be characterized by self-destructive behavior that may cause illness, disability, or a lower level of functioning. If the person is not fulfilling his or her needs properly, illness, disability, or poor health—symptoms of inability to fulfill health needs—may result.

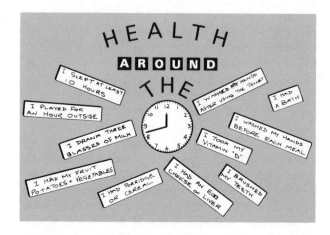

Fig. 1.7 "Health Around the Clock" theme for a bulletin board.

Elementary school teachers should be aware that children bring to school their good and bad habits of living. These habits reflect many alternative lifestyles in the United States today. Teachers should be aware that children attach themselves to a hero or subculture group and then emulate the habits, values, and behaviors of that group's lifestyle. For example, the lifestyles of Elvis Presley and the Beatles (clothes, hairdo, behaviors, etc.) were copied by many children and teenagers in the 1960s.

The message of this section is an obvious one. Optimal well-being accrues from one's style of living. Instead of emphasizing attainment of positive health habits and behaviors, elementary school teachers need to push for orthobiosis. Orthobiosis provides a lifestyle package that includes health and has built-in motivational opportunities for

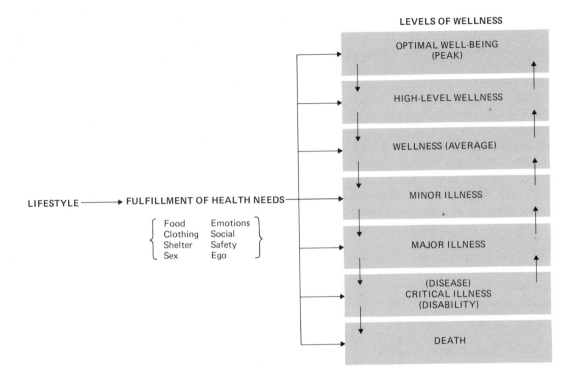

LEVELS OF WELLNESS

OPTIMAL WELL-BEING
(PEAK)

HIGH-LEVEL WELLNESS

WELLNESS (AVERAGE)

MINOR ILLNESS

MAJOR ILLNESS

(DISEASE)
CRITICAL ILLNESS
(DISABILITY)

DEATH

LIFESTYLE ⟶ FULFILLMENT OF HEALTH NEEDS

Food   Emotions
Clothing   Social
Shelter   Safety
Sex   Ego

quality and quantity of well-being. Although this approach breaks with traditional health-education philosophy of directly teaching health topics per se, teachers should be realistic about the failures of such traditional approaches. Today's American lifestyle dominates health behaviors. Instead of focusing on just the development of health habits, teachers need to give serious attention to helping children evolve constructive lifestyles. Teachers need to exemplify and illustrate orthobiotic lifestyles, for elementary school children are at an impressionable and idealistic age of molding lifestyles. They are a few years away from accepting specific lifestyles. Teachers should help children become aware that well-being is a consequence of lifestyle.

Teachers should also be aware that lifestyle has power. It is through our styles of living that we express ourselves and fulfill our basic human

Fig. 1.8 Relationships among lifestyle, human health needs, optimal well-being, illness, disease, and death. Human health needs are those suggested by Maslow (physiological, safety, social, ego, and self-actualization). Health, disease, and death are all a consequence of how human health needs are fulfilled through lifestyle.

needs. Once a commitment has been made to a lifestyle, a child is able to rule out many decisions that affect his or her well-being. A specific lifestyle excludes other health alternatives. Thus an early commitment to a lifestyle is a decision that identifies habits, behaviors, dress, food, drug use, activity, and so on. Teachers should provide classroom reinforcers for orthobiosis.

This chapter has explored the theory of health as it is related to a style of living. The prerequisite to teaching optimal well-being is for a teacher to have a good concept of health. We hope that this chapter has helped you to clarify your own theory of health, as well as your aspirations for a style of living.

REVIEW QUESTIONS

1. Can health be defined? Why?
2. What is the qualitative difference between optimal well-being and average well-being?
3. What is orthobiosis?
4. What is meant by levels of wellness?
5. What are the suggested fitness components of well-being?
6. What is health—process or state?
7. Does an overweight child have the same potentiality for optimal well-being as a child who is of average body weight?
8. What determines a child's well-being?
9. Explain the multicausation theory in terms of heart disease.
10. What is the relationship between basic human health needs and well-being?
11. Which is a consequence of the other—health or lifestyle?
12. List five characteristics of social fitness and spiritual fitness, respectively.
13. Why does a child need optimal well-being?

REFERENCES AND BIBLIOGRAPHY

Dubos, Rene. *Mirage of Health* (Garden City, N.Y.: Anchor Doubleday, 1961).

———. *So Human An Animal* (New York: Charles Scribner's Sons, 1968).

Dunn, H. L. "Points of Attack for Raising the Levels of Wellness," *Journal of the American Medical Association* (July 1957): 225.

———. *High Level Wellness* (Washington, D.C.: Mt. Vernon, 1961).

Fromm, Erich. *The Revolution of Hope* (New York: Bantam Books, 1968).

Glasser, William. *Reality Therapy* (New York: Harper & Row, 1965).

Hoyman, H. S. "Our Modern Concepts of Health," *Journal of School Health* (September 1962): 253.

Illich, Ivan. *Deschooling Society* (New York: Harper & Row, 1971).

McLuhan, Marshall. "Playboy Interview: Marshall McLuhan," *Playboy* (March 1969).

Maslow, Abraham H. *Religions, Values and Peak Experiences* (Columbus: Ohio State University Press, 1964).

———. *Eupsychian Management* (Homewood, Ill.: Dorsey Press, 1965).

———. "A Theory of Metamotivation: The Biological Rooting of the Value-Life," *Journal of Humanistic Psychology* (Fall 1967).

———. *Toward a Psychology of Being* (New York: Van Nostrand Reinhold, 1968).

May, Rollo. *Man's Search for Himself* (New York: New American Library, 1967).

Reich, Charles A. *The Greening of America* (New York: Random House, 1970).

Rogers, E. S. *Human Ecology and Health* (New York: Macmillan, 1960).

Rosen, G. *A History of Public Health* (New York: M. D. Publications, 1958).

Selye, Hans. *The Stress of Life* (New York: McGraw-Hill, 1959).

Sills, David L., ed. *International Encyclopedia of the Social Sciences* (New York: The Free Press, 1968).

Sorochan, Walter D. "Health Concepts as a Basis for Orthobiosis," *The Journal of School Health* (December 1968): 673-682.

Toffler, Alvin. *Future Shock* (New York: Random House, 1970).

Winslow, C. *The Conquest of Epidemic Disease* (Princeton, N.J.: Princeton University Press, 1943).

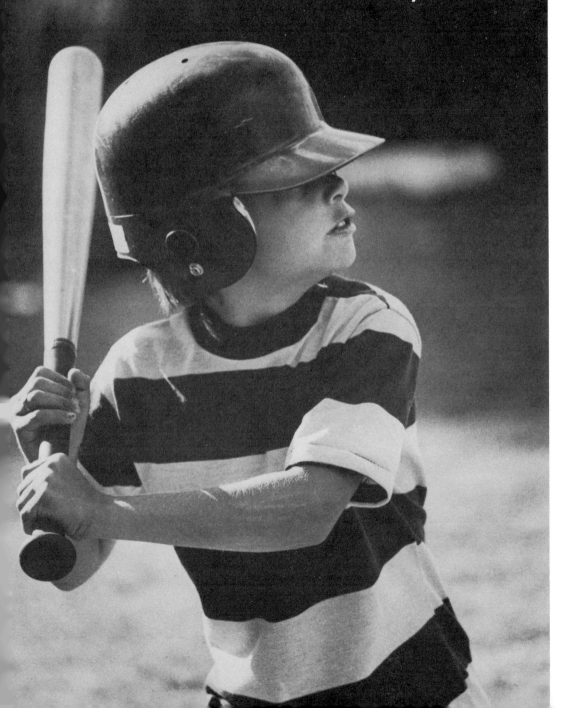

the health of the elementary child

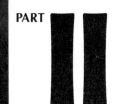

CHAPTER 2

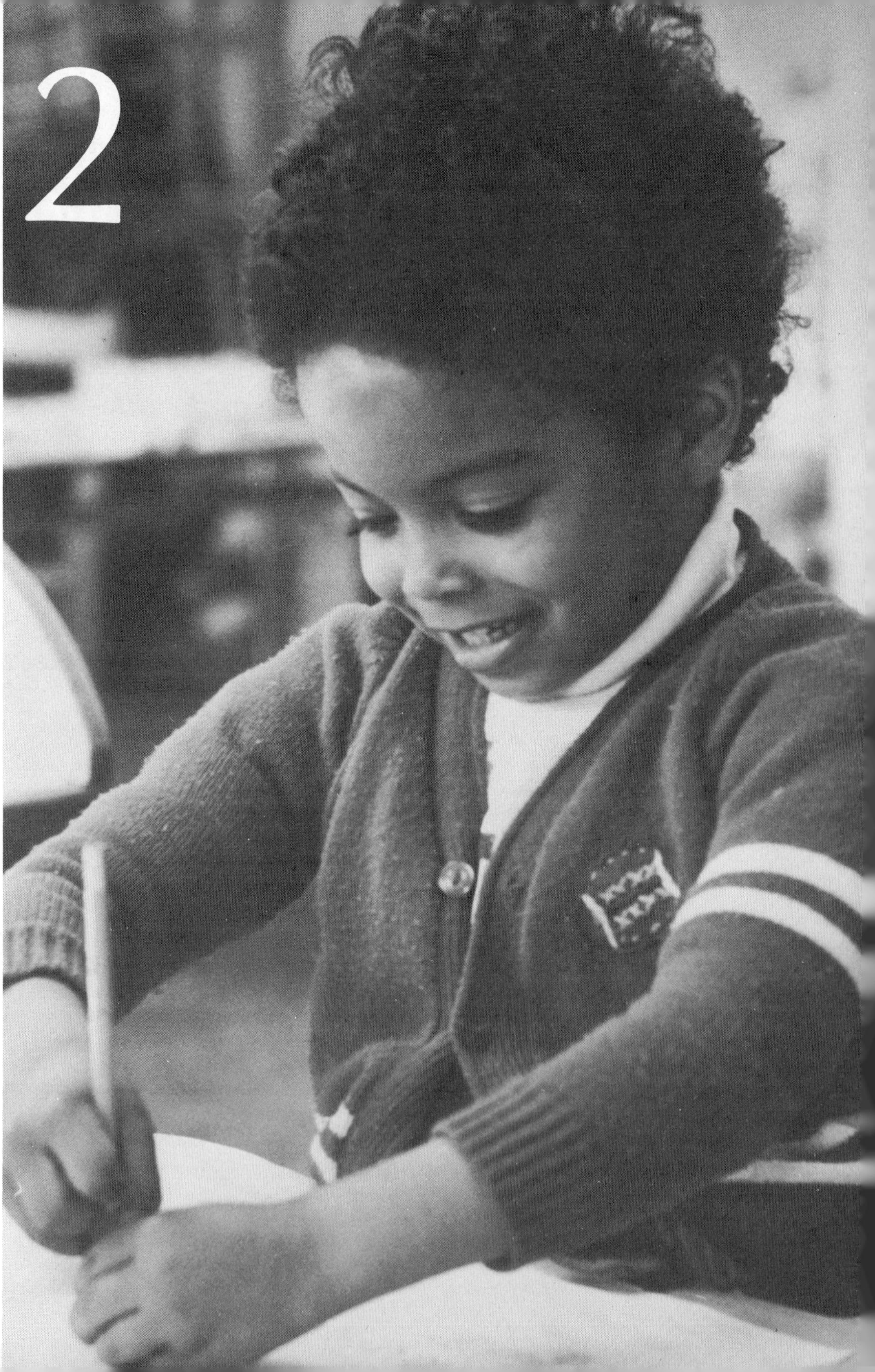

the elementary child

WHOLISTIC DEVELOPMENT: OVERVIEW

Childhood, an adorable stage of life, has been referred to as the latency period, a relatively quiescent and untroubled time for children ages 6-12. Excepting fatal accidents, death rates for children ages 6-12 are extremely low, involvement with the legal political system is limited, and severe problems of emotional disorders are rare. In a sociological sense this developmental period may be more accurately described as a "learning-the-ropes" period rather than as a latency period. It is a time when the child begins to cope with self-autonomy and a continuously expanding world. Before this time, the child was essentially a homebody, whose culture was confined largely to the family and to informal friendship groups. After entering school, the child comes into contact for sustained periods with children and persons other than the immediate family. He or she cannot escape the need to learn more with great speed in order to facilitate relations with strangers. The classroom is the child's first constant and highly organized group experience. Children become most aware of the necessity for learning and communicating and of the need for interpersonal, intellectual, and physical skills.

Preadolescence is also the time when the first signs and early warnings of personal and social inadequacies stemming from home life become evident and visible to others in the community. It is during the elementary school years that many children reveal for the first time the physical and behavioral problems that lead to their being tagged as "good or bad" and as "smart or dumb." On the other hand, it has been noted that the absence of psychiatric and behavioral symptoms in childhood virtually guarantees that a child will not be sociopathic as an adult (Freeman and Jones, 1971). It is during this time that new health-maintenance habits and behaviors are developed. Such health habits become the habits of life.

The attitudes that children pick up in school not only determine much of their early success or failure, but also influence the rest of their educational careers and adult attitudes toward work, responsibility, self, and later life in general. According to Erikson (1959, 1963), childhood is a crucial period for the development of a "sense of identity." An identity is structured through "industry" during childhood; it is through work that the child acquires

23

a sense of duty and achievement. The child makes subconscious commitments to both of these, thereby evolving an identity.

Perhaps equally important to structuring an identity and learning the "three Rs" is the child's need for standards of moral conduct and ethical behavior. The school setting offers unlimited supportive experiences for clarifying as well as acquiring values.

Teachers should observe children at all times of the school day and as they progress from grades one through six. During this time children's physical growth is slow, and their mental growth appears to go on quietly. By middle childhood, a child's ability to understand and to express self has progressed remarkably. In late childhood the child's reasoning becomes better, and this in turn allows him or her to progress from premoral selfish to conventional adolescent values.

In addition to observing children's physical and mental growth, teachers will also observe the children's state of health. They will note that children get sick less and less as they progress into late childhood. They also take better care of themselves, for they have learned many safe ways to live. But almost every day teachers will observe children with health, learning, and living problems. Such problems can be readily corrected or modified at a time when the problem is in its emergent stage and when children are most amenable to adjust and change.

It is during their elementary school years that boys and girls try out their own abilities and interests and begin to gain self-confidence and self-reliance. Although they still need and count on the friendly care and backing of their parents and family, they manage more and more of their own affairs. While becoming self-reliant, self-directing, and self-motivated adults, children still need appreciating attention, love, and sympathy.

Children love to play. Play is a way of not only making friends, but also expressing self, maintaining physical fitness, and clarifying values of life. Play, as activity, is also essential for the physical development of the body. It is through physical activities and play that the child acquires the good body balance, gracefulness, body coordination, muscular strength, and physical stamina that are the foundations of adult health and life. For example, children of ages six to ten delight in hopscotch and jacks. The intricate rhythm of skipping rope and the body control required in tumbling, gymnastics, and skating give children the thrill of new adventures and also the exhilarating new feeling of body control and management.

Children can't get enough of games that emphasize physical alertness—chasing, climbing, dodging. Swinging, whether from a safe swing, a rope, or a vine in the woods, gives children a chance to feel and identify their kinesthetic senses. Tag, run-sheep-run, cops and robbers, and other games in which there is a chance to avoid capture, appeal to children. Turning handsprings; balancing on a beam; bouncing a ball; catching, throwing, and batting a ball are all physical skills demanding control of big skeletal muscles.

While playing, children create their own rules and insist on playing by the rules. They enforce moral virtues of honesty and fair play much more harshly than a teacher does. Their play entails trying out values by which to play and live. These games and trying-out experiences are critical-period experiences, for they have great developmental meaning and payoff for adult maturity. All children need to play!

Once children, especially those in the primary grades, have acquired good control over their bodies, they have a great deal of energy to expend on learning and social skills and on developing their partially perfected abilities. Just as children's play develops their skeletal muscles and physical well-being, their efforts in learning to read and write demand exact adjustments of the smaller muscles and development of hand-eye coordination.

School-age children delight in putting their hands to work. With initiative and furor, children construct things—carts, kites, airplanes, and boats — weave, tie knots, carve, and cut out paper dolls with varying degrees of success. Intermediate-level children are very industrious. They like to work and to do things, finding it emotionally satisfying to accomplish things with their minds and bodies. It is through work that children discover how to become successful, feel good about themselves, and feel confident enough to "try it again."

Children try out new things. Experimentation challenges children to try out all of their senses. They discover the tastes of new foods and sweet grass and the pungent odors of perfume, flowers, and pine needles. They feel a kitten's fur, finger paint, and sift sand through their fingers. They burrow into snow and haystacks and fling themselves down slides. They enjoy going barefoot and feeling mud "squish" between their toes.

Children like guessing games, riddles, and jokes. Table games help children to learn that someone must be a loser.

Eating food is a joy, although children tend to gobble it. They get hungry between meals and snack—often on junk foods, thereby acquiring faulty eating habits.

Children often observe parents, teachers, and adolescents taking medicines, smoking tobacco and marijuana cigarettes, drinking alcoholic beverages, and abusing drugs. Such observations arouse their curiosity about habit-forming substances and medicines. Such curiosity motivates them to discover for themselves what it's like to be drunk and to inhale tobacco smoke. Ideally, such experimentation will satisfy children's curiosities before they drift into self-destructive behaviors.

Elementary school children are very conscious of the clothes that other children wear. Children want to look like their classmates.

Sometimes boys will be intolerant of girls, and girls will snub boys. Boys learn to become conscious of masculinity; girls of femininity. Boys learn to like looking and feeling rough, careless, and scruffy; girls often acquire the opposite characteristics.

Children are beautiful; they are naive and unspoiled, zestful, playful, and have boundless energies. They are eager to learn and discover, and they have undeveloped talents and abilities. Teachers are fortunate to be able to help children structure the foundations of life. Watching and helping children develop into unique, well-adjusted, successful personalities has to be one of the greatest rewards and joys of being a teacher.

This brief overview of the elementary school child has emphasized that children develop in many ways—physically, emotionally, socially, and morally—and gradually mature into healthy adult personalities. Their wholistic development is founded on their felt need to: (1) fulfill biological, safety, social, ego, and intellectual needs; and (2) develop skill competencies for fulfilling these human health needs. In essence, children attain optimal well-being when they are able to successfully develop skills that allow them to fulfill these basic needs. Conversely, children unable to develop skills to adequately fulfill most of their basic health needs suffer from minor illnesses and personality disorders. They are unable to become effective learners and successful in adult life.

DEVELOPMENTAL TASKS

The preceding generalizations about the development of elementary school children reflect a "wholistic" development. Such development is affected by not only the child's nutrition, genetic potentials, physical activity, and physical environment, but also the social milieu. Social and peer-group pressures greatly influence children's behaviors and habits. One such behavioral conditioner is the sociocultural environment. A culture creates aspirational needs: feeling a need to learn to read and write, to ride a bicycle or skateboard, to play team sports, to play a musical instrument, to go to college, to become a doctor or stockcar racer, to drive a car, to drink soft drinks, to chew gum, to drink beer, to smoke cigarettes, and so on.

By making children feel these needs, society "forces" them to behave in certain ways. The culture determines the manner in which children meet these socially defined, or developmental, needs. These developmental needs have been identified as socially expected behaviors, which Havighurst (1953, p. 2) refers to as "developmental tasks":

A developmental task is a task which arises at or about a certain period in the life of the individual, successful achievement of which leads to his happiness and to success with later tasks, while failure leads to unhappiness in the individual, disapproval by society, and difficulty with later tasks.

The developmental task of elementary school children can be summarized as follows:

1. learning physical skills necessary for ordinary games and activities;

2. building wholesome attitudes toward oneself as a growing organism;

3. learning to get along with peers;

4. learning an appropriate masculine or feminine role;

5. developing fundamental skills in reading, writing, and calculating;

6. developing concepts necessary for everyday learning;

7. developing a conscience, morality, and a scale of values;

8. achieving personal independence;

9. developing attitudes toward social groups and institutions.

Origin of Developmental Tasks

Developmental tasks arise from: (1) the physiological process of maturation; (2) social expectations; and (3) the child's personal values and aspirations. Thus some tasks arise mainly as a result of physical maturation, such as learning to walk, to control elimination, to skip, to throw and catch a ball, and to write. Other tasks are developed mainly from the cultural pressures of society, such as learning to read, to participate as a responsible citizen in society, and to assume appropriate sex roles. Still others grow out of personal values and aspirations, such as choosing and preparing for a vocation. Most developmental tasks arise from all three forces working together. For example, before a child can ride a bicycle, she or he must: (1) see others doing so (perceive a value and evolve an aspiration for attaining it); (2) feel pressure from peers and parents (social pressure); and (3) have reached a certain level of neuromuscular maturity (physiological) (see Fig. 2.1). Many sociohygienic tasks have similar origins.

The major developmental tasks for children and adolescents ages 0 to 18 are schematically illustrated in Fig. 2.2. This illustration identifies the developmental tasks of middle childhood (ages 6 to 12) as well as those that precede and follow this period.

Basis for Evolving Developmental Tasks

The key to understanding developmental tasks is to understand Erikson's theory of the development of a healthy personality (human life stages). Erikson (1963) has identified eight major life stages. For our purposes here, the most important stage of personality development is the fourth stage—becoming competent and acquiring skills. This stage coincides with the developmental tasks of middle childhood (ages 6 to about 12).

Developmental tasks evolve from three developmental thrusts in the child. First, the child is thrust out of the home and into the peer group by entering school. Second, while at school, the child is thrust physically into the world of games and work requiring neuromuscular skills. Third, the

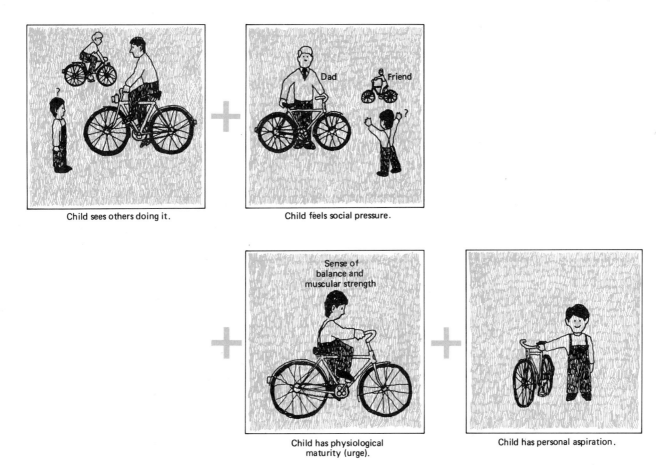

Child sees others doing it.

Child feels social pressure.

Child has physiological maturity (urge).

Child has personal aspiration.

Fig. 2.1 Example of how a developmental task (e.g., learning to ride a bicycle) originates.

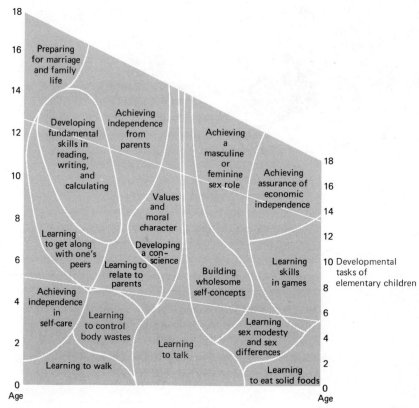

Fig. 2.2 The characteristics and continuity of developmental tasks for ages 0 to 18. The horizontal dimension of each task is a measure of the amount of development taking place. The vertical dimension of each task indicates the age at which development in such a task occurs.

school thrusts the child into the world of adult concepts, logic, symbolism, and communication. At the beginning of school, the child has all the potentials for realizing these possibilities. All developmental tasks have implications for optimal well-being and style of living. This is so because the child develops as a whole person—physically, emotionally, socially, culturally, and intellectually. Thus developmental tasks, because of their biological-sociocultural nature, are also developmental tasks for optimal well-being. The child needs to be well (healthy) in order to master the skills needed for abundant living and to be able to mature into a well-adjusted adult.

Developmental tasks occur at all ages. Society expects the child to successfully master the tasks appropriate to its age level. These tasks should be considered as active goals that all children, consciously or unconsciously, strive to achieve.

The number of developmental tasks for each stage is arbitrary. Thus a major task may be broken down into small tasks. Consider, for example, the child learning locomotion (a major developmental task). The minor tasks involved are as follows: The *infant* learns to sit up, crawl, stand, and walk; the *child* learns to walk, run, jump, skip, and ride a bicycle; eventually, the *adolescent* learns to drive a car. Furthermore, major developmental tasks may be broken into sequential and progressively smaller tasks. This has special significance for the selection of content for well-being by elementary school teachers.

All of the tasks to be learned are, in reality, ones that constitute healthful and satisfactory growth in our society. They are the things children must learn if they are to be judged, and to judge themselves, as reasonably happy and successful persons.

The timing of a developmental task is identical to the emergence of Erikson's life stages (1959, 1963). Failure to fully mature at one stage of development causes partial or complete failure to progress and to develop successfully in the subsequent stages. Developmental arrest of one or more developmental processes (physical, emotional, and social) upsets the functional harmony of the whole child, who eventually becomes a defective or deprived adult. Thus all development proceeds by critical steps—"critical" being characteristic of turning points or moments of decision between progress and regression. As a turning point, crisis should be interpreted as a crucial period of increased vulnerability and heightened potential and therefore a source of adjustment or maladjustment. Once a process or a part of it has been suppressed, it cannot develop at a later time. Such incomplete development hinders the development of future stages, so that a child often adjusts by evolving personality and behavioral aberrations during childhood, adolescence, and/or adulthood. Chapters 3, 4, and 5 provide more insight into such consequences—physical and psychoemotional-social problems.

GROWTH AND DEVELOPMENT

Definition of Terms

Three terms—growth, development, and maturity—are often used synonymously to describe the progress of the child toward adulthood. In reality, the terms are different, though inseparable; none takes place alone. *Growth* refers to quantitative changes—increase in size and structure. It indicates actual increase in size of either a part of the body or the whole organism in terms of multiplication of cells. A child grows in height and weight, and his or her brain increases in size.

Development, by contrast, refers to changes that are qualitative in nature. Development, as an organization of all the parts that growth and differentiation have produced, implies overall process of change, whereas growth implies change in one component of the body. For example, an increase in height is growth; an increase of small-muscle coordination in the fingers is development. Development depends in part on physical maturation—on growth. Development may also refer to emotional and social behavior.

Maturity marks the end of growth and development. However, when applied to children, it is used to connote potentiality. It is most often used to identify that process of inner growth and development by which the individual moves toward the attainment of his or her uppermost physical, emotional, intellectual, and social potentialities. It is a sort of ripening. Maturity also refers to growth and development that has reached its ceiling or that is greater than that expected for a child at a given age. A five-year-old child who resembles a seven-year-old in behavior, is said to be "mature for his or her age." The term may be used to describe either growth or development at any stage between the 0 and 100 percent mark, thereby expressing a definite point of arrival in a stated time sequence. For example, the child's ability to control elimination is dependent on development of the sphincter muscles. When these are fully developed, at about three years, the child can then begin to control elimination like other individuals.

The complex processes of growth, development, and maturation should be viewed as products of heredity, environment, self-concept, and cultural expectations. When the child is mature physically, emotionally, and socially, she or he is also ready to learn. Learning occurs most efficiently when the child is sufficiently mature for a particular learning experience.

Principles of Growth and Development

All growth and developmental processes of children, when studied in detail over a long period of time, follow basic patterns. These patterns reflect physical, emotional (psychological), social, intellectual, and behavioral traits of the whole child. All normal children tend to follow a general sequence of growth and development characteristic of their species and of their cultural group. Development follows a pattern that is little influenced by experience. The child matures when he or she is ready to mature. Such generalizing patterns are referred to as principles.

Teachers should use these principles as guidelines for understanding children, their growth and development, what to expect of them, when to expect it, and for handling children effectively. The following principles should be helpful to teachers:

1. *Growth is patterned.* Although some children mature early and others late, each child has a unique pattern that unfolds at his or her own characteristic rate.

2. *Growth is sequential.* Growth follows an orderly and predictable sequence, which in general is the same for all individuals. When age differentials are ignored, the growth pattern for boys and girls is the same. These progress from the general to the specific. One stage leads to the next. Deviations from the sequence provide clues to growth difficulties.

3. *Growth is cyclic.* Rapid accelerated growth is usually followed by an intervening period of slow, steady growth and development. These cycles are readily apparent in the curve of the growth of the body as a whole. Human life proceeds by stages. Each stage is distinguished by a dominant feature, a leading characteristic, which gives the period its unity and its uniqueness.

4. *Developmental rates vary.* Developmental rates are unique for boys and girls. After age ten, the growth rate for girls changes and is about two years ahead of that for boys. The tempo of development is not even. The feet, hands, and nose, for example, reach their maximum developmental level early in adolescence, whereas the lower parts of the face and shoulders are slower in reaching theirs. Likewise, the heart, liver, and digestive systems grow slowly in childhood, but rapidly during the early adolescent years.

5. *Developmental patterns show wide individual differences.* Each child's growth and development is unique. Children reach puberty at different ages. Because of genetic influences, each part of the body has its own particular rate of growth and development. Each child follows a predictable pattern in a way and at a rate that are unique. Physical development depends partly on heredity potentials and partly on environmental factors such as food, emotional stress, and so on. Personality development is influenced by attitudes and social relationships.

6. *Each stage of development has characteristic traits.* Each body system develops at a different rate when compared to another. Each body trait, such as physical, emotional, and social, has its own unique developmental rate and characteristics helping to identify the child's behavioral, chronological, and maturational levels. The developmental pattern is affected not so much by what the child can accomplish as by the way in which he or she behaves.

7. *Development is a product of the interaction of the child with his or her environment.* Growth and development are genetically, socioculturally, and environmentally determined.

8. *The body tends to maintain a stage of equilibrium,* called homeostasis. The body strives to maintain a constant internal environment despite changing conditions, whether internal or external.

9. *There is unity in growth patterns.* The child grows physically, emotionally, socially, morally, intellec-

tually as a whole being. All aspects of the child's development are interrelated. The stage of maturity in one trait affects the development of others. There is a marked relationship between sexual maturing and patterns of interest and behavior. Desirable traits complement one another and tend to go together.

10. *Development is continuous.* Cellular growth continues from conception to death. Likewise, emotional, social, spiritual, cultural, creative, and intellectual potentials exist and may be developed to high levels toward self-actualization. Because development is continuous, what happens at one stage has an influence on the following stage.

11. *Development proceeds from general to specific responses.* A baby sits before she or he walks. A child learns words that are abstract, like "doggie," before he or she calls the dog a specific name, like "Brownie."

12. *Development comes from maturation and learning.* Development of physical, emotional, and intellectual traits, for example, comes partly from an intrinsic maturing of those traits and partly from exercise and experience on the part of the child.

REVIEW QUESTIONS

1. Distinguish among development, growth, and maturation.
2. What is a developmental task?
3. List the nine developmental tasks outlined by Havighurst for elementary school children.
4. List the twelve principles of growth and development.
5. What is the purpose of play to a child?

REFERENCES AND BIBLIOGRAPHY

Dinkmeyer, Don C. *Child Development* (Englewood Cliffs, N.J.: Prentice-Hall, 1965).

Erikson, Erik H. "Identity and the Life Cycle," *Psychological Issues* **I** (1959).

_____ . *Childhood and Society* (New York: Norton, 1963).

Freeman, Howard E., and Wyatt C. Jones. *Social Problems: Causes and Controls* (Chicago: Rand McNally, 1971), pp. 287-288.

Havighurst, Robert J. *Developmental Task and Education* (New York: Longman, Green, Arnold, 1953).

Hurlock, Elizabeth B. *Child Development* (New York: McGraw-Hill, 1964).

Millard, Cecil V. *Child Growth and Development in the Elementary School Years* (Boston: D. C. Heath, 1958).

U.S.H.E.W. *Your Child from Six to Twelve* (Bronxville, N.Y.: Child Care Publishers, 1962).

Vincent, Elizabeth L., and Phyllis C. Martin. *Human Psychological Development* (New York: Ronald Press, 1961).

Watson, Ernest H., and George H. Lowrey. *Growth and Development of Children* (Chicago: Year Book Medical Publishers, 1962).

3

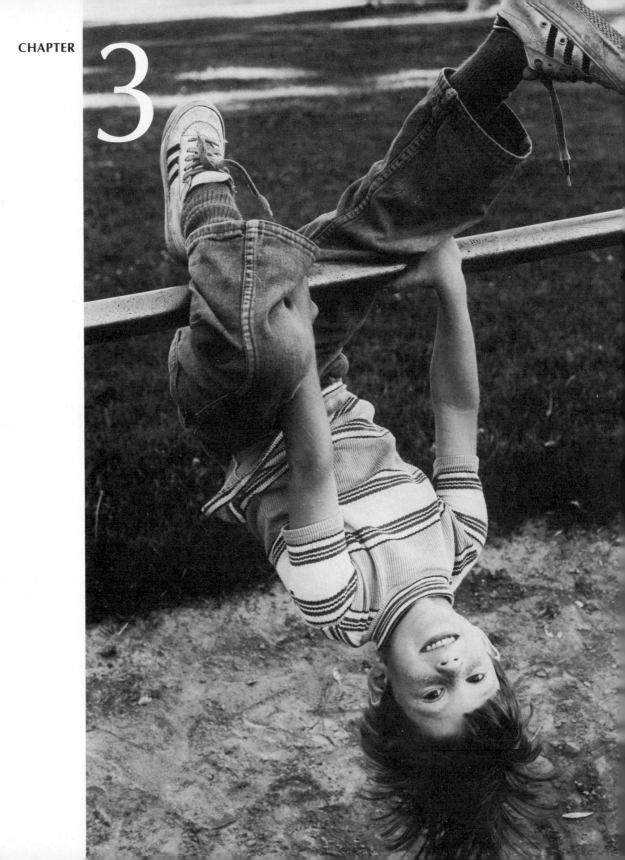

physical development

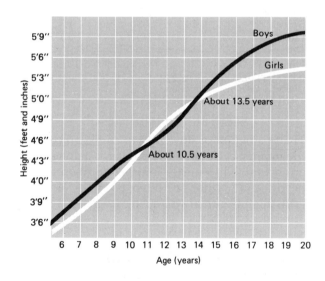

Fig. 3.1 Average height of 6–19-year-old boys and girls. (Adapted with permission from Elizabeth L. Vincent and Phyllis C. Martin, *Human Psychological Development*, The Ronald Press Company, New York, 1961, p. 225. Original source of data: F. K. Shuttleworth. Copyright © 1961 John Wiley & Sons, Inc.)

GROWTH CYCLES

Growth in height and weight reflects general physical progress in development of body systems and processes. It is an indication of progress toward the child's optimal well-being and maturity. Height and weight are only outward indicators of growth and development, for there is no correlation between body size and well-being. The organs and body systems within the body are also increasing in size and are developing their unique functions at their own speed.

Increases in height and weight progress at a slow rate for ages 6 to 12. Weight increases average approximately four to seven pounds a year, whereas height increases two or more inches a year (see Fig. 3.1). From ages five to ten years, boys are generally taller than girls. Then there is a short period, from ages ten to fourteen, when girls exceed boys in height. In general, children show a much steadier rate of gain in height than they do in weight.

Growth and development are rhythmic, not regular. A child does not gain a given number of pounds annually or grow a given number of inches.

33

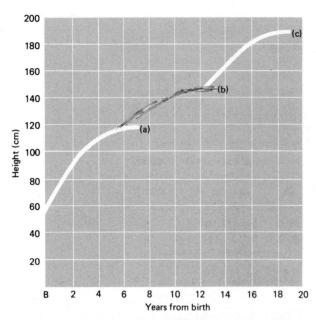

Fig. 3.2 The three cycles of growth in height: (a) infancy cycle; (b) childhood cycle; (c) adolescent cycle. (From Cecil V. Millard, *Child Growth and Development in the Elementary School Years*, Lexington, Mass.: D.C. Heath and Company, 1958, p. 65.)

Table 3.1 Average weights (in grams) of organs at different ages.

	Newborn	1 yr	6 yr	Puberty	Adult
Brain	350	910	1200	1300	1350
Heart	24	45	95	150	300
Thymus	12	20	24	30	0-15
Kidneys (both)	25	70	120	170	300
Liver	150	300	550	1500	1600
Lungs (both)	60	130	260	410	1200
Pancreas	3	9	. . .	40	90
Spleen	10	30	55	95	155
Stomach	8	30	. . .	80	135

From G. H. Lowrey, *Growth & Development of Children*, 7th edition. Copyright © 1978 by Year Book Medical Publishers, Inc., Chicago. Used by permission.

On the contrary, growth and development come in cycles or periods. Studies of growth and development have revealed that there are four distinct periods of growth—two characterized by slow growth and two by rapid growth. These periods are depicted by growth in height cycles in Fig. 3.2. From birth to two years, there is rapid growth. This is followed by a period of slow growth up to the time of puberty, or sexual maturing, which usually begins between the eighth and eleventh years. From then until 15 or 16 years, there is once again rapid growth. This in turn is followed by a period of fairly abrupt tapering off of growth to the time of full adult maturity.

The growth cycle for elementary school children is identified by the (b) cycle curve in Fig. 3.2.

This is a period of slow growth and is preceded by the infancy cycle. Because outward manifestations are presumed to mirror inner maturation as well, height and weight are often taken as indices of growth and normal well-being in general.

INCREMENTS OF GROWTH AND DEVELOPMENT

The measurement of various body organs at regular intervals during their periods of growth and development reveals certain trends in the rate of change common to all normal children. Table 3.1 presents such a summary. Such measurements may also be plotted on a graph to provide a visual summary of

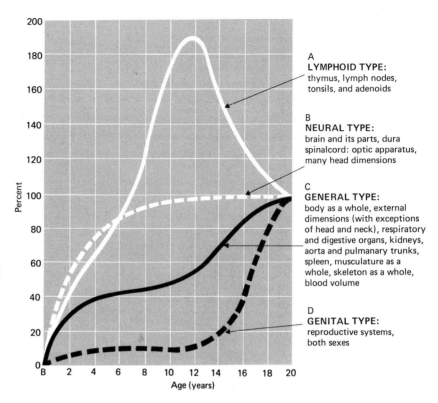

Fig. 3.3 Curves of organ growth drawn to a common scale by computing their values at successive ages in terms of their total (average) postnatal increments. (Adapted from J. A. Harris *et al.*, *The Measurement of Man.* Copyright © 1930 by the University of Minnesota Press, Minneapolis, Minn., and reprinted with permission.)

A
LYMPHOID TYPE:
thymus, lymph nodes, tonsils, and adenoids

B
NEURAL TYPE:
brain and its parts, dura spinalcord: optic apparatus, many head dimensions

C
GENERAL TYPE:
body as a whole, external dimensions (with exceptions of head and neck), respiratory and digestive organs, kidneys, aorta and pulmanary trunks, spleen, musculature as a whole, skeleton as a whole, blood volume

D
GENITAL TYPE:
reproductive systems, both sexes

the growth and development of the various parts of the body. This has been done in Fig. 3.3.

Four types of growth curves (A, B, C, D) are illustrated in Fig. 3.3. Curve A represents growth and development of the lymphoid type (thymus, tonsils, adenoids); curve B, that of the central nervous system (brain, nerves); curve C, that of the body as a whole (respiratory, digestive, muscular, skeletal, excretory, and cardiovascular systems); curve D, that of the reproductive, or genital, system. The growth curves for height and weight resemble the C, or general type, curve in Fig. 3.3.

In general, the body systems are increasing in size and are developing their unique functions at their own rate of speed. The increments of growth and development for each body system will be dis-

cussed in greater detail under the corresponding sections.

Development of Body Systems

The Central Nervous System

Neural maturity precedes the maturity of all other body systems. Because of its genetic endowment, the nervous system initiates the growth and development of the rest of the body. Neural maturity sets the stage for muscular development, which in turn allows psycho-emotional-social maturity to develop in the child. Brain growth is rapid during infancy and early childhood, but slows down after five years of age. Brain weight in ten-year-olds is as great as that of adults (see Table 3.1). Nerve fibers in the brain areas are nearly mature by about five years of age, thus equipping the child for complex learning experiences in school.

The growth of the central nervous system is most rapid in the first three years after birth, then slows down during childhood. This growth pattern of the nervous system is illustrated by curve B in Fig. 3.3. Such early postnatal growth consists primarily of the development of immature cells present at birth. Most of the special senses are well developed at birth, although their association with higher centers comes about gradually during early life. The eyeball, for example, reaches adult size at about 12 to 14 years of age. However, since there is continuous growth and development of the eyes, vision does not assume adult level until after the middle of childhood. The eyes are not biologically "ready" for reading in most cases before the sixth year. That is, the fine coordination required of the eye muscles for moving rapidly over a page of print is achieved partly as a result of nerve and muscle growth. Furthermore, most children are naturally farsighted in early childhood. Their eyes naturally take time to become normal-sighted and become best adapted to reading at about eight years of age.

The ear is fully developed at birth. Both the inner and middle ear have reached nearly adult proportions. The main difference in ear structure between the infant and the grown adult is in the Eustachian tube. In children this tube connects the ear with the throat and is a short, wide, straight passage. As a result, the young child is continuously threatened with ear infections which develop in the throat.

From ages three to ten, neuromuscular coordination and skills are developed. These are discussed briefly in the section on the muscular system.

Glandular (Endocrine) System

The glandular system, largely through specific hormones, regulates growth and development of the body in general. Hormones govern maturation. These concepts are not readily apparent from the organ growth curves in Fig. 3.3. All four types of curves probably represent some kind of glandular growth and function at one time or another. The numerous glands begin to influence body functions at various ages. Collectively, endocrine glands have a dynamic effect on the body. They regulate not only body growth and development during childhood, but also the functioning of body systems throughout life.

Four glands of internal secretion are concerned primarily with the regulation of growth: the pituitary, the thyroid, the gonads, and the adrenal cortex. Although the function of all the glands is determined by heredity, such function is often altered by nutrition and by physical and socioeconomic environments. All the glands reinforce and complement one another. Their synergistic action is essential for normal growth, development, and maturation.

The master gland in the body is not the pituitary gland. The pituitary is regulated by the hypothalmus (master gland) in the brain and directs the function of the other glands. Indirectly, the pituitary hormone influences growth of the skeleton, the muscles, and the viscera. General body size depends on the output of somatotropin, the principal growth hormone that also controls the pituitary gland. The gonadotropic hormone of the pituitary initiates and regulates growth and differentiation of the gonads. It also has a modifying effect on the energy metabolism and affects the growth pattern of the child.

The thyroid gland reinforces the work of the pituitary gland. It exerts a profound influence on growth and development of bones and governs the rate at which energy is used up.

The adrenal cortex, located at the tip of the kidneys, secretes hormones that promote metabolism and aid the body in stress adaptation. Cortin, the principal secretion of the adrenal cortex, affects the rate of maturation. There is a rapid decrease in the size of the adrenal glands after birth. Then they increase rapidly in size up to age 5, slow down in growth from 5 to 11 years, and then increase in size rapidly up to 16 years. Until growth in size has increased, there will be less adrenalin secreted. This has a marked influence on emotional states in childhood.

The gonads control the growth and development of the organs of reproduction and growth. Gonadal hormones bring about epiphyseal closure in bones and thus terminate growth. When gonadal secretion is inadequate during the period when normal epiphyseal closure should occur, the limbs may continue to grow in length, so that height becomes excessive, and body proportions may become abnormal.

The reproductive organs grow very little during early childhood, but develop rapidly from about age 10 to 14. This is illustrated in Fig. 3.3 by curve D. It is at this time that sex hormones bring about secondary sexual characteristics. The girl begins to ovulate, and the boy is capable of producing spermatozoa. Sexual development shows marked male and female differences. The cultural impact of sex-role expectation creates varied skill performances in boys and girls.

An awareness of the growth and development of the glandular system in elementary school children is most important for teachers. Many emotional and adjustment problems initially stem from the child's inability to cope with glandular changes at this time. Changing sexual development creates different and new roles, needs, and interests for boys and girls at various age levels. Such changes impose on the child numerous emotional stresses and adjustments. Children may in turn project their personal problems on their peers, parents, and teachers. Thus many emotional and health problems, as discussed in Chapters 4 and 6, initially stem from the impact of glandular growth and development on the child.

Skeletal System

Skeletal development and maturity follow a unique pattern. This is illustrated in Fig. 3.3 by the C, or general type, curve. In general, bone growth is rapid in the first five years and at the time of puberty when bones begin to harden, or ossify. Bone growth and ossification during childhood (ages five to ten) are slow, with various bones ossifying at various ages.

Children of different racial and geographic backgrounds have different skeletal-developmental rates. In general, the stage of osseous maturation correlates well with weight, height, and sexual development. That is, the child whose height and weight are less than average for age also has repressed bone maturation. A greater variation of this is found in girls. Longitudinal studies reveal that a boy or girl with advanced skeletal maturation will reach physiological maturity at an earlier chronological age than one with a relatively slow degree of maturation.

In comparison with the bones of the adult, the bones of the child contain a proportionately greater part of water and soft proteinlike materials and a considerably lesser portion of mineral substances. Likewise, the skeletal constituents contain much more cartilage and fibrous tissue during the early years. Therefore, the bones of the child are more pliable and elastic than those of the adult. Although this characteristic is desirable in that fracture is less likely, it does provide more opportunity for deformity and imperfection, since the bones resist less successfully the many stresses and strains of muscles and tissues.

From studying a series of X-ray pictures of a child's skeletal system as he or she matures, we can predict the sequence of physical maturation. We become aware that the bones in a young child are not firmly grown together. This is illustrated in Fig. 3.4 by the time schedule of appearance of ossification centers in the arms and legs. Figure 3.5 presents the normal maturation of the bones of the

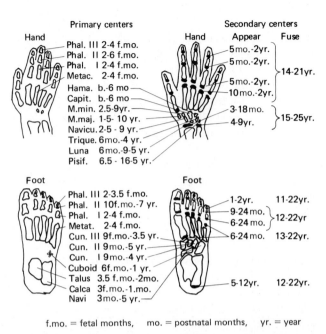

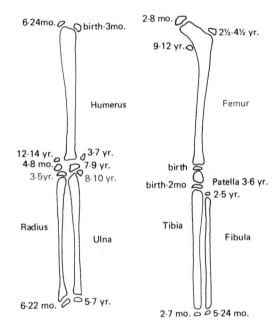

Fig. 3.4 Secondary ossification centers, showing average time of appearance.

f.mo. = fetal months,   mo. = postnatal months,   yr. = year

Fig. 3.5 Ossification centers of the hands and feet, showing time of appearance. Note the wide range of "normal." (From *Pediatric X-Ray Diagnosis*, 6th ed., by John Caffey *et al.* Copyright © 1972 by Year Book Medical Publishers, Inc., Chicago. Used by permission. Modified from Scammon in Morris's *Human Anatomy*.)

hands and feet in both sexes. Note the great amount of space between the ends of the bones. The amount of space is inversely proportional to age. Infant cartilage is gradually replaced by ossification of bone. Ossification, or fusion of the growth line of bones (epiphysis), follows a fairly definite pattern and time schedule from birth to maturity. The duration of the cartilaginous stage is a rough measure of the relative speed of general body development.

The number of teeth at given stages of development is another gauge of growth, development, and maturity. Figure 3.6 shows that tooth eruption follows the familiar pattern already illustrated by height and weight curves. The curve has a slow beginning, rapid acceleration, with a slowing down between ages 9 and 10, followed by a second rapid growth between ages 11 and 13.

A child entering school at six has usually lost some of his or her early teeth. At six years of age the child has 1 or 2 permanent teeth; at eight years, 10 or 11; at ten years, 14 or 16; at twelve years, 24 or 26; and at thirteen, 27 or 28. Growth of teeth is thus a continuing process.

There are individual differences in the time required for growth and in the ages at which teeth appear. Girls are more precocious, cutting their teeth a little earlier than boys do. Normally, as teeth appear, the jaw also grows so as to properly adjust to the number of teeth that it must accommodate.

Loss of teeth mars the child's appearance and makes him or her feel self-conscious. The child may become emotional about losing teeth and project such feelings toward others at this time.

Muscular System

Gain in musculature in childhood is related to the growth of other organs, systems, and tissues. As shown in Fig. 3.3, there are two rapid rates of muscle growth in general. One occurs before the age of five and the other after the age of ten. During the elementary school interval, there is less muscular growth taking place. Instead, muscular development replaces growth.

At birth, muscle fibers are present in an undeveloped state. No new muscle fibers develop after birth, but the ones that are present change in size, shape, and composition. Muscles increase in size by growth in length, breadth, and thickness of the fibers. With muscle growth comes an increase in body weight. Up to five years of age, muscles grow in proportion to the increase in body weight. The large skeletal muscles, as used for locomotion, become well developed. After the age of five, the smaller and finer muscles, which control the child's ultimate strength and manipulative capacities, begin to develop. During this primary period, there

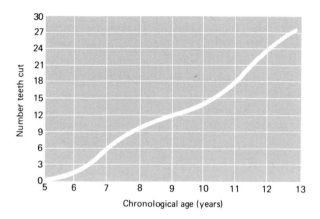

Fig. 3.6   The eruption of teeth as a form of growth and development. (From Cecil V. Millard, *Child Growth and Development in the Elementary School Years,* Lexington, Mass.: D.C. Heath and Company, 1958, p. 83.)

is a rapid spurt in muscle growth, at which time the child's weight gain is approximately 75 percent muscle weight. Now, as the small muscles develop, the child's ability to coordinate his or her body increases. As the child enters fourth grade, muscle development continues slowly until about age ten.

In general, as size and weight of muscle tissue increase, strength also increases. From age 3 on, a child's strength grows, doubling at about 11. It doubles again between 12 and 16 years of age. Because muscular development is relatively slow, the greatest increases in muscular strength take place during puberty. In boys and girls up to the age of ten, there is no difference in muscular strength.

Testosterone

However, after this period, muscular strength increases much faster in boys than in girls.

Exercise and physical activities seem to stimulate muscular growth (size) and development (neuromuscular coordination). The elementary child's need to move about is thought to be directly related to the building up of muscular tension resulting from physical growth. Activity not only relieves such tension and brings on a feeling of general well-being, but also stimulates further growth and development of large and small muscles. In addition to these benefits, exercise of large muscles helps to regulate body systems and processes. Exercise is thus essential to muscle growth and neuromuscular development.

From ages three to ten, neuromuscular coordination and manipulative skills are developed. During the first four or five years of life, the child gains control over gross movements—those involving the large muscle areas of the body used in walking, running, swimming, and bicycling. After five years of age, major development takes place in the control of finer coordinations—the neuromuscular development of the smaller muscle groups used in grasping, throwing and catching balls, writing, and using tools. Such neuromuscular maturity precedes learning and is related to the child's emotional and social adequacy. In general, girls mature more rapidly than boys do. Many neuromuscular differences between sexes, such as boys' greater proficiency in throwing a ball, are attributable to cultural influences. The changes in coordination during this time continue to follow the principle of movement toward increasing complexity. There are increases in speed, dexterity, and coordination ability for social purposes.

Cardiovascular System

Heart growth and development are characterized by two rapid growth spurts: between ages 1 and 5, and between ages 9 and 16 years. During the elementary school years, the heart grows slowly.

When compared to overall body size, the heart is proportionately smallest at seven years of age. Heart growth keeps pace with general body growth and development, as shown by curve C in Fig. 3.3.

Growth of the heart occurs at rapid increments after the first year. Such growth is summarized in Table 3.2. By age five it has increased fourfold; by age nine sixfold.

The heart rate is quite variable throughout the life of the child. Rates differ only slightly between sexes. Table 3.2 lists the average heart rates obtained from several sources for children at rest but not sleeping.

Blood pressure in a child may vary greatly from day to day, and the increase in blood pressure that occurs with age is not constant from year to year. In other words, each child has his or her developmental pattern. Table 3.2 presents the normal systolic blood pressures for various ages.

The growth in caliber of the arteries and veins seems related to the volume or weights of the regions to which they supply blood.

The child's heart is vulnerable to the stresses of life. Although heart growth keeps pace with general body growth and development, it is not ready to support all the activities in which the child's body participates, in addition to the growth and developmental needs of the body as a whole. Since it grows slowly during the early school years, the many activities imposed on it must be interspersed with periods of rest. Physical fatigue is nature's way of slowing the child down and protecting him or her from overworking the heart. A child who gets tired will naturally stop for rest. Teachers should keep these principles in mind when planning work and physical activities for their students.

Respiratory System

Growth and development of the respiratory system follow curve C, as shown in Fig. 3.3. With increased muscular mobility comes concomitant stress on development of the lungs after birth. Although the

Table 3.2   Comparison of heart growth and development from birth to adolescence, averaged for both sexes.

	Birth	1 yr	5 yr	7 yr	9 yr	10-16 yr
Heart size compared to birth		2×	4×	5×	6×	7×-20×
Heart weight (g)	20-24	38-45	82-90	100	125	135-220
Heart rate (at rest)	150	110-115	100	95	90-95	82-85
Average systolic blood pressure (mm Hg)	52	96	99	105	110	115-120

Table 3.3   Summary of variations in respiration with age.

	Birth	1 yr	5 yr	10 yr	20 yr
Lung weight (increases as compared to birth)	1	3×			20×
Respiratory rates (min)	30-80	20-40	20-25	17-22	15-20
Tidal air (cc)	19	48	175	320	500

number of air pockets, or alveoli, is the same at birth as in adulthood, the increase in respiratory exchange of gases is dependent on the growth in size of undeveloped alveoli as well as on the development of capillaries around each air sac to facilitate gaseous exchanges. As these changes take place, the oxygen-carrying capacity of the body increases with an increase in the number of red blood cells. Thus the lungs grow rapidly between birth and about five years and again with the advent of adolescence.

The young child breathes air by movement of the diaphragm until ages five to seven. Thereafter, the costal and other chest muscles begin to help out. The rate and depth of breathing are extremely variable in children (see Table 3.3). From studying this table, we can generalize that variations in respiration occur with changes in age. Respiration becomes slower, deeper, and more regular as the child gets older. Sexual differences in breathing are negligible during childhood. Lungs increase in size by

the utilization of more latent alveoli, thus increasing the volume of tidal air. It is during this time of alternating growth and development of the respiratory system that the child is most susceptible to respiratory infections.

Excretory System

Kidney growth is most rapid in infancy and during childhood. The kidney is five times its birth size by age five, and ten times its birth size by age ten. Bladder and bowel control in most children begins at about two years, when the sphincter muscles in the anus and bladder have matured and the child assumes willful control of these muscles. Such control is complete in most children when they enter school. In general, the excretory system follows the general growth curve as illustrated in Fig. 3.3. There is rapid growth up to five years, then a slow growth period during the elementary school period, and then an accelerated growth period during adolescence.

With the excretory system maturing in its capacity to function, at about five years, the entire body is brought into a higher state of homeostasis.

Lymphatic System

This is the protective system of the body and includes lymph nodes and tissue and the thymus gland. The number of lymph nodes and the amount of lymphoid tissue are considerable at birth. These increase steadily during childhood, but undergo a relative reduction after puberty. Such lymphoid growth is illustrated in Fig. 3.3. Tonsils, adenoids, and especially the thymus gland undergo marked hypertrophy from ages five to ten years, then atrophy to adult size. The hypertrophy of these structures is a normal physiological process.

The maximal development of these tissues during the time when acute infections of the respiratory and alimentary tracts are most common and during the period of greatest increase in weight and height has led to the conclusion that they are a part of a natural defense mechanism. The lymphatic system plays an important part in evolving body immunity during early and middle childhood. Formation of antibodies takes place in part or completely within this system. During infancy and childhood, lymphoid tissues characteristically respond to infection by rapid swelling and hyperplasia (increase in size of tissue). Hyperplasia is especially notable in the thymus gland.

The gradual building up of antibodies in the body reaches a peak at about 12 to 15 years of age. The buildup of such immunity also enhances body homeostasis.

Digestive System

Growth of the digestive system follows curve C as illustrated in Fig. 3.3. It is most rapid before the child enters school and during adolescence. There is a slow, gradual growth period while the child attends elementary school. In general, the digestive organs tend to resemble adult organs in appearance with advancing age.

Summary of Physiological Development

In general, physiological development is sequential, continuous, and unique. Body systems are interrelated in both function and development. One system affects the others. The child must mature physically before developing emotionally and socially. However, physical growth and development do not take place in a vacuum. They are nurtured by the child's environment.

REVIEW QUESTIONS

1. When do physical growth spurts occur? How many growth spurts do most elementary children have?
2. How do height and weight gains affect the child's running, hopping, balance, speed, coordination?
3. When is the brain physically developed in size?
4. When are the glands most active?
5. When do the large muscles begin to rapidly develop in bulk and strength?
6. When are eyes biologically ready for reading?
7. Why are primary school children susceptible to ear infections?
8. Which gland controls body height and bone length?
9. What is the function of the thymus gland?
10. Why are a child's bones more elastic than those of a teacher?
11. How may loss of teeth affect a child's personality?
12. Why are children usually fidgety?
13. What can you do to help children develp neuromuscular coordination?
14. When are children most susceptible to disease?

15. Do all children develop physically at the same rate?

REFERENCES AND BIBLIOGRAPHY

Anderson, C. L. *School Health Practice* (St. Louis: C. V. Mosby, 1960).

Blackfan, Kenneth D. *Growth and Development of the Child*, Report of the Committee on Growth and Development, White House Conference on Child Health and Protection (New York: Century, 1933).

Dinkmeyer, Don C. *Child Development* (Englewood Cliffs, N.J.: Prentice-Hall, 1965).

The Faculty of University School. *How Children Develop* (Columbus: Ohio State University Press, 1964).

Gordon, Ira J. *Human Development* (New York: Harper & Row, 1962).

Guyton, Arthur C. *Textbook of Medical Physiology* (Philadelphia: Saunders, 1966).

Hettinger, Theodor. *Physiology of Strength* (Springfield, Ill. Charles C Thomas, 1961).

Hurlock, Elizabeth B. *Child Development* (New York: McGraw-Hill, 1964).

Millard, Cecil V. *Child Growth and Development in the Elementary School Years* (Boston: D. C. Heath, 1958).

Nemir, Alma. *The School Health Program* (Philadelphia: Saunders, 1965).

U. S. Department of Health, Education, and Welfare. *Perspectives on Human Deprivation: Biological, Psychological and Sociological* (Washington, D.C.: U. S. Government Printing Office, 1968).

Vincent, Elizabeth L., and Phyllis C. Martin. *Human Psychological Development* (New York: Ronald Press, 1961).

Watson, Ernest H., and George H. Lowrey. *Growth and Development of Children* (Chicago: Year Book Medical Publishers, 1962).

4

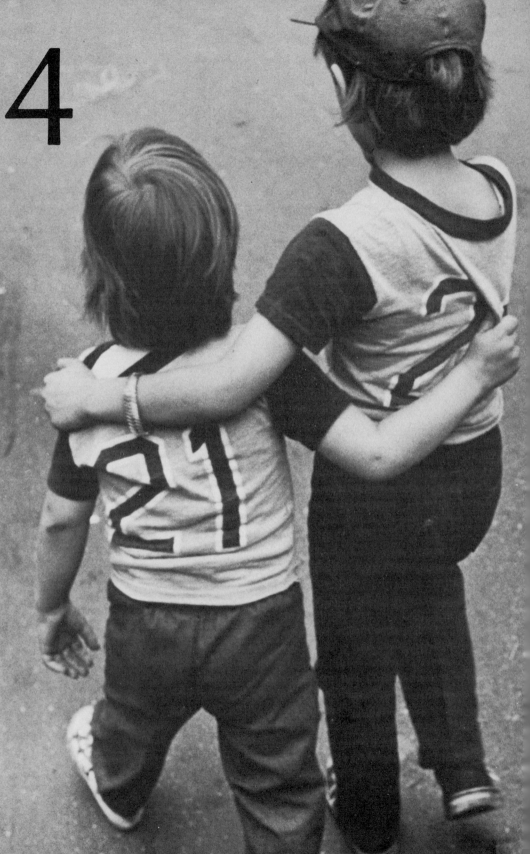

emotional-social development

INTRODUCTION

Children disturbed with the normal problems of growing up often experience difficulty in learning. If not resolved, their troubles—physical, emotional, and social tensions, anxieties, and frustrations—may become masked and later may erupt as antisocial behaviors. With each new group of kindergartners, some may be expected to develop serious emotional handicaps before completing the sixth grade. Such troubled children, often unrecognized when they start school, develop learning difficulties which in turn contribute to disciplinary problems and to dropouts. It is estimated that between 10 and 25 percent of elementary school children have emotional problems and maladjustments requiring psychiatric help. On the basis of these estimates, there must be, on the average, about three to eight emotionally handicapped children in each elementary classroom. At least one child in each classroom needs immediate psychiatric help.

Such children are problems to not only themselves, but also their peers and teachers. They often disrupt their classmates and exact a dispropor-tionate amount of their teacher's time and energy. The risk is substantially high that disturbed children in today's classrooms may become delinquent as adolescents or emotionally (mentally) ill as adults. More than 20 million Americans are mentally sick today. More than half of the adults consulting doctors have complaints related to emotional disturbances. Emotional illness is the major public health problem in this country today. The extent of such disorders may be put into better perspective when emotional disorders are interrelated to include drug abuse and misuse, alcoholism and social drinking, delinquency and crime, sexual aberrations, overweight and obesity, cigarette smoking, boredom and depression, and other deviant behaviors.

Physical problems such as asthma, poor posture, obesity, or poor vision or hearing all pose primary handicaps for the child. Likewise, family problems such as a bad home life, living with only one parent, parental neglect, sibling rivalry, being a battered child, lack of constructive home responsibilities, living in poverty, and lack of close emo-

Sexual inequities Issues

tional relationships with parents may constitute primary behavioral handicaps for the child. In addition to physical and family problems, the immediate social environment may spawn primary handicaps of an emotional nature for the child. For example, not being able to socialize with friends at the Saturday matinee, not belonging to the Boy Scouts or Brownies, being the only one without a bicycle, not playing by the rules of the game, and other social inequities may give the sensitive child a feeling of social deprivation and inadequacy.

When these and other social and family problems are not corrected, are not properly compensated for, are not resolved, or are not reinforced to the satisfaction of the child's immediate physical, emotional, and social needs, the child will feel insecure, rejected, and inadequate. Such a child often tries to cope with these feelings by adapting the original handicap to his or her social environment. Such forms of adaptation often result in secondary health problems such as emotional disorders and disturbances, disobedience, disrespect for law and order, dishonesty and cheating, promiscuity, and other forms of bizarre and self-destructive misbehaviors. Other environmental conditions that may create discipline problems are class size and grade level, the size of the school system, the availability of community services, transporting children by bus, and the school's administrative policies. Misbehavior arising out of unfavorable conditions in these areas often has origins which lie beyond the teacher's sphere of influence. Psychiatrists recognize these and other misbehaviors as unsuccessful attempts to fulfill the basic human needs to feel adequate and to love and to be loved.

DIFFICULTY IN INTERPRETING EMOTIONAL WELL-BEING

Emotional disturbances and abnormal behaviors are difficult to define. Various terms are used to describe them: mental illness, learning disabilities, behavioral problems, emotional disorders, emotional blocks, aberrations, social misbehaviors, psychopathologies, metapathologies, psychosomatic disturbances, psychoneurotic disorders, adjustive reactions, personality problems, maladjustments, and emotional handicaps. As symptoms, these may be secondary to a physical or a medical condition, although the etiology remains obscure. These terms are used interchangeably to denote conditions of tension or nervousness characterized by deviations in thinking, feeling, and acting. The more severe the disorder, the more radical are the disturbances, until a point is reached where the individual becomes almost incapable of adjusting to life.

The variety of terms used as reference to emotional well-being reflects the confusion that exists today among the professional groups and lay public. Emotional well-being appears to be interpreted as feelings (emotional), thinking (psychological), actions (adjustments), behaviors (social), and self-esteem (image). A very thin line often exists between normality and abnormality. More often than not, it is a qualitative difference. Many people pass back and forth over this line several times during their lives. Emotionally well persons tend to adapt to changes and conditions. Thus no person remains completely well adjusted for any great length of time. Adults are expected to conform to social standards of emotional behavior. On the other hand, children are in the developmental and maturational process of trying to fulfill their biological, psychological, emotional, and social needs. Much of their coping experiences are of a first-time nature. Therefore, children may pass back and forth over the normal-abnormal line several times a month. Their coping is often of a trial-and-error approach that is more readily tolerated in them than in adults. As with adults, the key to interpreting such coping behavior is whether the child is able to maintain a balanced and realistic orientation between needs and social expectations.

In conclusion, we should be aware that emotional well-being, like well-being itself, cannot be defined. Instead, it should be conceptualized. Various concepts and indices of the spectrums of emotional well-being and behavior are discussed in the section that follows.

CONCEPT OF EMOTIONAL WELL-BEING

Emotional well-being was conceptualized in Chapter 1 as feelings and thoughts reinforcing self-identity. We suggested that this state is characterized by the ability to: cope successfully with the stresses of daily living; be flexible in all social situations; experience feelings of being worthwhile and adequate as a person; feel content and happy; feel a sense of accomplishment and self-realization; face up to and accept reality; feel worthwhile as a member of society; have emotional stability; exercise self-discipline and self-confidence; accept responsibility for one's behavior and social roles; feel good about self and others; have worthwhile hobbies and recreational interests; have an adequate self-image; and be able to give, express, and accept love. Such feelings and thoughts may be interpreted as comprising an index of positive emotional well-being to be found among mature adults. Many of these traits may also be recognized in children.

At the other end of the spectrum of well-being are emotional disturbances. An emotionally disturbed child can be characterized as follows:

1. Seeming inability to learn which cannot be satisfactorily explained by intellectual, sensory, or health factors;

2. Unsatisfactory relationship with both peers and teachers;

3. Tendency to exhibit inappropriate behavior in normal circumstances;

4. Feeling of general unhappiness or depression;

5. Tendency to develop physical symptoms or fears in relation to personal or school problems.

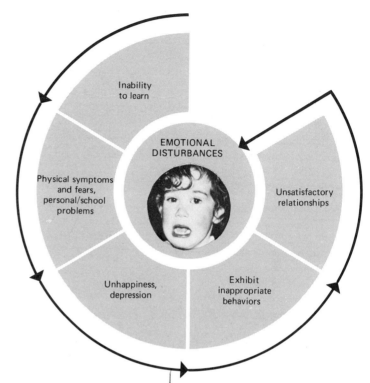

Fig. 4.1 A few characteristics of an emotionally disturbed child.

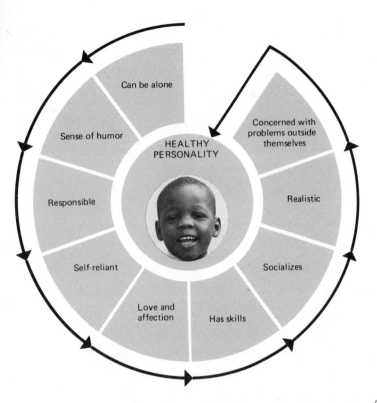

Labels in figure: Can be alone, Sense of humor, Responsible, Self-reliant, Love and affection, Has skills, Socializes, Realistic, Concerned with problems outside themselves, HEALTHY PERSONALITY

Fig. 4.2 Characteristics of a healthy personality. (Photograph by Bruce Anspach/Editorial Photocolor Archives)

Other indices may also be applied to the bipolar spectrum of emotional well-being and emotional illness. Erik Erikson (1964, 1968) has taken this approach in outlining human maturational life cycles. Thus, emotionally mature children have developed a sense of trust, autonomy (self-image), initiative, and self-assertion; they are industrious (have competence), accept responsibility, are interested in doing productive work, and feel adequate; they have evolved a self-identity (self-role image). Conversely, emotionally immature children often develop the opposite feelings and behaviors: mistrust, shame and doubt, guilt and overaggression, inferiority (inadequacy), and identity diffusion.

Emotional well-being may also be conceptualized as a component of a sound personality. The indices of a "healthy, multi-valued personality" have been abstracted by Rucker *et al.* (1969) from Adler, Fromm, Blotz, Horney, Rank, Sullivan, Rogers, Maslow, Allport, and Jourard. Their collective thinking suggests that healthy persons have the following characteristics:

1. They acknowledge *personal responsibility* for their own actions (high rectitude status).

2. They are *self-reliant* (high status of self-respect). They are more independent in solving their problems than are average or ill persons.

3. They deal *with their environment* in a creative manner (enlightenment and skill). They use their own skills and understanding to do those things necessary for their health and happiness.

4. Their *concepts about other people are realistic* and are not distorted by past experiences. Such people are aware of these relationships and that their beliefs about themselves and other people are accurate (enlightenment and skill).

5. They have *social feeling* (love and respect). Such persons are identified with humanity. The unhealthy person concentrates on competing for power in order to escape from feelings of insecurity,

whereas the healthy person is free to love and to respect others.

6. They tend to *realize their latent potentials* in everyday activities (skills). They are not afraid to try out new ways of doing things for fear of failure (with consequent loss of respect).

7. They tend to *see reality as it is* and to be comfortable in their relationship with it. Such persons can more easily distinguish between the true and the false, the honest and the dishonest person. They do less "wishful" thinking than emotionally ill persons. They have less fear of the unknown and thus are relatively free to create new ways of doing things and to try them out with confidence (self-respect and skill).

8. They *think and often act spontaneously*. While inwardly despising the conventional, they will often accept it in order to avoid hurting people. Such persons can thus be said to have a social consciousness which forces them to think before they may act unconventionally (rectitude).

9. They are *concerned with problems outside themselves* rather than with self, as are insecure people (rectitude, enlightenment, and skill). As adults, such people are concerned with the basic issues of life and work in the broadest frame of reference in thinking about values and their achievement.

10. They can be *alone without discomfort* (self-respect). Such people even have need of solitude or privacy more so than the "average" or ill person, who is usually uncomfortable when alone.

11. They continue to *get pleasure from the beauty of their environment throughout life*. They respond aesthetically and with pleasure to a beautiful flower, even though they have seen one almost exactly like it many times before (high status of aesthetic skill). This attitude of continuing appreciation is an index of good mental health.

12. They have *democratic personalities*. They demand that all values be shared. This is an index of high rectitude status. They will learn from the experiences of any person of good character regardless of political belief, class, religious persuasion, or nationality (respect and affection). They treat people courteously, have respect for people on the basis of merit rather on family or other unearned status. They are ethical in their interpersonal relationships. They demand that others have the same access to values that they demand for themselves (rectitude).

13. They are *able to distinguish between means and ends* (enlightenment and skill). They always place the goals they seek above the means by which they seek to achieve them. This trait may often be displayed in the judicious management of personal finances.

14. They have an *unhostile sense of humor* (respect), do not laugh at misfortunes of others, and do not attempt to make people laugh by hurting others. Such people, however, are quick to see the humor in the errors of human beings in general, such as trying to feel important when this feeling is not justified. They can laugh at their own mistakes. Their humor is spontaneous rather than planned (well-being).

15. They *offer intelligent and responsible resistance* to many aspects of the cultural mold (rectitude). They conform with many of the observable symbols of conventionality, but are really not conventional in the dependent sense. They accept conventional practices only to the degree to which they think they are good.

People with these personality characteristics have mature values guiding their behavior. Such persons are positive, purposeful, enthusiastic, and proud.

The indices of a healthy, multivalued personality are reinforced by the characteristics of people with good mental health as outlined by the National Association for Mental Health (1965). Such people: feel comfortable about themselves; feel right about other people; and are able to meet life's demands.

Emotional feelings and thoughts are often fused into overt actions and behaviors. Consequently, understanding, interpreting, and identifying behavioral problems in children becomes a complex and difficult task when the child's thoughts and feelings, as reactions to tensions and anxieties, are masked by and transformed into overt actions and behaviors. Such behaviors are usually not perceived as being related to emotions. Because of this lack of association, teachers are often unable to recognize the early symptoms of emotional disturbance or the latent signs of maladjustment and misbehavior. As a result, disturbed children may be overlooked by a teacher and receive no assistance until their problems become so acute that they attract the attention of clinical or law enforcement agencies.

The variety of behavioral problems teachers encounter in school requires them to make some discriminatory judgments and interpretations. It is quite important that teachers be able to distinguish forms of behavior that are harmful or destructive to the child and/or to society from those that are temporary and that are consequences of environmental upsets, are by-products of normal growth, or are expressions of emotional release. Also, they must be able to predict which characteristics may be outgrown and which can be expected to become progressively worse and lead to serious behavioral problems.

These judgments are not always easy to make. However, various research studies and clinical reports reveal certain clusters of symptoms to be indicators of chronic maladjustment. The following list, adapted by Kaplan (1959) from a compilation made by the Minneapolis Public Schools, indicates some of the behavioral *characteristics commonly associated with serious adjustment problems*:

1. *Nervous behavior:* habitual twitching of muscles, scowling, grimacing, twisting the hair, continuous blinking, biting or wetting the lips, nail biting, stammering, blushing or turning pale, constant restlessness, frequent complaints of minor illnesses, head banging, nervous finger movements, frequent crying, rocking the body, frequent urination;

2. *Emotional overreactions and deviations:* undue anxiety over mistakes, marked distress over failures, absentmindedness, daydreaming, meticulous interest in details, refusal to take part in games, refusal to accept any recognition or reward, evasion of responsibility, withdrawal from anything that looks new or difficult, chronic attitude of apprehension, lack of concentration, unusual sensitivity to all annoyances (especially noises), inability to work if distracted, lack of objective interests, frequent affectations and posturing, inappropriate laughing, uncontrolled laughing or giggling, explosive and emotional tone in argument, tendency to feel hurt when others disagree, unwillingness to give in, shrieking when excited, frequent efforts to gain attention, sudden intensive attachments to people (often older), extravagant expressions of any emotion;

3. *Emotional immaturity:* inability to work alone, tendency to cling to a single intimate friend, inability to rely on own judgment, unreasonable degree of worry over grades, persistent inferiority feelings, unusual self-consciousness, inability to relax and forget self, excessive suspiciousness, overcritical of others, too docile and suggestible, persistent fears, indecision, compulsive behavior, hyperactivity;

4. *Exhibitionist behavior:* teasing, pushing or shoving other pupils, trying to act tough, trying to be funny, wanting to be overconspicuous, exaggerated courtesy, marked agreement with everything the teacher says, continual bragging, frequent attempts to dominate younger or smaller children, inability to accept criticism, constant efforts to justify self, frequent blaming of failures on accidents or on other individuals, refusal to admit any personal

Table 4.1 Erikson's stages of human development.

Age	Stage	Characterization of stage	Value strengths
0-1	oral-sensory	basic trust vs. shame	hope and drive
2-3	muscular-anal	autonomy vs. shame, doubt	willpower and self-control
4-5	locomotor-genital	initiative vs. guilt	purpose and direction
6-12	latency	industry vs. inferiority	competence and method
13-19	puberty and adolescence	identity vs. role confusion	fidelity and devotion
20-30	young adulthood	intimacy vs. isolation	love and affiliation
30-64	adulthood	generativity vs. stagnation	care and production
65 +	maturity	ego integrity vs. despair	wisdom and renunciation

Adaptation of Epigenetic Chart from *Childhood and Society*, 2nd Edition, Revised, by Erik H. Erikson, is reprinted with permission of W. W. Norton & Company, Inc. Copyright 1950, ©1963 by W. W. Norton & Company, Inc.

lack of knowledge or inability, frequent bluffing, attempting either far too little or far too much work;

5. *Antisocial behavior:* cruelty to others, bullying, abusive or obscene language, undue interest in sex (especially efforts to establish bodily contact), telling offensive stories or showing obscene pictures, profound dislike of all school work, fierce resentment of authority, bad reaction to discipline, general destructiveness, irresponsibility, sudden and complete lack of interest in school, truancy;

6. *Psychosomatic disturbances:* reversals or complications in toilet habits, enuresis, constipation, diarrhea, excessive urination, feeding disturbances, overeating, nausea or vomiting when emotionally distressed, various aches and pains.*

Most teachers will recognize many of these characteristics as appearing in the behavior of normal children. Whenever combinations of these symptoms appear frequently and consistently or are not outgrown in time, however, the teacher

---

*This listing is reprinted from pp. 283-284 in *Mental Health and Human Relations in Education* by Louis Kaplan. Copyright © 1959 by Louis Kaplan. By permission of Harper & Row, Publishers, Inc.

should suspect a serious problem. A child may also be suspected of having an adjustment problem whenever his or her behavior is exaggerated beyond what is customary for youngsters of that age.

Emotional-social well-being may also be interpreted according to Erikson's theory of the development of a healthy personality, or human life stages. Erikson has proposed eight emotional-social development stages, as summarized in Table 4.1. In order to develop into a well-adjusted adult, a child needs to progress through the various stages in positive rather than negative ways. Stage four, concerned with acquiring competence and skills, occurs from ages 6 to 12 and is therefore of direct concern to elementary teachers because it is a time when the teacher can help children to acquire the sociohygienic skills of life. Many of the later skills of life are rooted in and are dependent on mastery of the sociohygienic skills in the formative years of the child's life. The preceding stages are also relevant, but the elementary teacher is not in a position to help the child during them. The focus of attention in this chapter, therefore, centers on the stage relevant to the elementary school child and school teacher.

The first three stages of life as outlined by Erikson should prepare the child for the fourth period. Hopefully, by the time the child attends school, he or she will have progressed through all of the developmental stages successfully. Thus the child will have developed hope and trust from security as an infant; will have developed a will from autonomy between two and three years of age; and will have picked up a purposefulness from his or her initiative in play between ages four and five. The child is ready to acquire skills that will help him or her to become socialized and a self-realizing person.

In addition to all of the behavioral and emotional concepts just reviewed, the teacher should be aware of the possibility of value deprivation in some elementary school children. Such a condition appears when the new values of today are in conflict with the traditional values of the child. The usual values that normally guide the child in making decisions about his or her behavior do not appear to be present. The child's behavior may appear irrational, abnormal, and without purpose. Maslow (1967) interprets this condition as "valuelessness." The feelings of such children are described as a lack of something to believe in and to be devoted to, amorality, rootlessness, anhedonia, anomie, emptiness, hopelessness, and other metapathologies. No doubt, today's rapid and numerous changes of technology have affected our lifestyles dramatically. People unable to cope successfully with changes have been described by Toffler (1970) as being in a state of "future shock." A modern concept of emotional well-being would be incomplete without an appreciation of human value needs and an understanding that a person's physical, emotional, social, spiritual, and cultural needs and reactions are mediated by his or her value needs.

Finally, the picture of emotional and social well-being would be incomplete without an awareness of Maslow's hierarchy of human needs (1967, 1968). Children, like adults, have basic human health needs (see Chapter 1). Hountras (1961, p. 99) points out that people who have been satisfied in their basic needs throughout their lives, particularly in their earlier years, develop exceptional power to withstand present and future thwarting of these needs. They have strong, healthy character structures as a result of satisfaction and fulfillment of their basic human health needs. Children have a strong motivation to fulfill physiological, safety preservation, social love, and status, or ego (emotional), needs. Fulfillment of these needs early in life optimizes well-being and a happy and well-functioning person. Acquisition of many skills early in life increases the child's facility for more adequately fulfilling these needs in adulthood.

EMOTIONAL PROBLEMS

Etiology

Physical problems and the feelings and thoughts that children use in their attempts to cope with stress are not the only conditions causing emotional disturbances and misbehaviors. Teachers and schools may unknowingly contribute to the adjustment difficulties of children. The etiology of behavioral problems has traditionally been viewed as stemming from causative factors such as rejection, marital discord, and adverse parental attitudes that begin early in the child's life. The family has always been assumed to be the cause of tensions within the child that influence his or her interpersonal relationships, perception of self and others, and impair his or her effectiveness in learning and in behavioral control. Such a child has been referred to as "emotionally disturbed." But because this model has focused attention on personality development, it has failed to consider why some children do not do well in school. Significantly, assessment of the child's areas of competence or weakness in skills has been left out. The interactions between the child's competence levels and the demands made by the school situation have not been taken into account. Nonetheless, the root cause of an emotional problem is often hidden and masked by precedent physical or social skills that may be undeveloped or lacking.

The latency stage in Erikson's theory has important implications for elementary school teachers. Characterized by the child's learning to become industrious, this stage requires teachers to help the child develop both numerous skills and competencies in these skills. This stage coincides with entrance into school and lasts until about the age of 12. It is a prelude to entering adult life and the world of work. The child sublimates previous feelings of "making" people respond by direct attack and instead learns to win recognition by producing things. Work provides the child with the satisfaction of doing and teaches him or her the pleasure of work completion. Along with work, play not only helps the child learn to share things with others, but also fulfills the needs to be useful, to feel a sense of involvement from participation in the group, and to feel able to do well and to make things with quality. The child garners prestige and status and structures his or her self-image by becoming self-reliant in work and play, receiving self-esteem and joy from the social recognition of the things produced. The variety of skills mastered helps to reinforce the child's need for feeling adequate. She or he is motivated to face new tasks with confidence and anticipated pleasure. Thus successful work-play experiences in the elementary school help the child to structure positive self-esteem and a wholesome personality. It is vital for teachers to nurture children's competence in many different kinds of skills. Development of such skills is an essential prerequisite to the development of not only positive emotional well-being, but also readiness to learn.

The danger of the primary school stage is that the child may encounter more failures than successes at work. Such failure may also be a consequence of immature development in the preceding preparatory life stages. Then, too, family life may not have prepared the child for school life, or school life may fail to sustain that which the child has already learned to do well. Discouragement with work deters the child from identifying with signifi-cant modelers of jobs. Besides tool skills, the child needs to develop competencies in physical, play, social values, emotional, hygienic, and learning skills. All of these skills are dependent on the maturity of neuromuscular, glandular, and other body systems. Lacking these skills when he or she needs them will make the child feel incompetent in work or play or dissatisfied with his or her status among peers in the work-play context. Such a child may develop a sense of inadequacy and inferiority, which may become a lifelong hindrance.

The damaging effects of such emotional deprivation may be reflected in the child's behavior. He or she may withdraw from becoming involved with other children (a possible carry-over into adult life). Lack of emotional warmth toward the child at these critical times may also stifle his or her intellectual growth. If the teacher provides only intellectual stimulation, autism, or a state of "emotional refrigeration," may result, in which the child has no interest in people. A warm, emotional classroom atmosphere, generated by a perceptive teacher, becomes crucial in nurturing the emotional development of all children.

Children failing to acquire essential skills readily acquire poor self-esteem, inadequacy, and emotional disorders. They are unable to function optimally in school and society. They become poor learners and "early loosers" in life. If this negative development continues, they become nonfunctioning or low-performing adolescents and adults. There are millions of people with these disorders in this country. Inability to function is the number-one social health problem today. Many adults who do work do so at a low level of proficiency, and many others are unhappy in their work.

Teachers have the marvelous opportunity to help children develop competencies in health, work, and life skills during this critical elementary school period. If such skills are not developed at this opportune time, they will probably not be developed later on. The child grows into a "skills-deprived adult," unable to function adequately in society. Thus it is vital that teachers nurture children's competence in many different kinds of skills—health and life maintenance, self-discipline, values and social skills, the three Rs, and just learning to work and achieve success at accomplishing things. Personal competence means that one can accomplish something with a high level of quality and to the satisfaction of others. Personal skills are essential for optimal mental health.

Research supports the view that many emotionally disturbed children have moderate to severe cognitive motor deficits. Such children are especially vulnerable to failure and maladjustment, showing symptoms of anxiety, avoidance, low achievement, low motivation, poor self-concept, low frustration tolerance, and poor emotional control. Research also indicates that at least 40 percent of children identified by their teachers as having moderate to severe behavioral problems also show signs of gross inadequacy in cognitive, perceptual, or motor-skill development.

Rubin (1970) develops these ideas in his "social competence" model, which he feels can help teachers to identify maladjusted children. The model emphasizes effective functioning in school as a measure of the child's ability to ultimately function in society (see Fig. 4.3). Academic failure or inability to learn effectively may thus be a manifestation of a lack of proper emotional, social, or physical (motor) skills. Collectively, lack of such skills programs a child for failure. If the teacher were to backtrack from the observed behavior (e.g., academic failure), he or she would discover that a tertiary (emotional), secondary (social), or primary (physical) problem was probably at the root of the observed failure (see Fig. 4.3(b). Figure 4.3(a) suggests that progressive development of essential physical, social, and emotional skills prepares the child to not only succeed in life, but also learn effectively. Both models (success/failure) point out that academic failure and inability to function in life may have hidden, or latent, causes.

The primary grades construct a crucial social environment in which to establish a momentum toward development of essential life skills. These skills, in turn, can provide reinforcers for positive emotional, social, and intellectual development. The intermediate grades become an extension of the kind of momentum and enthusiasm generated in the primary grades. Ideally, the child has received continual satisfaction and emotional pleasure from successfully coping with skills and so is capable of integrating his or her feelings, thinking, and behavior. When a child has not achieved satisfactorily the developmental tasks of his or her age level, we can expect to observe symptoms of emotional maladjustment. Violent drives and frustrations of this stage remain dormant (latent) only to explode and become "the storm of puberty"—the next step in the life cycle of the child.

Awareness of the etiology of emotional disturbances has implications for teachers and schools in planning appropriate early programs that adapt to individual differences in cognitive, perceptual, social, hygienic, value, emotional, and motor skills. In different grades different achievement demands should be made, and different skills should be required for adequate and challenging performances. Rubin (1970, p. 491) illustrates this approach as follows:

In the primary grades when materials are presented in a concrete fashion, there is a high dependence on visual perception, eye-hand coordination, and visual and auditory memory. By the time the child reaches the third or fourth grade, it is assumed that basic skills have been acquired and there is then an increasing demand on conceptual skills. In social studies and science the child is asked to read to gain facts and ideas and see the relationships between these. In arithmetic, story problems call upon the child's learned number facts but the method for the solution of the problem must be inferred. There are some children successful in the primary grades who learn well by rote, make perceptual discriminations easily, and have adequate visual and auditory memory who, lacking

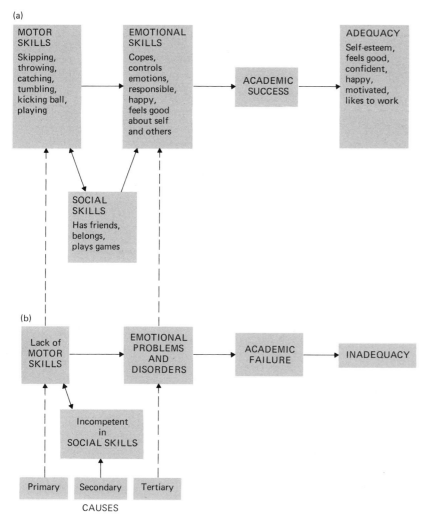

Fig. 4.3 A personal-social competence model illustrating failure/success in the classroom: (a) success track; (b) failure track.

adequate conceptual skills, experience frustration in the later elementary grades. *

Despite the fact that handicapped children may tend to have more than their share of emotional and learning problems, with proper help and training they are capable of becoming happy and useful persons. Studies have shown that a handicap will not stop a youngster from achieving vocational success and social acceptance, provided he or she develops the appropriate skills and the ability to work harmoniously with others. This suggests that schools can best serve the emotionally disturbed child by helping him or her gain social acceptance, by promoting his or her feelings of personal adequacy, and by encouraging him or her to develop his individual potentialities as fully as possible. In addition, provisions must be made for helping such a child to achieve satisfying personal and social adjustments. The disturbed child needs to be shown how to cope with everyday problems and how to retain a flexible attitude toward life in general.

General Symptoms of Emotional Problems

Teachers should be aware that a child's feelings and thoughts about self and others may evolve into primary emotional disturbances. If these are not resolved, they may be transformed into more serious secondary disorders such as maladjustments and antisocial behaviors. The classroom teacher does not need to discriminate between the symptoms of each of these disturbances in order to identify children with such problems. Instead, emotionally disturbed and maladjusted children may have similar overt symptoms that are easily observable.

Children may be suspected to be emotionally disturbed and maladjusted when they exhibit a group of the following general symptoms that constitutes a syndrome of emotional disturbance.

Appearance

1. Physically tense body
2. Worried look
3. Overweight
4. Sudden change in appearance or personality
5. Pallor
6. Rapid breathing
7. Depression
8. Sloppy appearance

Behavior

1. Infantile speech
2. Nail biting
3. Thumb sucking
4. Temper tantrums
5. Daydreaming
6. Restlessness
7. Frequent or near-accidents
8. Overtalkative
9. Highly excitable
10. Tattler
11. Overdaring or excessively shy
12. Overaggressive
13. Overdomineering
14. Excessive bragging
15. Overanxious to secure approval
16. Teases other children constantly
17. Cruelty to other children and animals
18. Marked hostility
19. Overinterest or complete indifference in sex matters
20. Easily upset
21. Extreme sensitivity to criticism

---

* Reprinted by permission from Eli Z. Rubin, "A Psycho-Educational Model for School Mental Health Planning," originally published in *Community Mental Health Journal*, Vol. 6, No. 1, February, 1970.

22. Resistance to authority
23. Poor sportsmanship
24. Constant quarreling with others
25. Always a spectator on the sidelines
26. Inability to relate to others
27. Inability to make decisions
28. Low achievement motivation
29. Low frustration tolerance
30. Poor emotional control
31. Clumsy in fine or gross motor movements
32. Impatient
33. Inability to solve or face problems
34. Stutters
35. Cheats
36. Lies
37. Always late
38. Absent or truant from school often
39. Breaks school rules often
40. A nonacademic achiever
41. Jealous of others
42. Bizarre behaviors and expressions
43. Cigarette smoking and drug abuse
44. Running away from home
45. Hyperactive
46. Preoccupation with own problems

Typical Complaints

1. Being picked on
2. Others are cheating
3. Fear of failure
4. Feeling inadequate and lack of confidence
5. Poor self-concept
6. Headache
7. Sore eyes
8. Has no friends
9. Can't be on time
10. Doesn't care about school
11. Doesn't want to go home (after school is dismissed)
12. Insomnia
13. Phobias
14. No one cares
15. Often suffers from excessive fatigue
16. Difficulty in concentration
17. Despair and hopelessness
18. Unable to make decisions
19. Cannot solve simple problems

Suggestions for Helping Children with Emotional Problems

1. Give child recognition when appropriate and possible.
2. Be friendly and warm but firm.
3. Be a good listener.
4. Create a warm, friendly atmosphere in the classroom.
5. Call students by name.
6. Ask for volunteer helpers.
7. Involve "wallflowers."
8. Demand everyone's attention before teaching.
9. Respond to inattention, disorder, and disobedience in classroom through body language. Do so quickly (evolve self-discipline).
10. Give clear and explicit directions.
11. Provide for intrinsic instead of extrinsic rewards and behavioral reinforcements.
12. Arrange for frequent rest periods.
13. Arrange for a balance of rest, sleep, and exercise.
14. Encourage interests such as hobbies, art, crafts, drama, music.

15. Allow for individual differences in academic assignments.
16. Provide for more successes than failures.
17. "Do with the child" certain complex tasks and then gradually withdraw. Show the child how to work.
18. Emphasize each child's developing emotional self-control and self-discipline.

Remedial Approaches

The primary responsibility of the classroom teacher to maladjusted and emotionally disturbed children should be to identify them early. In addition, the teacher should provide a climate favorable to the development of optimal emotional well-being. However, the teacher should refrain from correcting deep-seated behavioral problems without having the necessary training in therapy. In making such an attempt, the teacher may intensify a child's problem. After identifying an emotionally disturbed or maladjusted child, the teacher should refer the child to the proper professional or school authorities.

REVIEW QUESTIONS

1. How may childhood problems of growing up erupt as antisocial behavior?
2. How many emotionally handicapped children should you expect to find in your classroom?
3. How may emotional well-being be interpreted?
4. What are the indices of emotional well-being?
5. List 15 characteristics of a healthy, multivalued personality.
6. List Kaplan's six behavioral characteristics commonly associated with serious adjustment problems of children.
7. How may lack of skill and accomplishment help to create an emotionally disturbed child?

8. What childhood behaviors might lead you to suspect valuelessness in a child?
9. What is Rubin's social-competence model?
10. How can you, as a teacher, best help an emotionally disturbed child?
11. What symptoms of appearance, behavior, and complaints form a syndrome of emotional disturbance?
12. Suggest ten things classroom teachers can do to help children with emotional problems.
13. What is the primary responsibility of the classroom teacher for maladjusted children?
14. How does the child's need for adventure and risk taking relate to good emotional well-being?
15. Can emotionally sick parents and teachers infect children with their malaise?

REFERENCES AND BIBLIOGRAPHY

Caplan, Gerald. "Opportunities for School Psychologists in the Primary Prevention of Mental Disorders in Children," in *The Protection and Promotion of Mental Health in Schools*, Publication No. 1226 (Washington, D.C.: U.S. Department of Health, Education and Welfare, 1965), pp. 9-22.

Coelho, George, David A. Hamburg, and John E. Adams. *Coping and Adaptation* (New York: Basic Books, 1974).

Erikson, Erik H. *Childhood and Society* (New York: Norton, 1964).

_____. *Identity, Youth and Crisis* (New York: Norton, 1968).

Glasser, William. *Reality Therapy* (New York: Harper & Row, 1965).

_____. *Schools Without Failure* (New York: Harper & Row, 1969).

Hountras, Peter T. *Mental Hygiene* (Columbus: Charles E. Merrill, 1961).

Jones, Edward V. "A Public Health Approach to Emotional Handicap in the Schools," *Journal of School Health* (November 1969): 627-632.

Kaplan, Louis. *Mental Health and Human Relations in Education* (New York: Harper & Row, 1959).

Maslow, Abraham H. "A Theory of Metamotivation: The Biological Rooting of the Value-life," *Journal of Humanistic Psychology* (Fall 1967): 93-126.

———. *Toward a Psychology of Being* (New York: Van Nostrand Reinhold, 1968).

Mental Health (New York: National Association for Mental Health, 1965).

Radin, Sherwin S. "Mental Health Problems of School Children," *Journal of School Health* (June 1963): 250-257.

Rubin, Eli Z. "A Psycho-Educational Model for School Mental Health Planning," *Journal of School Health* (November 1970): 489-493.

Rucker, W. Ray, V. Clyde Arnspiger, and Arthur J. Brodbeck. *Human Values in Education* (Dubuque, Iowa: Wm. C. Brown, 1969).

Toffler, Alvin. *Future Shock* (New York: Random House, 1970).

Vincent, Elizabeth L., and Phyllis C. Martin. *Human Psychological Development* (New York, Ronald Press, 1961).

5

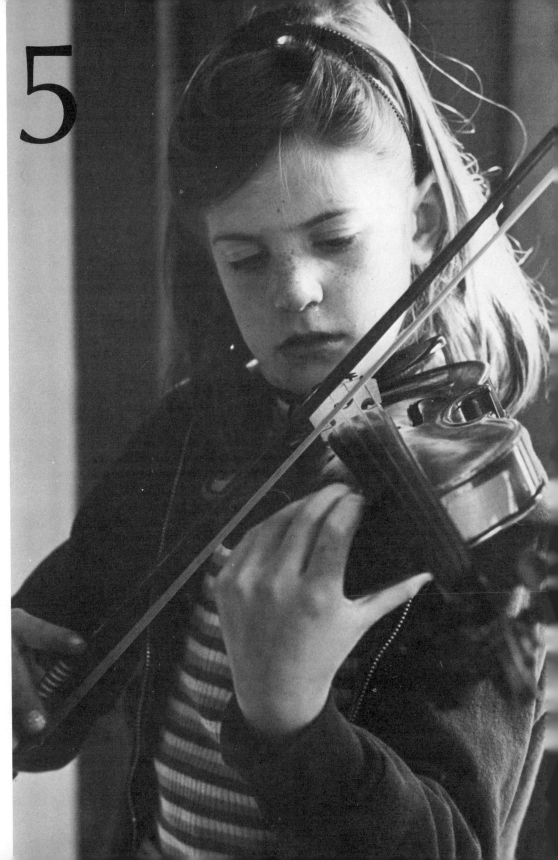

development of values

*Education should consist, as it has always done in Greece, of music and gymnastics. Music is considered first. The early education is of most importance, and that must be imparted at first by means of tales which are untrue. For the aim of early education is not to impart information, but to produce a certain type of character. But if the historical truth of stories told to children is unimportant, the moral effect which such stories are likely to produce is of utmost consequence.**

HISTORICAL PERSPECTIVE

The quote above from Plato (Lindsay, 1950, p. xxxiii) reminds us of the great emphasis placed on character (values) development in ancient Greek society. Character education has been an integral part of education in all past civilizations. The ancients recognized that values—such as love, trust, joy, truth, honesty, beauty, goodwill, cooperation, and understanding—are essential for good living. These values† must be taught because they are the key to human survival. Indeed, civilizations have risen and fallen on the virtues of their value systems. Human beings have been able to survive by adapting values that mediate their actions and behaviors. Teaching human values is really teaching survival skills. This chapter focuses on values development, for children are at a prime and critical time for evolving values by which to live as adults.

Values should be taught primarily at home and in the community. However, many parents do not have this skill or don't have the time to do it, and our technological lifestyle has eroded the once "rooted" community as a place for developing values; therefore, the schools need to assume responsibility for helping children to develop values. Schools should not replace the parental role in

---

*From *The Republic* by Plato, translated, with an introduction by A. D. Lindsay. An Everyman's Library Edition. Published in the United States by E. P. Dutton, and reprinted with their permission.

† "A value is a characteristic or attribute of some general realm of human experience which is considered desirable by an individual or group (Dalis and Strasser, 1973).

value development; instead, schools should complement the parents' efforts.

Shortly after World War II and with the escalation of technology, character and morals were deemphasized in the schools of the United States. Teachers were sensitized not to impose their values on their students. Values education was left up to the family. Unfortunately, parents have not been able to effectively assume such responsibility. Consequently, as Maslow and others have pointed out, young people have been growing up in a values vacuum. In Maslow's words: "We have evolved a 'valueless' society."

During the early 1970s, "values clarification" became a popular approach in this country (Raths, 1966). Obviously the pendulum had swung back to values education. The greatest emphasis and need for such education is at the elementary school level, where the groundwork in values is initiated. With the child developing cognitive ability in abstract thinking, he or she is able to rationalize about values and moralize about human conduct on a personal and social basis. Because of this cognitive development and involvement with developmental tasks, all children have a great need for clarifying their values. This need is a psychological one and reflects a need for self- or ego identity—an essential prerequisite to optimal emotional and social well-being.

Values are the intermediates applied to alternative decisions about living. Children discover very early in life that they are expected to acquire a "workable" understanding of the meaning of life. The values that children develop become the organizing core of their thinking lives. Values enable the youngster to maintain a sense of direction in fulfilling his or her basic human needs and in daily living. Values should enable the child to feel self- and societal-directed excellence.

The elementary school child develops inner controls that regulate his or her "right" and "wrong" behavior. These inner controls reflect the culture's values and standards as imposed on children by parents. The young child accepts such values, but the adolescent begins to question them and to select values that help him or her give a better meaning to life.

Teachers have traditionally taught moral, or values, development by drilling students in a set of fixed virtues, such as honesty, helpfulness, willingness to obey, washing hands before eating, and so on. The teacher would display the virtue by precept and example and moral tales and then reward those students who conformed to the virtue and punish those who did not. This time-honored method was successful for many civilizations before World War II, but it has not been successful in the United States since then.

STAGES OF MORAL DEVELOPMENT

Recently, a newer approach to moral-judgment training has emerged, theorized initially by Jean Piaget and more recently by Lawrence Kohlberg. These men have assumed that the formation of moral judgment is a process of development through stages of knowing—that is, a growing awareness of the external world. Development of moral judgment is recognized as a cognitive process and not one of absorbing an imposed set of standards. Let us briefly review Kohlberg's research on how values are developed.

Kohlberg (1968) studied the development of moral judgment and character of the same group of 75 boys from early adolescence through young adulthood—a period of over 12 years. His findings are supplemented by a series of studies on moral development in other cultures. On the basis of theoretical and philosophical considerations and from listening to children of all ages and backgrounds explain their judgments about hypothetical moral dilemmas, Kohlberg originally identified six stages of moral thought, summarized in Fig. 5.1.

Stage 1. *Obedience and Punishment Orientation*

The child avoids trouble because of the consequences. The physical consequences of an action determine its goodness or badness, regardless of the human meaning or value of these consequences. The child perceives no difference between the moral value of life and its physical or social value.

Decisions result from a blind obedience to power, an attempt to avoid punishment, or an attempt to seek rewards.

Stage 2. *"Naively Egoistic" Orientation*

Right action is whatever satisfies one's own needs and, occasionally, the needs of others. The operating principle is: "You scratch my back and I'll scratch yours." Such reciprocity is not one of loyalty, gratitude, or justice. Rather, human life is perceived as an instrument for satisfying the needs of its possessor or other persons.

Decisions result from a desire to satisfy one's own needs and, occasionally, the needs of others.

Stage 3. *Good Boy–Nice Girl Orientation*

The next stage is characterized by a search for approval by helping others. Good behavior is that which *pleases or helps others* and is approved by them. Conformity often gets the feedback "he or she means well," and one earns approval by being "nice."

Decisions result from a desire to please and help others and to receive their approval in return: "Please others." Human life is valued on the basis of empathy—affection of family members and others toward its possessor.

Stage 4. *Law-and-Order Orientation*

In late childhood the adolescent is oriented toward authority, fixed rules, and the maintenance of social

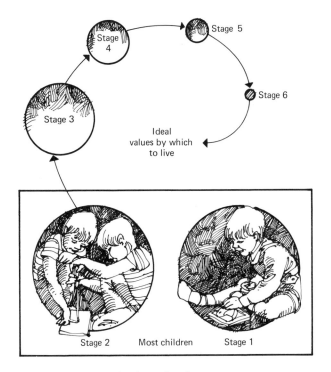

Fig. 5.1 Stages of values development.

order. Right behavior consists of doing one's duty, showing respect for authority, and maintaining the social order.

Decisions result from a desire to maintain the existing authority, rules, and social order: "Do and obey." Human life is conceived as sacred in terms of its place in a categorical moral or religious order of rights and duties. The value of life is partly dependent on serving the group, state, God, and so forth.

Stage 5. *Social-Contract, Legalistic Orientation*

The adult behaves appropriately even in the absence of law and authority. Right action tends to be defined in terms of general rights and standards

Pages 63-67 are adapted from Walter D. Sorochan and Stephen Bender, *Teaching Secondary Health Science,* New York: Wiley, 1978. By permission.

that have been critically examined and agreed on by the whole society. There is a clear awareness of the relativism of personal values and opinions and a corresponding emphasis on procedural rules for reaching consensus. Aside from what is constitutionally and democratically agreed on, right or wrong is a matter of personal "values" and "opinion." The result is an emphasis on the "legal point of view," but with an emphasis on the possibility of changing law in terms of rational considerations of social utility rather than freezing it in terms of stage 4, "Law and order." Outside the legal realm, free agreement and contract are the binding elements of obligation.

Decisions result from recognition of an individual's rights within a society that has a social contract. Human life is valued in terms of both its relation to community welfare and as a universal human right.

Stage 6. *Universal Ethical-Principle Orientation*

This stage has recently been combined with stage 5. Right behavior is guided by one's conscience in accord with self-chosen ethical principles appealing to logical comprehensiveness, universality, and consistency. These principles are abstract and ethical (e.g., the Golden Rule, the Categorical Imperative); they are not concrete moral rules like the Ten Commandments. Instead, they are universal principles of justice, of the reciprocity and equality of human rights, and of respect for the dignity of human beings as individuals.

Decisions result from an obligation to universal ethical principles that apply to all humanity: "Operate with a consciousness." Human life is valued as sacred and as representing a universal value of respect for the individual.

These six stages fall into three levels: Stages 1 and 2 are premoral (no values as yet) in nature; stages 3 and 4 are conventional (cope with life); and stages 5 and 6 are based on principles (ideal values for all). They represent a developmental sequence that illustrates an increased movement through the stages toward an increased universality of moral valuing of human life. At stage 1, only important persons' lives are valued; at stage 3, only family members; at stage 6, all lives are equally morally valued. Such transitions provide not only a psychological explanation of why the child moves from stage to stage, but also a philosophical basis of why one stage is "better" than another. The progression of moral development is further illustrated by the "Miracle Drug" dilemma and the responses of children to this dilemma.

The Miracle Drug

A woman was suffering from an extremely rare, painful disease. According to the most qualified doctors, there was a 95 percent chance that in three months she would become nearly completely paralyzed and thereafter would suffer a very painful bedridden existence. There was one medicine that offered a 50 percent chance of a cure.

The only medicine presently available was developed by a physician who spent several years in the research and development of the substance. Furthermore, he financed the development with his own money. For a complete treatment the medicine cost the doctor $100. However, he charged each patient $2000 (20 times his cost in time and ingredients), donating $1600 to an orphanage.

The woman's concerned husband lacked the $2000 needed to buy the treatment. Selling their household goods and automobile raised only $800. His efforts to acquire loans or welfare aid proved fruitless. The husband pleaded with the physician to give him the medicine for the $800. He promised to pay the remaing $1200 on installment payments. The physician rejected the offer, saying "I developed this substance after years of financial sacrifice, and because there are never more than two or three cases of this disease a year, I must demand the full amount in cash."

The husband felt desperate. His wife needed the medicine now, but there was no way he knew of to get it for her except to steal it. He turned to his minister for advice. The minister told him that stealing is against the Ten Commandments and that because his wife's suffering was God's will, he shouldn't interfere with what God had willed. His best friend refused to advise him, not wanting to get involved. His wife pleaded with him to steal, even murder if necessary, to get the medicine.

One night, the husband broke into the doctor's office, stole the medicine his wife needed, and in a fit of anger destroyed the remaining medicine and the formula.

The reactions of children and adolescents to this moral dilemma are summarized in Table 5.1. Their reactions, when classified into stages, reflect their level of moral maturity.

Many aspects of how values develop and change have already been pointed out. Other aspects reflecting such development are summarized below.

1. Children do not make all of their moral judgments at the same time. As a child develops, 50 percent of his or her judgments are at one stage, which can be designated as the child's current stage of moral development (Conger, 1973, p. 309). The remainder of the child's judgments are divided between the preceding and following stages.

2. A child must experience and attain a lower-order stage before being able to move on to a higher-order stage.

3. A child develops *sequentially* upwards from a lower-order stage to a higher-order stage. Moral reasoning of the conventional, or stage 3-4, kind never occurs before the preconventional stage 1 and 2 thought has taken place. No adult in stage 4 has gone through stage 6, but all stage 6 adults have gone at least through stage 4.

4. Two adjacent stages may overlap. A developing person may moralize at stage 3 in certain situations, then moralize at stage 4 in another situation, then revert to stage 3 thinking.

5. There are wide individual differences in the ages at which particular children or adolescents reach or pass through various stages.

6. An individual may cease to progress beyond a given stage. That is, a person's moral development may become fixated or arrested at a specific level in a stage.

7. Values/moral formation is born out of an interacting process between the individual and his or her surrounding social system.

8. Types of moral judgments or the stages are not related to age.

9. There is universality of sequence among various cultures. The last two stages are not present in preliterate villages or tribal communities.

10. An individual's morals are shaped by complex factors, especially his or her family, friends or peer group, games and sports or playing, social experiences, mass media, sex role, military service, and so forth.

11. Moral development is related to personality development and personal adjustment. For example, it has been observed that maladjusted persons are less mature in moral judgment and base their judgments more on concepts of absolute authority than do well-adjusted persons.

12. Moral development is related to cognitive development, intelligence and mental traits, or the ability to reason. Moral development thus has a cognitive core.

13. Children and adolescents comprehend all stages up to their own, but not more than one stage beyond their own. They prefer this next stage.

14. Moral judgments in all societies have certain features in common. That is, since societies are made up of social institutions (family, health, education, religion, economics, politics,

Table 5.1 Responses of children to ethical dilemmas at various stages of moral development.

Stages	Statements on "the basis of worth of human life"
Stage 1: The value of a human life is confused with the value of physical objects and is based on the social status or physical attributes of its possessor.	*Tommy, age 10* (Why should the druggist give the drug to the dying woman when her husband couldn't pay for it?): "If someone important is in a plane and is allergic to heights and the stewardess won't give him medicine because she's only got enough for one and she's got a sick one, a friend, in back, they'd probably put the stewardess in a lady's jail because she didn't help the important one." (Is it better to save the life of one important person or a lot of unimportant people?): "All the people that aren't important because one man just has one house, maybe a lot of furniture, but a whole bunch of people have an awful lot of furniture and some of these poor people might have a lot of money and it doesn't look it."
Stage 2: The value of a human life is seen as instrumental to the satisfaction of the needs of its possessor or of other persons.	*Tommy, age 13* (Should the doctor "mercy-kill" a fatally ill woman requesting death because of her pain?): "Maybe it would be good to put her out of her pain, she'd be better off that way. But the husband wouldn't want it, it's not like an animal. If a pet dies you can get along without it—it isn't something you really need. Well, you can get a new wife, but it's not really the same."
Stage 3: The value of human life is based on the empathy and affection of family members and others toward its possessor.	*Andy, age 16* (Should the doctor "mercy-kill" a fatally ill woman requesting death because of her pain?): "No, he shouldn't. The husband loves her and wants to see her. He wouldn't want her to die sooner, he loves her too much."
Stage 4: Life is conceived as sacred in terms of its place in a categorical moral or religious order of rights and duties.	*John, age 16* (Should the doctor "mercy-kill" the woman?): "The doctor wouldn't have the right to take a life, no human has the right. He can't create life, and he shouldn't destroy it."
Stage 5: Life is valued both in terms of its relation to community welfare and in terms of being a universal human right.	*Bob, age 16* (Should the captain order the soldier on a suicide mission to save the company?): "If nobody wanted to volunteer, I don't think he has the right to make someone go. I don't know if the army rules give him the right not to go, but as a person in the world I think he has the right not to go. But if it would save so many other lives, he really should go. The captain would have to decide to send him if it's necessary to save all their lives."
Stage 6: Belief in the sacredness of human life as representing a universal human value of respect for the individual.	*Steve, age 16* (Should the husband steal the expensive drug to save his wife?): "By the law of society he was wrong but by the law of nature or of God the druggist was wrong and the husband was justified. Human life is above financial gain. Regardless of who was dying, if it was a total stranger man has a duty to save him from dying."

technology, and mass media) helping people to fulfill their needs, the basic values of the social institutions are similar.

15. Opportunity to participate in roles of persons in different social situations (as in social institutions) is vital to the child's advancing morally from one stage to the next. Values emerge as a consequence of social interaction.

The child should progress from premoral selfish to conventional adolescent values toward universal values. As was pointed out earlier, a child initially observes the consequences of his or her behavior and judges the severity of transgressions with respect to their visible damage or harm. As the child becomes older, he or she tends to reason about values from a perception of imminent justice, observing that punishment follows from principles that take into account consequences for other people. Gradually, the preadolescent perceives that application of rules is established and maintained through reciprocal social agreements.

Not all persons in our society will attain formal operational thinking (reasoning). Even fewer should be expected to attain the postconventional level of moral development. Only about 10 percent of adolescents over age 16 may be expected to attain stage 5 or 6 thinking (Clarke, 1968, p. 458). Most people become arrested in stages 3 and 4.

DEVELOPMENT OF VALUES

Values are obviously evolved very early in life. As preschoolers observe and interact with family members, people outside the family, and their own peer groups, they become aware of what others expect of them. Social values, such as sharing possessions and getting along with others, are probably developed through playing with other little boys and girls between ages three and five. Such awareness of expectations serves as a set of "ground rules" that children use in response to different health-life situations. Moral virtues, or the

dispositions to behave in morally desirable ways (e.g., honesty, fair play, loyalty, courage, and so on), are also taught by precept and example. Parents serve as models of behavior for preschoolers and elementary-age children, gradually being replaced by teachers. Children need to be taught certain "survival-social" values (such as taking turns, not pushing, brushing teeth) early in life. Hamm (1976) points out that such values need to be carried out as learning experiences if children are to learn these behaviors: "If children don't or can't understand the reasons for socially desirable moral rules, then they should be encouraged to live by those rules for purposes of their own safety and security, and for protecting them from their own misconduct." Thus teachers need to identify specific survival values and moral virtues that need to be structured in children at various levels of development and evolve rules and school practices that temporarily safeguard the well-being of children.

Values may be developed in other ways. Eight approaches to values education have been identified by Barrs (1975):

1. Evocation—help students to express their values through free, open classroom in which content tends to be overlooked.

2. Inculcation—instill or internalize certain desirable social values into students. Students are told to act according to certain values which teachers and society deem valuable. Teachers can provide positive or negative reinforcements to help students shape their values.

3. Awareness—help students to become aware of and to identify their values.

4. Moral reasoning—help students to develop a higher level of moral reasoning. A dilemma story is utilized to expose students to a stage of moral reasoning that is one stage higher than their own.

5. Analysis—allow students to use logical thinking and a scientific procedure in dealing with value issues. This approach requires students

to acquire facts about a social issue, case study, or dilemma.

6. Clarification—help students to use both rational thinking and emotional awareness to distinguish their personal behavior patterns and to clarify and actualize values.

7. Commitment—help students to partake in personal and social action in relation to their values, e.g., working on Saturdays as a volunteer in a home for the aged.

8. Union—help students to perceive themselves as parts of a larger whole, rather than as separate entities. This approach may be too difficult to implement, however.*

Thus there are numerous ways to help children develop values. Not all of these will be applicable to elementary school classroom settings.

Kohlberg emphasizes role playing as a values-developmental experience. Opportunities in a variety of socially useful roles should be selected so that the student will be able to see a moral decision from a number of different perspectives. The wider the range of role experiences, the more likely the student is to make a moral decision that will be just and satisfactory to many people instead of only to self. The critical factor in role taking appears to be empathy. The more an individual is able to empathize with others, the more likely she or he is to make a just moral decision.

A natural setting for role playing exists in all elementary schools. Students can serve as teacher aides, as cooks, as blackboard cleaners, as planners of activities, as referees of games, and so on. If such settings are not opportune, teachers may help pupils to simulate roles through role playing in skits and plays. In addition, children should be provided with learning experiences that are social in nature and not just personal or individual. Children should play many socially useful roles through which they can both expand their awareness of their world and also increase their scope of empathy.

Minor games, such as prisoner's base, dodge ball, and even low-level competitive sports games, all have built-in values as well as natural appeal to both boys and girls. The few rules of a simple game gradually become transferred into the rules by which youngsters live. Teachers should not overlook the silent and hidden values inherent in sports, games, and play. Children need to play in a variety of games and situations. Such play not only structures values, but also clarifies existing ones.

Although many teachers and counselors have popularized values clarification as a values-development experience, there is virtually no research evidence to support its use over other methods. Many teachers are using values clarification without any specific classroom behavioral objectives and without their accountability.

Values clarification can take place without the teacher or pupils actually doing a values-clarification strategy. It can begin with the challenge of varying viewpoints that can come through literature of all types, films and television, sports, traveling, resource people, field trips, and action projects. Traditional school activities, such as fact, concept, and skill-building activities and homework assignments, can be part of the process. Reading and discussions, writing assignments with a value focus, and community-action projects are all examples of values-clarification strategies that one can use year after year in many schools. Such strategies are simply good education.

Cultural Values

Eight kinds of cultural values have been identified by Rucker *et al.* (1969):

1. affection—love, friendship;

---

* Summarized from an article by Stephen Barrs which appeared in *The School Guidance Worker* **31**,2 (November/December 1975), pp.21-25 with the permission of the Guidance Centre, copyright The Governing Council of the University of Toronto.

2. respect—recognition of status and accomplishment;

3. skill—feel competent in motor activities, thinking, communication, job, social customs, social/personal accomplishment;

4. enlightenment—feel knowledgeable about some things;

5. power—feel that one has influence over self and others, make sound decisions;

6. wealth—a service, goods, or contributions to make (not materialism);

7. well-being—health and life, attaining and maintaining it;

8. rectitude—sense of right and wrong, moral ethical values and conduct.

Although this list identifies important values for teachers, most school boards of education (and teachers) have yet to adopt guidelines for classroom instruction of these values. In addition to establishing such guidelines and identifying priorities for values, there is an immediate need to clarify Kohlberg's first four developmental stages in terms of helping teachers to identify the stage a child is in. This is most essential if teachers are to help children take the next step in the direction toward which they are already tending, rather than imposing fixed virtues. Finally, more information is needed on the kinds of learning experiences that best match the developmental levels of children and adolescents. Such educational experiences should aim primarily at communicating at a level one stage above the child's own and secondarily, at the child's own level. The behavioral demands made of children must also be correlated to their already existing moral values.

A key need for all schools and teachers (as well as parents) is to clearly identify enduring values that not only are socially acceptable, but also have withstood the test of time. Enduring values are "orthodox" and are essential to survival and optimal living, e.g., health and sanitary habits and lifestyle behaviors. There should be little, if any, dispute over these values. On the other hand, there may be considerable disagreement over emergent values, which result from technological progress and are often more personal than social. There may be considerable disagreement over emergent values, but there should be no argument over enduring social values. Enduring social values help us to survive. They are really essential skills.

VALUES EDUCATION

Finally, we need a way to assess the competence of a values education. Although there are shortcomings in the development of values, teachers and others should be aware that children will develop values of one kind or another with or without the help of parents and teachers.

Very little good research on values education, aside from Kohlberg's, has been conducted. Recently, moral-education experiments in the Canadian provinces of British Columbia and Ontario have been helpful in clarifying the process of values education. Sullivan *et al.* (1975) worked with Ontario elementary schools in an attempt to help fifth-grade pupils, typically at the preconventional level of focusing mainly on the needs of self, to progress to a conventional-level concern for the expectations and needs of others. Teachers experimented with two distinctly different approaches: a deductive discussion method, moving from general principles to specific applications, and a more inductive method of deciding what to do about a hypothetical moral "event." The researchers found that: (1) increases in maturity of moral reasoning did not show up until a year after the classroom experiences had ended; (2) there is a definite need for all teacher-training institutions to systematically prepare teachers to be moral educators; and (3) moral education curriculum needs to involve children in the decision making of the total life in the school and community.

Perhaps the greatest need in values education is that teachers need to be certain of their own values. They need special preparation in teaching strategies for values development. Teachers can do the following to prepare themselves for values education:

1. Begin a reading program so as to acquire a background in this area. The references at the end of this chapter are a good start.

2. Get some tested dilemmas and try these out:

    a) Sidney Simon, *et al., Values Clarification,* New York: Hart Publishing, 1972

    b) Beverly Mattox, *Getting it Together,* San Diego: Remnant Press, 1976

    c) Alan Lockwood, *Moral Reasoning: The Value of Life,* Columbus, Ohio: American Education Publications, 1972

    d) Edwin Fenton, ed., *Teacher's Guides to Value Education,* New York: Holt, Rinehart and Winston, 1973

    e) Film strips for elementary teachers: *First Things: Values.* Order from Guidance Associates

3. Attend classes, workshops, and conventions featuring moral education.

4. Subscribe to moral-education publications:
    Moral Development Forum
    221 East 72nd Street
    New York, New York 10021

As was pointed out earlier in this chapter, values are closely related to decision making, self-identity, and emotional, social, and spiritual well-being. These topics are discussed more fully in Chapters 1, 5, and 15-25. All of these chapters should be integrated with the topic of values.

REVIEW QUESTIONS

1. How do values mediate in health/life decisions?

2. Identify and discuss Kohlberg's six stages of moral development.

3. At what stage(s) of moral development are elementary school children?

4. Explain how values are developed (as perceived by Kohlberg).

5. List the various ways in which values may be developed.

6. What are the weaknesses of the value-clarification technique as it has been used in the past?

7. List Rucker's eight kinds of values.

8. List ten enduring values essential for survival and life. Compare your list of values with those of other students and teachers.

REFERENCES AND BIBLIOGRAPHY

Arbuthnot, Jack. "Modification of Moral Judgment Through Role Playing," *Developmental Psychology* (May 1975): 319-324.

Association for Values Education and Research. *Final Report of a Study in Moral Education at Surrey, British Columbia* (Vancouver, B.C.: Faculty of Education, University of British Columbia, November 1975).

Barrs, Stephan. "What is the Most Desirable Value Education Approach in the History Classroom?" *School Guidance Worker* (December 1975): 21-24.

Clarke, Paul A. *Child-Adolescent Psychology* (Columbus, Ohio: Charles E. Merrill, 1968).

Conger, John J. *Adolescence and Youth* (New York, Harper & Row, 1973), pp. 454-479.

Dalis, Gus T., and Ben B. Strasser. "A View of Values Education," a paper presented to the Los Angeles School District, 1973.

Developmental Psychology Today (Del Mar, Calif.: CRM Books, 1971), pp. 303-319.

Engeman, T. S. "Practical Possibilities in American Moral Education: A Comparison of Values Clarification and the Character Education Curriculum,"

Journal of Moral Education (October 1974): 53-58.

Galbraith, Ronald E., and Thomas M. Jones. *Facilitating Classroom Discussion of Social and Moral Problems: A Teacher's Handbook* (Pound Ridge, N.Y.: Sunburst Communications, 1974).

Goldiamond, Israel. "Moral Behavior: A Functional Analysis," *Psychology Today* **2**,4 (September 1968).

Guidelines for Drug Education Programs in the Schools (Sacramento: California State Board of Education, 1974).

Hamm, Cornel. *Moral Education Forum* (April 1976): 3-7.

Hawley, Robert C., and Isobel L. Hawley. *Human Values in the Classroom* (New York: Hart, 1975).

Hurster, Madeline. "The Identification of Value Orientations of Sixth Graders, with Specific Reference to Health Concepts in the School Health Education Study Curriculum," *American Journal of Public Health* (January 1972): 82-85.

Kohlberg, Lawrence. "The Child as a Moral Philosopher." *Psychology Today* **2**,4 (September 1968): 25-30.

Konopka, Gisela. "Formation of Values in the Developing Person," *American Journal of Orthopsychiatry* **43**,1 (January 1973): 86-96.

Lindsay, A. D., trans. *Plato: The Republic* (New York: Dutton, 1950).

Mattox, Beverly. *Getting it Together: Dilemmas for the Classroom* (San Diego: Remnant Press, 1976).

Peck, R., and R. Havighurst. *The Psychology of Character Development* (New York: Wiley, 1960).

Piaget, Jean. *The Moral Judgment of the Child* (Glencoe, Ill.: Free Press, 1948).

Program of Studies for Elementary Schools of British Columbia (Victoria, B.C.: Department of Education 1947).

Raths, Louis et al. *Values and Teaching* (Columbus, Ohio: Charles E. Merrill, 1966).

Rogers, Dorothy. *The Psychology of Adolescence* (New York: Appleton-Century-Crofts, 1972).

Rucker, W. Ray, V. Clyde Arnspiger, and Arthur J. Broadbeck. *Human Values in Education* (Dubuque, Iowa: Wm. C. Brown, 1969).

Simon, Sidney *et al. Values-Clarification: A Handbook of Practical Strategies for Teachers and Students* (New York: Hart, 1972).

Simpson, Elizabeth Leonie. *Democracy's Stepchildren* (San Francisco: Jossey-Bass, 1971).

Strong, Ruth. *An Introduction to Child Study* (New York: Macmillan, 1959).

Sullivan, Edmund *et al. Moral Learning: Findings, Issues and Questions* (New York: Paulist Press, 1975).

Thornburg, Hershel D. "Behavior and Values: Consistency or Inconsistency," *Adolescence* **8**,32 (Winter 1973); 513-532.

Valuing Process
1) Choose freely from alternatives
2) Understand consequences
3)
4) Prize
5) Affirm
6) Act on it
7) Repeat

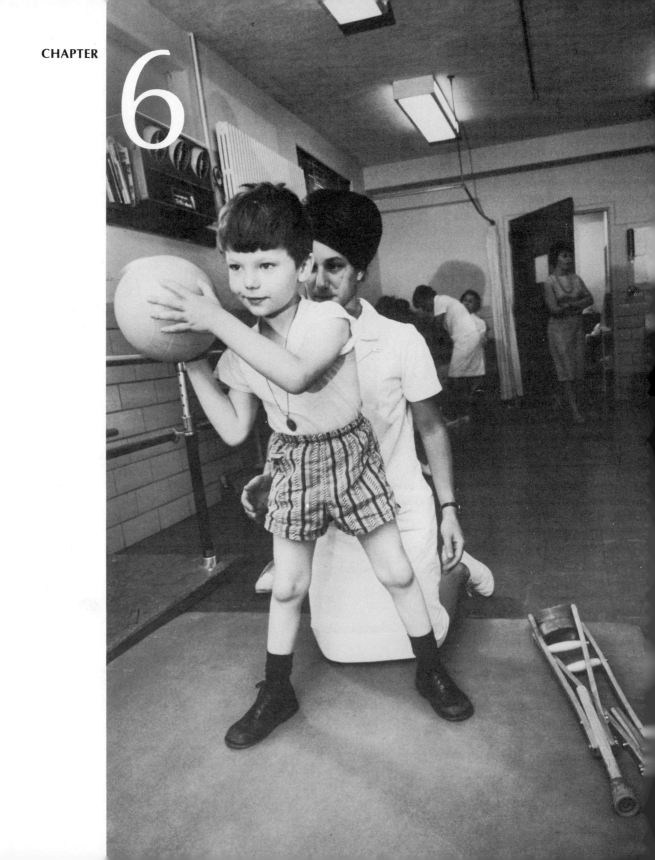

health and developmental problems of the child

INTRODUCTION

The vast majority of elementary children are able to fulfill their culturally expected tasks, resolve their needs, and continue to mature satisfactorily. However, a few children do encounter difficulty in fulfilling these tasks and are unable to achieve satisfactorily in school because of specific health impediments. Such children are therefore in need of special help and counseling services. In this chapter we deal with the most common health problems and disorders of school children. In addition to providing background information about the nature of a health problem, we will describe symptoms of the problem and outline suggestions for helping the child.

The prudent teacher should be aware that the child is a whole being, bringing to school all of his or her problems and feelings. Helping the child to overcome his or her problems is, in fact, rendering an integral service to the child in the school. This approach, ideally, complements the efforts of the parents at home.

The physiological health problems of elementary school children can be grouped into four broad categories:

1. Physiological disorders
   a) vision
   b) hearing
   c) dental
   d) posture

2. Metabolic disorders
   a) overweight or obesity
   b) diabetes

3. Neurological disorders
   a) epilepsy

4. Communicable diseases and allergies
   a) communicable (respiratory)
   b) rheumatic fever
   c) allergies

These are the problems and disorders that occur most often in elementary school children and that most elementary school teachers will sooner or later encounter in the classroom.

All of these problems are important because they have the potential to evolve into grave emotional problems for the child. The danger of emotional problems in the child, in turn, is that they may often interfere with the child's ability to:

1. learn effectively;

2. mature physiologically, psychologically, and sociologically in a manner that allows the child to fulfill his or her developmental tasks and progress in a manner of readiness from one maturational life stage cycle to another;

3. develop a wholesome, balanced personality;

4. maximize his or her potentials for self-actualization;

5. mature into a responsible member of society; and

6. graft roots for a proper lifestyle, or orthobiosis.

A child may be considered to have a health problem or disorder if she or he cannot, within limits, play, learn, work, or do the things that peers can do. Teachers should be aware that all children will have health problems to some degree. Indeed, all adults encountered some degree of emotional-social-physical problems or aberrations in their childhoods as part of the natural process of growing up.

Most adults eventually outgrew their childhood health problems, learned to cope with these problems and the realities of life, and became responsible and productive adults. On the other hand, a few adults never outgrow their childhood health problems, because they failed to receive proper attention and guidance. Their handicap escalated into a disabling lifetime health problem. About 15 to 20 percent of the people in our society have thus become socially dependent. A greater proportion function at work and in society at a lower level of existence, unable to realize their potentialities. Although they are unhappy and feel frustrated and unfulfilled, they perform their family and social roles, albeit in diminished ways. Such

results have implications for elementary health education.

Teachers should also be aware that a continuing health problem may persist for years as a handicap that can interfere with the child's learning and maturation. Such children lose years that are difficult, if not impossible, to reclaim. Unable to progress satisfactorily from one maturational stage to another, they can develop serious emotional and personality disorders and become socially maladjusted. Later, as adolescents and adults, they often "cop out" of school and society. One wonders whether elementary school teachers could have been instrumental in preventing or changing the destiny of such persons.

Before the child can learn, he or she must be physically, emotionally, and socially well. To ensure such well-being, the teacher's role is simply to locate, through observation, children in the class who may have unusual and peculiar symptoms, signs, appearances, or behaviors. It would be wrong for the teacher to diagnose the problem, much less prescribe medical treatment or therapy. These are medical concerns. The teacher's primary responsibility is to discover such children and then, with the guidance of professional personnel, help them to overcome their problems. Such a preventive approach can be extremely rewarding in that perhaps teachers' greatest happiness accrues from helping children, seeing them mature successfully, and fully sharing their happiness with them.

A useful technique for helping the teacher identify children with growth and developmental problems is the Wetzel Grid. The Grid shown in Fig. 6.1 (adapted from Grueninger, 1961; *The AAU-Wetzel Grid Growth Project*; Wetzel, 1941) is made up of 9 physique channels and 20 isodevelopmental levels for assessing a child's growth and development. When weight, height, and age are plotted on the Grid over a period of time, they project a graphic profile of the child's progress. The Grid summarizes the physical growth and developmental

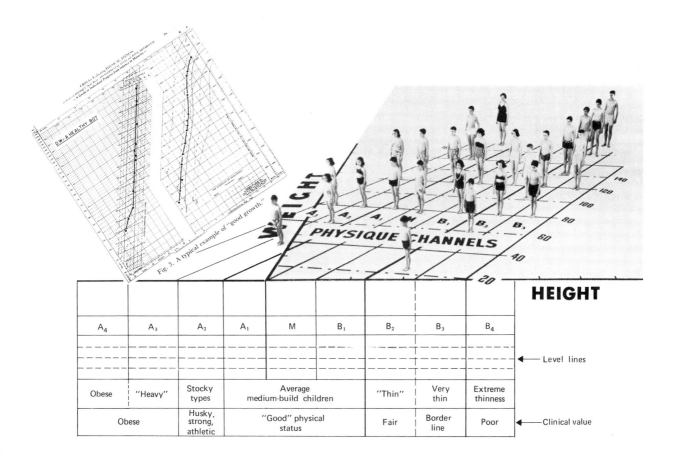

A₄	A₃	A₂	A₁	M	B₁	B₂	B₃	B₄
								← Level lines
Obese	"Heavy"	Stocky types	Average medium-build children			"Thin"	Very thin	Extreme thinness
Obese		Husky, strong, athletic	"Good" physical status			Fair	Border line	Poor	← Clinical value

progress attained, forecasts the progress to follow, and affords a means of judging individual performance by comparison with standardized guidelines of achievement. The Grid makes appropriate allowances for the great individual physical differences that are commonly found among children of the same age. Such age differences are also illustrated in Fig. 6.1. Obviously, teacher observations and suspicions about the physical health and behavior of a child may be confirmed by use of the Wetzel Grid. The Grid is also an aid to justifying referrals and follow-ups.

Fig. 6.1 Variations and progress in growth and development of children of different ages are conceptualized by the Wetzel Grid. Inset Grid shows data plotted over a seven-year period for a boy. (Adapted and presented with permission of the author, Dr. Norman C. Wetzel, and NEA Services Inc. Photograph by Francis Miller, Life Magazine, © 1950, Time Inc.)

TECHNIQUE OF OBSERVATION

Teacher observation is still the best and most reliable way to locate children with health problems and disorders. It is with the teacher that the child spends a large part of the day. The child's life in the school reveals his or her reactions and feelings to others. It is also to the physical and social environment of the school that changes in the child's appearance and behavior take place. Because of familiarity with the pupils, the teacher is in a strategic position to observe and to detect variations that may indicate a child's deviations from normal development, maturation, and well-being.

The teacher should observe children for health problems at the beginning of each school year. The sooner that children with problems are located, the sooner they may be helped and the greater the likelihood of their achieving more in school. Observations should be conducted at different times of the day. Each child should be observed under different stress situations. Teachers should watch children: while they play at recess, noon hour, during physical education class, and after school; while they eat their lunches; while they study in the classroom; and while they participate in social activities. The pupil's well-being may change from minute to minute or from hour to hour or from day to day. Teachers must be constantly on the alert for these changes.

The teachers should act like a detective, observing the child for: (1) physical-personal appearance; (2) behavior; and (3) complaints about how the child feels or is. Each of these factors will provide many clues about the child's possible problem. Understanding and/or employing the Wetzel Grid technique would be especially helpful with respect to item (1) above.

Observation of a single symptom or "clue" does not mean that the child has a health problem or disorder. Nor does a single observation of an unusual behavior indicate something is wrong with the child. It is only when the symptom or the unusual behavior recurs over a long period of time that the teacher should suspect that something is wrong. Health problems are expressed as recurring symptoms and interrelated behaviors. Collectively, these form an identifiable syndrome. Thus once having located a child with a possible problem, the teacher needs to reconfirm any suspicions. The teacher should observe the appearance-behavioral syndrome in the child for a period of two to four weeks. If the child does not outgrow the problem during this period or resolve the disorder, the teacher should refer the child for further examination and proper attention. Such referral and follow-up steps are suggested at the end of this chapter.

PHYSIOLOGICAL DISORDERS

The physiological disorders most often encountered with developing children and which the teacher can detect through observations are: (1) poor vision; (2) defective hearing; (3) dental caries; and (4) poor posture. If not corrected, these initial problems may manifest themselves in secondary emotional and behavioral disorders.

Vision

Vision is the child's most precious sense. The preschooler's eyes allow the child to explore and to relate to the surrounding physical and social world. Upon entering school, the child discovers that somehow he or she must begin to use vision as an instrument through which to learn. Then as the child progresses, the eyes sensitize the mind to the complexities of the larger world. Eyes are the most precious of all the senses; without them, the world takes on a dark sensuality and mars the child's development and progress. Defective vision may account for slow scholastic achievement, impairment of normal psychosocial progress, and numerous emotional problems. The earlier that visual defects are identified and corrected, the greater the child's chances for a normal life.

Some 80 percent of the work a child does in the elementary school is built around visual acuity within arm's reach. Obviously, it becomes important that visual difficulties be corrected as early as possible in the primary grades. Some 20 to 25 percent of all school children have eye defects. School surveys show that less than half of the children who need glasses actually have them.

Normal seeing involves both eye optics and brain development. Young children are normally farsighted and see large objects, large print, and pictures fairly well. The eye and its muscles need to be trained to adjust to close-up work. Eye muscles especially need to mature in order for visual acuity to be considered normal.

The most common visual difficulties have to do with refraction errors. In the eye without refractive error, parallel light rays focus on the retina. Objects at a distance of 20 feet project rays that are so nearly parallel that they focus on the retina without any accommodation on the part of the eye. Because of this natural phenomenon, this distance has been accepted as a measure of normal vision acuity, or emmetropia. A child has 20/20 vision if he or she can see at 20 feet what other children with normal vision can see at 20 feet.

Four main eye defects prevail among elementary school children. The child may be nearsighted, farsighted, have astigmatism, or poor binocular or two-eyes vision, such as double vision (strabismus).

Myopia – nearsighted

Variations in refraction are referred to as refraction errors (see Fig. 6.2). If parallel light rays come to a focus before reaching the retina, the image is formed in front of the retina, a condition called myopia, or shortsightedness. Although the myopic eye cannot focus distant objects distinctly on the retina, near objects are focused sharply. Because of this accommodation, the child may develop the habit of holding objects close to the eyes, as when reading a book. Often, the child compensates for nearsightedness by "squeezing" the eyelids to-

Squinting

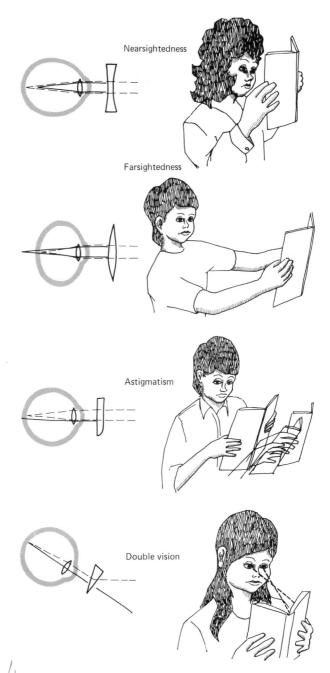

Fig. 6.2 Four main types of defects of the eyes and the lenses needed to correct these conditions.

gether. This symptom may be observed by the teacher as squinting or frowning.

Hyperopia – farsighted

On the other hand, if the rays reach the retina before coming to a focus, the condition is called hyperopia, or farsightedness (see Fig. 6.2). The image is formed behind the retina. About 80 percent of children are born with hyperopia, 5 percent with myopia, and about 15 percent with emmetropia (normal vision).

The teacher should be aware that the refractive status of the eye is continually changing; hence the elementary school child is most susceptible to eye and reading problems. There is a need to assess the child's visual acuity from time to time.

Astigmatism

Another possible refractive condition of the eye is astigmatism (see Fig. 6.2). The curvature of the lens or cornea or both may vary so that light rays are refracted, or bent, differently. The result is a blurred image on the retina. The child with astigmatism tends to frown and hold work near.

Strabismus

This condition occurs when one eye looks in a different direction from the other eye and is caused by lack of small–eye muscle coordination. That is, one eye fixates and the other eye turns out when an object is brought near the eyes. There is a lack of clear vision, lack of single vision, and lack of coordination between clearness and singleness of vision. Hence this disorder is often referred to as cross-eyes. On inspection on the eyes, the teacher will notice a slight "crossing" of the eyes. This is more noticeable when the child is fatigued or under great emotional stress.

Color-blindness

A less frequently occurring optical disorder is color-blindness. This is a sex-linked characteristic among boys; girls are almost never affected. Most of these children have difficulties distinguishing red-green colors accurately. Children have difficulty in identifying colors in the classroom may be confused about traffic signals.

Eye infections

Other eye problems the teacher should be aware of are common infections of the eye. A stye is an infection of a hair follicle in the lower eyelid and is characterized by swelling, pain, tenderness, and redness. In most cases a core of pus gradually develops. A similar infection in the upper eyelid is referred to as a shalazion. Such infections often erupt from eye strain and irritation. Excessive redness of the thin mucous membrane, or conjunctiva, lining the eyelids and eyeball may be due to irritation or infection of the blood vessels in the conjunctiva. This condition is referred to as conjunctivitis. Such irritation may be caused by smoke, dust, smog, excessive glare from the sun, snow, or bright light, or it may be associated with colds, hay fever, or allergies.

General symptoms of eye problems

No one single physical symptom, behavior, or emotional disorder identifies the child with an eye problem. Usually, there is more than one "tell-tale" symptom when the child has seeing or learning difficulty. A syndrome of behaviors, when found observable in the child, helps the teacher to suspect that the child may have an eye problem. The following physical symptoms and behavioral conditons, occurring usually as syndromes, will help teachers in locating children with eye problems:

A. *Appearance*
    1. *Lids:* crusting, swollen, red; skin at outer corner cracked
    2. *Eyes:* sunken, protruding, crossed, bloodshot, styes, watery, presence of discharge, swelling, irregular pupils

B. *Behavior*

1. Attempts to brush away blur
2. Blinks continually when reading
3. Cries frequently
4. Has frequent temper tantrums
5. Holds the book far away from face when reading
6. Holds face close to the page when reading
7. Holds body tense when looking at distant objects
8. Reads for only a brief period without stopping
9. Reads when should be at play, as compensation
10. Rubs eyes frequently
11. Squints face when reading
12. Screws up face when looking at distant objects
13. Shuts or covers one eye when reading
14. Thrusts head forward to see distant objects
15. Tilts head to one side when reading
16. Poor alignment in penmanship
17. Tends to look cross-eyed when reading
18. When reading, tends to frequently move book farther away and closer
19. When reading, tends to lose place on the page
20. In reading and spelling confuses: o's and a's; e's and o's; n's and m's; h's, n's, and r's; f's and t's
21. Makes apparent guesses from a quick recognition of parts of the word in easy reading material
22. Proneness to accidents; stumbling over objects in path or failure to appreciate height of steps, getting fingers caught in machines, etc.
23. Frowns
24. Dislikes tasks requiring sustained visual concentration
25. Unusual fatigue after completing a visual task
26. Uses finger or marker to guide eyes
27. Says words aloud or lip reads
28. Moves head rather than eyes while reading
29. Has difficulty in remembering what is read
30. Has poor hand-eye coordination, as in catching a ball or skipping rope

C. *Typical complaints*

1. Headaches
2. Nausea or dizziness
3. Burning, pain, or itching of eyes
4. Blurring of vision at any time
5. Sensitive to light
6. Cannot see well

Suggestions for Helping the Child with Vision Problems

1. Rearrange seating plan to give preferential seating to those students who need it.
2. Rearrange desks and location of teacher so pupils do not face the light.
3. Provide adjustable desk tops to ensure better light reflection on work, no glare from desk tops.
4. Permit child to sit as near as possible or as close as necessary to obtain best view.
5. Provide adequate lighting: replace burned-out lights in classroom; avoid glare and shadow.
6. Always provide clean blackboards: use yellow chalk on gray-green or blue-green color; avoid glare.
7. Provide clean, pastel-colored walls and white ceilings to avoid glare.

8. Select reading materials to ensure: clear type and pictures; adequate spacing between lines, words, and letters; adequate margins; good-quality paper with nonglossy finish.

9. Teacher's writing on chalkboard should be large and clear.

10. Amount of homework assigned should be limited for all children, but especially for those with severe visual loss.

Hearing

After the eyes, our ears are probably the second most important sense we have. Not only do we learn by hearing, but we also learn to understand the sounds we hear. In addition, our sense of balance is located in the inner ear. When a child has a hearing defect, the inability to hear is only a sequel to speech disorders, communication gaps, and emotional disturbances.

It is estimated that 1 out of 20 Americans has some degree of hearing loss, with about 0.6 percent of the school population having educationally significant losses. Hidden ear damage threatens as many as one in ten American youngsters. Some 400,000 children begin school each year handicapped by unrecognized hearing loss. The elementary classroom teacher can expect to find about two children in the classroom with a hearing problem in one or both ears. Most children who have some hearing loss acquire it gradually.

All hearing difficulties can be divided into two classes: (1) *conduction hearing losses,* associated with the conductive structures of the outer or middle ear; and (2) *sensorineural hearing losses,* associated with the ear's sensory receptors in the middle ear or fibers of the auditory nerve. Relatively few of the hearing problems found in children of school age are of the sensorineural type. Sometimes both conductive and sensorineural losses are present, in which case the impairment is termed *"mixed."*

The most common cause of conductive impairment involving the outer ear is an accumulation of ear wax that blocks the canal. Conductive disorders of the middle ear are a more serious matter. Almost all middle ear disease in childhood is due to malfunction of the Eustachian tube. A watery fluid, or transudate, may fill the air space of the Eustachian tube, resulting in pain and high fever. This condition is identified as *otitis media.*

Children with hearing losses may be described as either hard of hearing or deaf. The *hard of hearing* include those pupils in whom the loss of hearing is educationally significant, but whose residual hearing is functional for acquiring language—often with a hearing aid. The *deaf* include those whose sense of hearing is insufficient for understanding speech. Fortunately, most of the hearing problems that the teacher encounters in pupils are no more than hard of hearing.

Profound deafness is usually identified in early infancy. Any hearing impairment acquired before language has been mastered affects the entire child, not just the sense of hearing. Mild to moderate hearing loss is difficult for parents to detect. Often it is recognized only after several years of school. Meanwhile, it handicaps the normal growth of the child—at the age when speech, thought development, learning, and social relationships all depend on normal hearing. Because a hearing loss reduces or cuts off normal acquisition of language, hearing-impaired pupils not only tend to score less as a group on tests of intelligence, personality, adjustment, and social competence than those with normal hearing, but also are most likely to be under-achievers academically.

General Symptoms of Ear Problems

The teacher should be cognizant of any or all of the following conditions in a child:

A. *Appearance*
   1. Discharge or odor from an ear
   2. Strained facial expression
   3. Cotton in ear

4. Favoring one ear over the other

5. Appears mentally retarded

B. *Behavior*

1. Difficulty in talking and pronouncing

2. Inability to localize sound

3. Turning head to one side when spoken to

4. Persistently inattentive

5. Asks questions repeatedly

6. Fails to answer or answers incorrectly when called on

7. Watchful of the teacher

8. Slurs word endings

9. Speaks loudly

10. Turns volume up on radio or TV

11. Watches lips of other pupils as they speak

12. Slow learner

13. Written work better than oral work

14. Looking at someone else's work before starting assignment

C. *Typical complaints*

1. Earache

2. Ringing or noise in ear

3. Inability to hear

4. "Speak louder"

5. "Repeat the question, please"

Suggestions for Helping the Hard-of-Hearing Child

1. Face the pupil as much as possible.

2. Move around the room as little as possible while carrying on a conversation.

3. Secure the child's attention before addressing him or her.

4. Talk slowly and enunciate clearly.

5. Ask child to clarify or repeat what you said.

6. Prescribe advance reading on the subject to be discussed in class.

7. Appoint a "buddy" friend to help the hard-of-hearing child.

8. Develop understanding and awareness in the pupils in the classroom toward the hard-of-hearing child.

9. Place child near front of room.

10. Avoid competing and distracting noises (air conditioners, fans) in classroom.

Dental Problems

Dental cavities occur more frequently in school children than any other disorder or health problem. About 95 to 99 percent of all children suffer from dental problems. The times of greatest carious activity are at ages five to eight in the primary teeth and twelve to eighteen in the permanent set.

Good, healthy teeth are essential to the child for several reasons. They provide the hard chewing surfaces so necessary for the mastication and proper digestion of food. Teeth are also necessary for good speech, and they mold the contour of the lower part of the face. More important, teeth help to project the child's appearance and personality. Good breath accompanies healthy teeth. Loss of several teeth, dental caries, poorly aligned teeth (or malocclusion), and poor breath (or halitosis) may interfere with the child's normal development and achievement in school. More important, these disorders often are masked by emotional disturbances.

Dental Caries

The most common defect is decay. The causes of dental decay are multiple and include: inherited susceptibility to caries, poor nutrition during the years that teeth are being calcified, prevalence of acid-forming bacteria in the mouth, and eating too many sugar sweets and starches. The progress of decay is initiated by bacteria acting on carbohydrates. Research findings indicate that acids form within five minutes after sweet foods are eaten. Harmful acid levels build up within 15 minutes. The acids produced from fermentation combine with saliva in the mouth to cause erosion of tooth enamel. Calcified tissue is destroyed, and a small carie, or hole, is started. When the decay is limited to enamel and dentin, the tooth is sensitive to heat, cold, and sweets. When the pulp is involved, a toothache develops. When the nerve is destroyed, pain ceases.

Halitosis, or Bad Breath

This may indicate that the child is in poor health. The causes of bad breath may be dental caries, poor dental habits, eating strong-smelling food, gastric disorders, or infected mouth and/or gum tissues.

Malocclusion

Poorly aligned teeth may be caused by heredity, loss of a primary tooth and a drifting of adjoining teeth toward the empty space, chronic mouth breathing, poor oral habits such as thumb or finger sucking, impacted teeth, or congenital problems such as cleft palate.

Malocclusion interferes with proper cleansing of teeth, disturbs chewing, increases the likelihood of injury to protruding teeth, and alters facial appearance. Such conditions may cause unfortunate psychological and social effects. Often "buck teeth" become an emotional stigma for life.

Gum Infections

Gingivitis is inflammation of gum tissue; the gums appear red and swollen, feel tender, and tend to bleed if pressure is applied. The condition occurs most often whenever oral hygiene and dental care are neglected. Faulty brushing neglects to agitate bacteria and prevent plaque formation. Failure to remove plaque, a sticky bacterial deposit, from the teeth near the gum line leads to the formation of calculus, or tartar. Removal of this calculus by the dentist, as in cleaning teeth, is important in avoiding gum trouble.

Neglected gingival disease may result in an advanced disease called *pyorrhea.*

General Symptoms of Tooth and Mouth Problems

A. *Appearance*
   1. Cavities in mouth
   2. Excessive tartar at necks of teeth
   3. Malocclusion
   4. Irregular teeth
   5. Bleeding or inflamed gums
   6. Swollen jaw
   7. Cracking of lips and corners of mouth

B. *Behavior*
   1. Keeps mouth closed, refrains from smiling
   2. Sensitive about missing teeth
   3. Does not brush teeth regularly
   4. Speech defect
   5. Difficulty in mastication
   6. Thumb sucking
   7. Rubs gums
   8. Constant picking of teeth

C. *Typical complaints*
   1. Toothache
   2. Sensitivity to hot, cold, or sweets
   3. Complaint about sore gums
   4. Mouth feels sore
   5. Others don't want to play with him or her

Suggestions for Helping the Child with Dental Problems

1. Provide time to brush teeth after snacks and lunches.
2. Have those children who do not brush teeth in school rinse mouth out with water.
3. Discourage eating of sweets and drinking soft drinks.

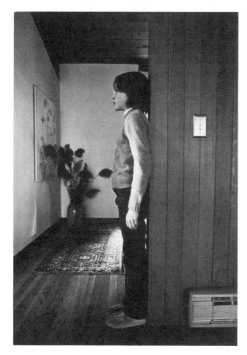 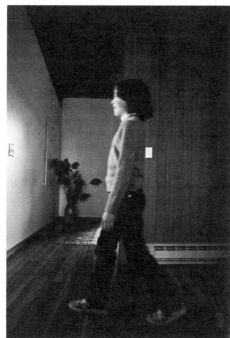

Fig. 6.3 Illustration of good posture.

4. Discourage finger sucking.
5. Demonstrate proper brushing technique.

Posture Problems

Postural habits established in the early years carry over to adulthood, with corresponding difficulties of vertical alignment and body movement. Various studies have found a significant association between poor posture and numerous physical, mental, and emotional disorders. Children with habitually poor posture have been observed to: be more susceptible to diseases, tire easily, be often underweight, be more self-conscious, have hearing defects, be more restless, be more timid, and have a greater incidence of asthma. Actually, 70 to 80 percent of all children and adults have varying degrees of postural malalignment.

Fortunately, most childhood postural disabilities may be corrected with a minimum of difficulty. When body mechanics improve in children with postural problems, there is almost always a corresponding improvement in health, physical efficiency, school work, and the child's self-image.

Good standing posture may be interpreted as an imaginary straight line (plumb line), projected alongside a person's (1) ear lobe, (2) center of the shoulder, (3) through the hip joint, (4) just behind the kneecap, and (5) through the outside ankle on the floor (see Fig. 6.4). A child's posture may be subjectively appraised as either being normal or deviating from the normal by observing where the plumb line falls relative to the child's five body landmarks.

In addition to the status of posture from the side position, the child's lateral body alignment should

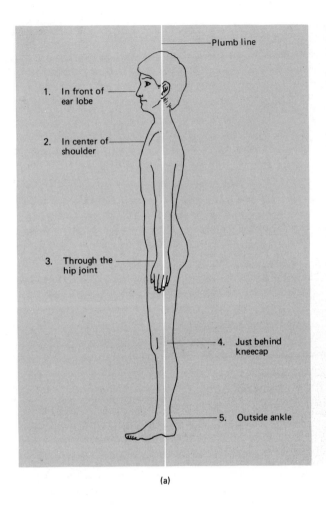

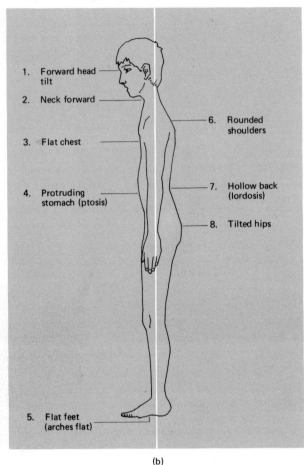

Fig. 6.4 (a) Side view of good posture and body alignment with imaginary straight line, or plumb line. (b) Side view of poor posture and malalignment of body and observable posture defects.

be assessed as well. The alignment of the head, neck, shoulder blades, spine, and hips should be balanced (see Fig. 6.5). Feet should naturally point straight ahead while standing and walking.

One observable posture defect is usually accompanied by one or more defects located in other parts of the human frame. For example, lordosis (exaggerated curve in the lumbar region, giving the appearance of a hollow back), is usually accompanied by such compensatory deviations as for-

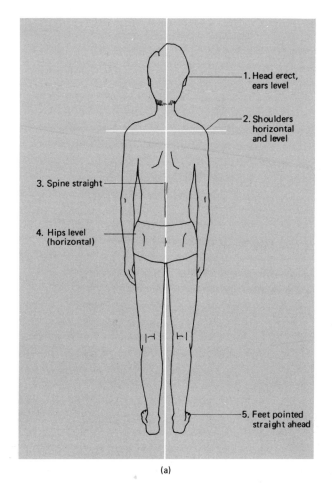

1. Head erect, ears level
2. Shoulders horizontal and level
3. Spine straight
4. Hips level (horizontal)
5. Feet pointed straight ahead

(a)

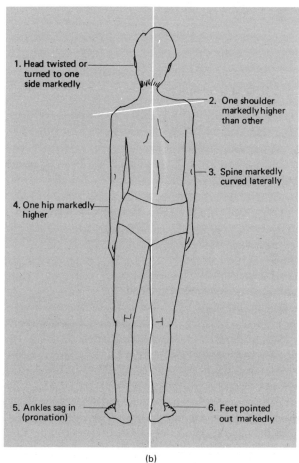

1. Head twisted or turned to one side markedly
2. One shoulder markedly higher than other
3. Spine markedly curved laterally
4. One hip markedly higher
5. Ankles sag in (pronation)
6. Feet pointed out markedly

(b)

ward head, cervical lordosis, round shoulders, flat chest, knees bent backward, or flat feet.

Fig. 6.5 (a) Back view of good posture and body alignment with postural landmarks. (b) Back view of poor posture and malalignment of body and observable postural defects.

General Symptoms of Posture Problems

A. *Appearance*

1. Head tilted forward, chin-in appearance
2. Exaggerated front-to-back spinal curves
3. Lateral spinal curves (scoliosis); one shoulder lower than the other

4. Flat chestedness
5. Flat feet (no arch)
6. Cramped toes
7. Ptosis (protruding stomach) (obesity)
8. Losing balance
9. Hands and shoulder-joint leaning in front of ears and hips

B. *Behavior*
1. Slouching forward
2. Lack of energy
3. Withdrawal from strenuous activity
4. Clumsy and uncoordinated
5. Desire to go barefoot or take off shoes
6. Restlessness
7. Changing sitting positions

C. *Typical complaints*
1. Sore feet
2. Sore back
3. Fatigue
4. Lack of sports skills

Suggestions for Helping the Child with Postural Defects

1. Encourage all children to sit and walk properly.
2. Feet flat on floor when sitting.
3. Keep head up, chest out.
4. Use backrest of chairs so that buttocks and back are resting against backrest.
5. Provide many stretch periods, interspersed with corrective exercises.
6. Encourage coordination and graceful movements.

METABOLIC DISORDERS

The two related metabolic disorders often handicapping children and adults are overweight and diabetes. Overweight is often a manifestation of diabetes. These are also interrelated conditions in that both disorders are suspected of having a common origin. Teachers need to anticipate confronting such disorders in children.

Overweight and Obesity

Next to dental caries, obesity is probably the most prevalent health disorder in the United States. Approximately 20 million Americans are overweight or obese. At least ten percent of elementary age children are overweight or obese. The teacher must be concerned about overweight and obese children, for obvious reasons.

Obese children are a major reservoir for obesity in adult life. Fat children tend to remain fat as adults. Adults who were excessively heavy children have more difficulty in losing excess weight and in maintaining fat loss than do the people who become obese as adults.

Obesity is the presence of excess adipose tissue in contrast to a measure of total body weight which includes bony structure, muscular tissue, and body fluids as well as fat tissues. A normal child should have average weight for his or her height, sex, and physiological maturity. A child with 15 percent or more in excess of average weight may be considered to be overweight. A child with 30 percent or more in excess of average weight may be considered to be obese. Overweight and obese children are less active physically than nonfat children, tend to be withdrawn, and often copy the faulty eating habits of their obese parents.

The psychological aspects of obesity are most complex. Obesity and overweight expose youngsters to difficult situations and damaging pressures. The child's adaptation ability, ability to successfully cope with problems, and self-image may all be part of the obesity syndrome. Many obese children and adults have been found to be unhappy and frustrated, although they may not relate such feelings to their disorder.

Obesity runs in families, and children most susceptible to this disorder have genetic and cultural predispositions. Obesity developing before age ten has a somber prognosis for eventual weight reduction. At least a third of all fat adults were formerly overweight children. A fat person tends to remain fat. Weight-reduction programs for such people have not been successful or effective.

Obesity at any age is a hazard to well-being. It interferes with normal body functions; increases the risk of developing certain diseases, such as diabetes and heart disease; has a detrimental effect on established diseases; and has adverse psychological reactions on the child. Obese adults tend to die sooner than do persons of normal weight. For these many reasons, the teacher's role in the classroom becomes one of preventing obesity in the students.

Warning signs of obesity are somewhat more difficult to recognize in children than in adults. In general, any change in the developmental channel in a child's auxodrome (as in the Wetzel Grid) is cause for careful medical examination. Post pubertal obesity is sometimes mistaken in its early stages for the normal "filling out" of early adulthood. Such a condition may be temporary, in which case there is no need to bring this to the attention of the child. On the other hand, the obese and overweight condition may persist and become irreversible and permanent if the child moves toward passivity, inactivity, and overeating.

General Symptoms of Overweight and Obesity

A. *Appearance*
   1. Fat and excess weight
   2. Ptosis (protruding abdomen)
   3. Padded waistline
   4. Large body frame
   5. Clumsy gait

B. *Behavior*

   1. Withdrawn from participation in physical activities
   2. Inactive
   3. Eats a lot
   4. Lazy and apathetic
   5. Self-conscious

C. *Typical complaints*
   1. Difficulty in normal breathing
   2. Exercises too difficult
   3. Play is too long—need rest

Suggestions for Helping the Child with a Weight Problem

1. Become involved and interested in the child as a human being.
2. Provide challenging alternatives to coping with problems of living.
3. Relate to child's emotional needs.
4. Involve the child in a lot of physical activity and exercise.
5. Discourage nibbling, snacks, and overeating.
6. Help child to identify his or her own self-image.
7. Allow for rest periods, but do not let rest become apathy.
8. Arrange social activities that are fun for everyone.
9. Help the child to meet many new friends.

Diabetes

Many children may be potential diabetics in the elementary school. They may have diabetes and not know it, or this metabolic disorder may develop as time goes on. It is estimated that 1 American in every 50 has diabetes and that 1 child in 2500 under the age of 15 suffers from this disturbance. The incidence of diabetes in the average elementary school is less than one percent. The classroom teacher's role in locating the diabetic child becomes very important when we realize that diabetes runs in families. Nearly 50 million Americans are believed to be capable of transmitting diabetes to their offspring, although most "carriers" are themselves free of the condition.

Unfortunately, the first signs of diabetes go unnoticed. The affected child and his or her parents may not be aware of the condition until well after the process has begun and the child is gravely ill. Diabetes is usually more severe in children than in adults.

Diabetes is a hereditary metabolic disorder in which the body is unable to break down and use food properly. This defect results in increased amounts of sugar in the blood and in the urine. The condition is aggravated when the pancreas cannot regulate the secretion of insulin. Insulin, in turn, regulates the storage and use of the body's sugar, or glucose.

Diabetes mellitus involves two opposite reactions, referred to as *diabetic coma* and *insulin shock.* Diabetic coma occurs when the pancreas fails to produce sufficient insulin. Because the child's normal use and storage of glucose is impaired, extra amounts of glucose accumulate in the blood (hyperglycemia) and are excreted in the urine. When the body is not utilizing sugar normally, fat is burned to supply energy; a by-product of this burning of fat is the formation of ketone bodies, which are acid in nature. Even though the body makes every effort to neutralize them, eventually they produce an acid condition in the blood and other body fluids. Insulin shock, a severe hypoglycemic state, occurs when an excess of insulin is administered to the known diabetic child. Body sugar is used up very quickly, and the blood sugar may drop far below normal.

Both types of diabetic reactions may be controlled by a carefully maintained program of proper diet, exercise, and medication. There is no known cure for diabetes. It is a lifetime disorder. However, when diabetes is controlled, the diabetic child can lead a normal life.

Diabetes may be detected by assessing the amount of sugar in the urine or in the blood. A medical examination is required to confirm the presence of diabetes.

General Symptoms of Diabetes

The signs and symptoms for diabetic coma and insulin shock are different and need entirely different treatment. Although the teacher's job is not to diagnose or treat, an awareness of the signs and symptoms will help the teacher to observe for potential diabetics and to recognize the critical needs of known diabetics in the classroom:

		Diabetic coma	Insulin shock
A.	*Appearance*		
	1. Skin	Red, dry, flushed	Moist, pale (cold sweat)
	2. Breath	Fruity color (acetone)	Normal
	3. Tongue	Dry	Moist
	4. Fever	Frequent	Absent
	5. Tremor	Absent	Frequent
	6. Convulsions	None except when lapsing into coma	In last stages
	7. Vomiting	Common	Rare
	8. Breathing	Deep and labored	Normal to rapid, shallow
	9. Pulse	Weak and rapid	Full and normal
B.	*Behavior*		
	1. Alertness	Drowsy	Excited
	2. Attention	Inattentive	Inattentive
	3. Walking	May stagger	Lacks coordination

	Diabetic coma	Insulin shock
4. Irritability	Incoherent as drunk person	Irritable

C. *Typical complaints*

		Diabetic coma	Insulin shock
	1. Thirst	Intense	Absent
	2. Urination	Frequent	Not affected
	3. Hunger	Absent	Intense
	4. Activity	Sluggish	Tires easily
	5. Vision	Dim	Double vision (blurred)
	6. Headache	Yes	Yes

D. *Clinical*

		Diabetic coma	Insulin shock
	1. Onset	Slow to gradual	Sudden
	2. Sugar in urine	Large amounts	Absent or slight
	3. Improvement	Gradual	Rapid following administration of carbohydrate

The teacher should be aware that the child who knows that he or she is diabetic will be aware of the symptoms. On the other hand, the child who is unaware of having diabetes will not be conscious of the symptoms. Such a child may not have pronounced symptoms, and the first sign will probably go unnoticed.

The symptoms listed in tabular form are symptomatic of the diabetic who is actually experiencing the disorder. Children with latent diabetes may not have all of the prevalent symptoms. Thus although many of the specific symptoms may prevail, the following general indicators of excessive thirst, frequent urination, overweight, constant hunger, loss of weight, fatique, drowsiness, vision changes, and a history of diabetic relatives should be clues for the observant teacher.

Suggestions for Helping the Child with Diabetes

1. Through conferences, involve the entire family in the maintenance of the child.
2. Help the child adhere to recommended medical therapy.
3. Do not demand too much of the diabetic.
4. Do not allow class to focus attention on the child.
5. Encourage the child to participate in normal play as much as possible.
6. Make the child feel adequate at all times.
7. Help the child to become self-accepting.
8. Help the child to check weight regularly.
9. Help the child to follow medical advice regarding the amount of exercise and physical activity that may be safe for him or her.
10. Have the child eat regularly in school.
11. Insist that the child follow a medically prescribed diet.
12. Have the child avoid strenuous exercise immediately before meals, since this is the period of lowest blood sugar levels.
13. Don't overtreat the child, who simply has different eating requirements from other people.

NEUROLOGICAL DISORDERS

Epilepsy

Elementary teachers will not be confronted very often with an epileptic child. A teacher who does come in contact with such a child is often psychologically unprepared to deal with such a situation. The teacher's initial shock is often so overwhelming that it creates adjustment problems for the child. It is for these reasons that epilepsy is dealt with in this chapter.

A child with epilepsy can lead a normal, healthy life. Yet when such a child has a convulsive seizure in school, it is often a dramatic and frightening experience for the teacher and the pupils. The epileptic child becomes more self-conscious and ashamed of his or her condition. Lack of understanding and failure of social adjustment by the pupils and teachers cause the development of a social stigma toward the epileptic child. Such a stigma is unwarranted, for the epileptic child has emotional, physical, and social needs similar to those of other children.

Epilepsy is not a disease, but rather a sign or symptom. It results from an underlying neurological disorder; a seizure occurs when a group of brain cells becomes overactive, and the well-ordered cooperation within the brain breaks down. This overactivity may remain in one area or spread to other areas of the brain. Most seizures do not last longer than two minutes. After the seizure has ended, harmonious activity is restored among the brain cells.

Convulsions are much more frequent in children than in adults. The exact cause for brain cells becoming suddenly overactive is not certain. In some children the brain cells seem to be more than usually sensitive to chemical irritation. In other children seizures may be caused by any of the following: brain damage before, during, or shortly after birth; infections of the brain (encephalitis and meningitis); emotional disturbance; metabolic disorders (hypoglycemia); tetanus; temper tantrums; overdosage of drugs such as aspirin and tobacco; inhalation of gasoline or alcohol fumes; snake bites; and allergies. Everyone is capable of having a seizure if his or her brain cells are irritated enough.

There are at least two million known epileptics in the United States. Between 10 and 20 percent of the population may be latently epileptic. About 1 in every 400 school children may be expected to have epilepsy. The predisposition toward epilepsy may well be inherited.

The age of onset of epilepsy varies and is important in determining the resulting psychological changes. Approximately one-eighth of all epileptic persons begin to have their attacks between the ages of 1 and 3, and approximately 75 percent between 12 and 20. About 70 percent of the epileptics are gripped by only one type of seizure; the remaining 30 percent have two or more types.

At the present time the seizures of 80 to 90 percent of children and adults can be controlled by a healthful lifestyle and with medication. In many cases the seizures will disappear, and the former epileptic can lead a normal, healthy life.

Epileptic children often need to take medication to control their convulsions. Such therapy may dull the child's responses just enough or cause the child to be irritable enough so that special learning problems occur. Memory may be affected. Such children may need to have restricted or limited participation in physical education and social activities in the school. All of these social conditions may affect the emotional and mental thinking of the epileptic child. It should not be too surprising to the teacher to find that such children have numerous emotional and personality problems. Such problems become secondary handicaps in that they interfere with learning. Emotional disturbances or difficult behaviors in a child with seizures are usually not due to the seizures themselves.

Despite what it may seem when a child has a convulsion, he or she does not suffer any pain. Despite the violent movements, deep and slow breathing, breath holding, paleness, or blueness, the unconscious child is not going to die and is unlikely to suffer any serious damage to the brain or body. The teacher should also remember that a convulsion will be over in a few minutes and can never harm the onlooker.

General Symptoms

There are five types of epileptic seizures. Each has a specific pattern and identifiable symptoms. In order for the teacher to be able to locate potential epileptic children and then be aware of when a child has a mild seizure or has a warning attack, or aura, only general symptoms are presented here. Specification of identifiable symptoms for each kind of seizure and its prognosis is a medical matter. Therefore, the symptoms for grand mal are presented separately from the rest of the seizures. The following symptoms suggest the possibility of epilepsy:

Grand mal	Petit mal/psychomotor convulsions (occur most frequently)

A. *Appearance*
  1. Aura (felt by child)

Tingling skin	Staring
Tension	Confusion
Blinking eyes	Blinking eyes
Staring	Rage/anger
Confusion	Sluggishness
Loss of con-	
sciousness	
(1-2 min)	

  2. Convulsions

Eyes roll up	Slight jerking
Difficulty in	of arms and legs
breathing	Chewing movement
Muscles tighten	with mouth
Frothing at mouth	Stares into space
Pale bluish skin	Temporary blackout
Convulsions begin	
with cry, jerky	
movement of	
whole body	
Possible involuntary	
urination and	
defecation	

  3. After convulsions

Deep coma	Sleep
Noisy breathing	

B. *Typical complaints*
  1. Aura stage

Feeling of fear	Abdominal pains
Unpleasant odors	Headache
Funny sounds	Spots before eyes
Spots before eyes	Buzzing and ringing
Feeling sick	in ears
	Dizziness

  2. Upon waking
     Confused

Headache	Inability to
Feeling malaise	remember what
Feeling nausea	happened

Suggestions for Helping the Child with Epilepsy

1. If a child has a seizure, administer suggested first aid procedures.
2. Help the child to be active by adhering to the commonsense rule of "nothing in excess."
3. Encourage the child to participate with peers.
4. Limit participation in body-contact sports and swimming.
5. Discourage riding a bicycle until the child is declared free of seizures.
6. Avoid overprotection.
7. Reassure the child that all is well.
8. Keep the child mentally active.
9. Provide the usual amount of discipline.
10. Encourage regulated physical activity.
11. Encourage regular meals.
12. Provide for rest periods.
13. Help the child to take medication regularly as directed by a physician.
14. Avoid emotional stresses.
15. Do not let the child become fatigued.

16. Make the child feel worthwhile.
17. Give the child recognition.
18. Encourage a wholesome, regular diet.
19. Encourage the child to establish regular bowel habits.

DISEASES AND ALLERGIES

Communicable Diseases

Communicable diseases today are no longer the threat they were to the survival of the child prior to 1940. With the advent of antibiotics and the use of immunizations, serious bacterial and viral complications have been greatly reduced. However, viral infections such as colds and influenzas are still not under control.

Communicable diseases are those in which the causative microbes may pass or be carried from one person to another either directly or indirectly. The usual childhood diseases are caused by bacteria or viruses. Almost all children will be exposed to respiratory infections early in childhood. Ideally, they will build natural immunity to the invading organism or have their inherited immunity reinforced when exposed to a communicable disease.

Respiratory

About 46 percent of the common childhood diseases fall into the respiratory group and occur in childhood at a time when the child attends elementary school. Consequently, an ill child becomes physically debilitated and does not attend school regularly. Although effective immunizations are available for most communicable diseases, with the exception of colds and influenzas, most elementary school children are susceptible to the following diseases: chicken pox, diphtheria, German measles, Rubella measles, mumps, whooping cough or pertussis, streptococcal infections of the respiratory tract, poliomyelitis, and tetanus. The symptoms of these diseases are common and similar in nature.

Most states legally require that parents have the child immunized for most of these diseases before the child enters kindergarten or the first grade. The teacher should observe the students for general symptoms indicative of illness. The child with several or many of these symptoms should be suspected of illness and referred immediately to the school nurse, principal, and/or the parents.

General Symptoms of Communicable Diseases

A. *Appearance*
   1. Flushed face
   2. Nasal discharge
   3. Persistent sneezing
   4. Persistent coughing
   5. Profuse sweating
   6. Watery eyes
   7. Red throat
   8. Swollen glands
   9. Rash or skin eruption
   10. Diarrhea
   11. Earache
   12. Nausea or vomiting
   13. Pallor (in skin of the Caucasian)

B. *Behavior*
   1. Loss of appetite
   2. Lack of interest in playing
   3. Irritability and restlessness (illness, fatigue, hunger)

C. *Typical complaints*
   1. Sore throat
   2. Headache
   3. General body soreness
   4. Difficulty swallowing (sore throat)
   5. Dizziness
   6. Stiff neck

7. Chills, fever
8. Pain
9. Fatigue
10. Itchiness

Suggestions for Helping the Child with a Communicable Disease

1. Arrange to have the child lie down in the first aid room.
2. Arrange to transport the child home.
3. Keep surveillance for other sick children.
4. Instruct pupils on proper use of handkerchief during a cough or sneeze.
5. Insist that the child wash hands and face with soap and water after using washroom.
6. Help the child to catch up on lost school work.
7. Enforce the practice of keeping hands and unclean articles away from the eyes, ears, nose, mouth, genital areas, scratches, and sores.
8. Encourage the concept of voluntary immunizations.

Rheumatic Fever

Most heart disease in childhood is the result of rheumatic fever, which usually begins between the ages of 5 and 15. It causes more longtime crippling illness in children than does any other disease. Although rheumatic fever is no longer the threat it once was, it has a way of repeating itself, and each attack increases the chances for heart damage.

Rheumatic fever occurs as a sequel of streptococcal infection. The initial illness starts with a group A streptococcal infection (strep throat, streptococcal tonsilitis, or scarlet fever) that occurs about four weeks before the onset of rheumatic fever. Not all tonsilitis is streptococcal, and only about one to three percent of such streptococcal infections are followed by rheumatic fever.

Because of this one- to four- week interval between the streptococcal infection and the onset of rheumatic fever, it is possible to prevent rheumatic fever in those with the initial infection. If not treated in time, rheumatic fever can cause extensive and permanent disabilities and a shortened life. Teachers can help to locate pupils with suspected streptococcal infections and follow suggested preventive procedures as a way of intervening with the rheumatic fever cycle.

The final phase of rheumatic fever occurs when the streptococcal toxins irritate the heart-valve areas on the left side of the heart, causing inflammation of the surrounding tissue. A fever usually accompanies the inflammation. The inflammation subsides in about two to three weeks, and a scar is formed in place of the inflammation. The scar(s) interferes with the proper opening and closing of the heart valve, thus interfering with the normal blood flow through the heart. This chronic condition is then referred to as rheumatic heart disease.

Rheumatic fever is a recurrent disease. Streptococcal infection can precipitate a recurrence in 25-30 percent of children with a past history of rheumatic fever. About 90 percent of the first attacks occur in the age 5-15 age group. The age of peak risk seems to be about 8-10 years.

The signs and symptoms listed below do not necessarily indicate rheumatic fever; they do, however, signal the need for a visit to a physician.

General Symptoms of Rheumatic Fever

A. *Appearance*
   1. Pallor
   2. Unexplained nosebleeds
   3. Sore throat
   4. Running nose and frequent colds
   5. Twitching or jerky motions

B. *Behavior*
   1. Failure to gain weight
   2. Unusual restlessness

3. Irritability

4. History of previous rheumatic fever or strep throat

5. Behavior and personality changes

6. Decreasing accomplishment in school

C. *Typical complaints*

1. Poor appetite

2. Unexplained fever

3. Pain in joints of arms and legs

Suggestions for Helping a Child with Rheumatic Fever

1. Involve the child in classroom activities.

2. Provide rest periods.

3. Allow slow progressive involvement in activities after the child has recovered from streptococcal infection.

4. Direct the child into creative activities.

Allergies

An allergic child is one who is hypersensitive to one or more substances harmless to most children. About one child in ten will be allergic to something. For children under 15 years of age, one in five may suffer a major allergy, and normally it can be expected that four out of five allergic conditions will appear before the age of 15. Childhood is a time when children are most sensitive to substances in their environment. Certain types of food, house dust, animal dander, feathers, cosmetics, soaps, medicines, and even sunlight may cause reactions in the body. Such substances can enter the body by being swallowed or inhaled, coming into contact with the skin, or being injected as with drugs. Predisposition to allergies may be inherited, or they may be induced, but all are usually complicated by psychosomatic factors. Children with emotional problems who are overworked or under stress tend to be more susceptible to allergies. The emotional aspect of allergies is not understood at the present time.

There are many, many types of allergy. The teacher should observe allergic reactions as illnesses in children. The most common types are nasal allergy, hay fever, asthma, food or intestinal allergies, and skin allergies.

Nasal allergy is characterized by swelling of the mucous membranes of the nose, watery secretions resulting in a "runny" or stuffed-up nose, and red and itchy conjunctiva with tearing. Sneezing is a dominant sign.

Hay fever is a seasonal nasal allergy to pollens from trees, weeds, and grasses. Such sensitivity usually starts in childhood. About 1 child in 20 may be expected to have sensitivity to hay fever. About one child in three who suffers from hay fever will develop asthma.

Asthma is characterized by swollen mucous membranes of the bronchial tubes in the lungs, the presence of a sticky mucus in the tubes, and a spasm of the muscle surrounding the tube. The result is a narrowed air passage obstructed by mucus, causing difficulty in breathing. Since there are at least three million people in the United States with asthma, the classroom teacher can expect to find 1 child out of 50 with asthma. Asthma is the most serious of the allergies.

Food allergies are caused by sensitivity to one or more foods. The symptoms, which can appear shortly after the food is eaten, may affect the skin, the digestive tract, or the respiratory system.

Skin allergies are caused by the contact of certain substances on the skin, such as the oil resin from the leaves of the poison ivy plant. Allergic conditions may also be caused by insect or sea-animal stings.

Children vary in their reactions to allergies. Such reactions are seldom fatal, but they are always distressing, and the discomfort will interfere with work, sleep, recreation, and naturally the learning process.

General Symptoms of Allergy

A. *Appearance*

1. Wheezing

2. Running nose
3. Red eyes
4. Nausea or vomiting
5. Skin rash
6. Inflammation of skin—redness, oozing
7. Shock

B. *Behavior*
1. Nose rubbing
2. Nose wrinkling
3. Sneezing
4. Self-consciousness
5. Absence from school
6. Inability to participate in strenuous activities

C. *Typical complaints*
1. Insomnia
2. Difficulty in breathing
3. Headache
4. Difficulty in hearing
5. Loss of appetite
6. Abdominal pain
7. Itchy skin

Suggestions for Helping the Child with Allergies

1. Encourage the child to participate in activities and play.
2. Avoid stressful conditions and situations that bring about allergic symptoms.
3. Arrange day for breathing exercises.
4. Perform prescribed exercises with asthmatics.

Skin Problems

Everyone, including elementary school children, is susceptible to skin problems. Although skin disorders are often approached as specific disorders, they are often a part of or mask other diseases (measles, scarlet fever, cold, or fever), emotional disorders, allergies, and insect bites. A great deal of clinical confusion appears to exist about skin disorders. The best advice for teachers is to look for rashes, boils, warts, ringworm, and acne on any part of the child's body, then follow the suggested referral procedures outlined at the end of this chapter.

SUGGESTED REFERRAL AND FOLLOW-UP PROCEDURES

Specific teacher responsibilities for helping a child with a health problem or behavioral disorder include the following:

1. *Check* the medical, family, school, and life history files of each child at the beginning of each school year. Observe for written symptoms and signs.

2. *Observe* for physical, emotional, and social deviations and manifestations (see Table 6.1). Relate these to the academic progress. Is the child progressing normally in school and toward maturity? Does the child enjoy optimal well-being? Do any of the signs and symptoms noted in the history file

Table 6.1 Techniques for observation.

1. Conduct initial observation on each child at beginning of school year.
2. Observe child at different times of the day.
3. Observe child during different stress situations (play, recess, physical education period, lunch, etc.).
4. Observe for:
   a) personal physical appearance
   b) unusual behavior
   c) complaints
5. Observe for a syndrome of appearances, behaviors, feelings, and complaints. These should be interrelated and recurring.
6. Confirm your observation and suspicions over a time period of two to four weeks.

recur? How often and under what conditions? Make notes of the appearance, behavior, and complaints of the child.

3. *Confirm* your original observations by further detection over a period of two or four weeks. Is the child outgrowing these and adapting, or are these health problems and behavioral disorders becoming established patterns?

4. *Refer* the child suspected of a problem or disorder for medical examinations and proper attention. Use the proper channels in the school for such referrals. The school nurse is the logical person to assume referral responsibilities from the teacher. The teacher should confidentially share his or her observations and suspicions with the school nurse, the child's parents, and the principal.

5. *Follow up* on the referral:

a) *Receive* from the physician and school nurse a medical appraisal and an evaluation of the referral.

b) Then *visit* with the school nurse, physician, and parents and decide with them on the initiation of a *corrective program*. Emphasis in such a program needs to be placed on the handicap of each child. The teacher is probably the best person to *coordinate* the corrective program, being in a unique liaison position and in daily contact with the child.

c) *Administer* the school aspect of the corrective program. Consult with the parents, physician, nurse, and others periodically.

d) *Evaluate* and record the progress the child is making as the year progresses. This should be done three or four times during the school year.

These suggested steps should be followed by all prudent and responsible teachers. No doubt, most school districts already have similar remedial approaches for dealing with the health problems and disorders of children. The teacher should realize that the most important aspect of the corrective program will be the carry-over value that such a program may have for the child. Improved well-being should result in improved learning as well as in a well-adjusted, responsible, and self-actualizing adult.

REVIEW QUESTIONS

1. What physiological disorders should you, as a teacher, anticipate finding among children?
2. Of what value is plotting height and weight on a Wetzel Grid?
3. What technique of observation will be helpful in locating problem children?
4. What should you observe children for?
5. How many children in your classroom should you expect to have vision, hearing, dental, and postural problems, respectively?
6. What are the general symptoms of eye problems?
7. Does "squinting" alone imply that a child has a vision problem?
8. List ten things you can do in the classroom to help children with vision and hearing problems.
9. How can you quickly assess a child's posture?
10. What are the general symptoms of communicable diseases?
11. What is rheumatic fever?
12. What is the problem of a child who suddenly develops the following symptoms: running nose, sneezing, watery eyes? What should you do to help that child?
13. What procedures should a teacher follow in helping a child with a health problem or with a behavioral disorder?
14. What techniques can a teacher use to confirm a child's unusual behavior?
15. What can a teacher do to help a child with diabetes?

REFERENCES AND BIBLIOGRAPHY

Allergy, Pamphlet No. 168 (Washington, D.C.: U.S. Public Health Service, 1963).

Allergy—A Story of Millions, Pamphlet No. 253 (New York: Committee on Public Affairs, 1957).

The AAU-Wetzel Grid Growth Project, NEA Service Inc., 100 West Third Street, Cleveland, Ohio.

Barrows, Howard S., and Eli S. Goldensohn. *Handbook for Parents* (Epilepsy) (New York: Ayerst Laboratories, Ltd.).

Betts, Emmett Albert. *Visual Readiness for Reading* (St. Louis: American Optometric Association).

Brunner, L.S., *et al. Textbook of Medical-Surgical Nursing* (Philadelphia: Lippincott, 1964), p. 954.

Current Information on Epilepsy (Washington, D.C.: The Epilepsy Foundation, 1966).

Dental Health Facts for Teachers (Chicago: American Dental Association).

Engh, Jeri. "Are You Sure Your Child Can Hear?" *Readers' Digest* (March 1968): 137-140.

Epilepsy—The Teacher's Role (Washington, D.C.: The Epilepsy Foundation, 1965).

Facts About Diabetes (New York: American Diabetes Association).

Facts Not Fancy About Allergy in Childhood (New York: Allergy Foundation of America).

Grueninger, Robert M. *Don't Take Growth for Granted* (NEA Service Inc., 100 West Third Street, Cleveland, Ohio, 1961), pp. 1-16.

Guyton, Arthur C. *Textbook of Medical Physiology* (Philadelphia: Saunders, 1964).

Hammond, Eva. "Hearing Defects of School Age Children," *Journal of School Health* (October 1970): 405-409.

Handbook for the Asthmatic (New York: Allergy Foundation of America, 1964).

Harlin, Vivian K. "Experiences with Epileptic Children in a Public School Program," *Journal of School Health* (January 1965): 20-24.

Hay Fever (New York: Allergy Foundation of America, 1962).

Heart Disease in Children, Pamphlet EM-56 (New York: American Heart Association).

Mortimer, Edward A. "Heart Diseases—Rheumatic in Children," *Traumatic Medicine and Surgery for the Attorney* (Reprint), Vol. VIII (1962): 673-696.

Nemir, Alma. *The School Health Program* (Philadelphia: Saunders, 1965).

An Opportunity for Schools Detecting Diabetes among Children (New York: American Diabetes Association, 1965).

A Pocket Reference for the Diabetic (Indianapolis: Eli Lilly and Company, 1961).

Pryor, Ray, ed. *Heart Disease in Children*, Publication No. 1314 (Washington, D.C.: U.S. Public Health Service, 1962).

Research Explores Dental Decay, Pamphlet No. 1483 (Washington, D.C.: U.S. Public Health Service, 1966).

Scholl, M. L. "Treatment of Seizure Disorders," *New England Journal of Medicine* (December 26, 1963): 1420.

The Skin and Its Allergies (New York: Allergy Foundation of America, 1962).

Teacher's Guide to Vision Problems (St. Louis: American Optometric Association, 1963).

Top, F. H. *Communicable and Infectious Diseases* (St. Louis: C. V. Mosby, 1964).

Vaughan, Daniel, Robert Cook, and Taylor Asbury. *General Opthalmology* (Los Altos, Calif.: Lange Medical Publications, 1962), p. 13.

Wetzel, Norman C. *Instructional Manual for Use of the Grid for Evaluating Physical Fitness* (NEA Service Inc., Cleveland, Ohio, 1941).

What Teachers Should Know About Children With Heart Disease, Pamphlet EM-25 (New York: American Heart Association, 1965).

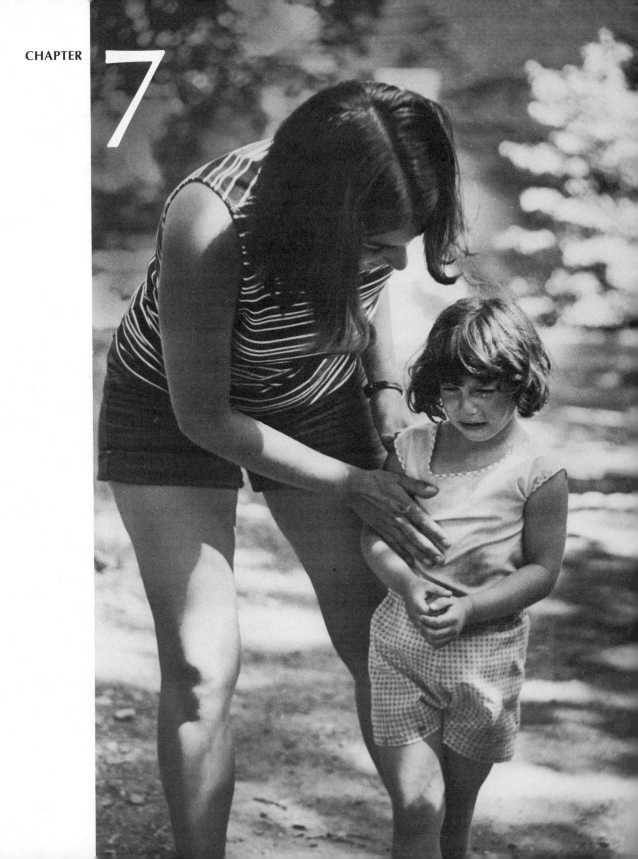

guidelines for emergency care

△ bandage dowl

One of the more seriously neglected aspects in the preparation of future elementary teachers on a national basis is their training and skill in the handling of emergency-care situations that might arise in the classroom. Perhaps the most traumatic moment for a teacher occurs when a student has been seriously injured or has taken ill while under the teacher's jurisdiction. With such thoughts in mind, the paramount question becomes one of whether or not you are capable of performing reasonably and prudently if and when you are faced with what might be a life-or-death emergency-care situation. If your answer is no, it is imperative that you make an effort to prepare yourself adequately in advance of your teaching assignment, because accidents are by far the leading cause of death among the age group you will be teaching.

The Standard Red Cross First Aid Course offered by most institutions of higher learning is an excellent approach for preparing oneself for the emergency-care eventualities that all prospective elementary teachers will invariably face. After completing such a course, it will be apparent to you that there is actually little one can do even in the most critical of emergency-care situations. However, skill in administering the minimum emergency-care procedures may very well be the difference between life and death for a seriously injured or sick child.

BASIC PHILOSOPHY

Emergency care can be defined simply as that aid administered immediately and temporarily to the victim of an accident or sudden illness. This care most often ceases as soon as trained medical help can be obtained. The definition above implies that the victim has been involved in a serious mishap or illness. Obviously this is not always the case in a school situation. In fact, the vast majority of accidents and illnesses that confront the elementary teacher in the daily routine are minor and require a minimum of expertise in their handling. It is when a major catastrophe strikes that the teacher must be prepared to assume the responsibility of efficiently administering first aid to the victim. The teacher is not only morally responsible for the care of an injured student, but also perhaps legally.

LEGAL IMPLICATIONS

Specific responsibilities and liability for school accidents and illnesses vary from state to state. It is highly recommended that as soon as possible after being appointed, the fledgling teacher become cognizant of the specific rules and regulations regarding emergency care in the school system. In some states certain circumstances constitute liability for teachers in injury cases. A teacher can actually be sued and, if found negligent, ordered to personally pay damages. In other states teachers can be held responsible for accidents, although they are not necessarily held financially liable. However, negligence in such a situation is often excellent grounds for dismissal. Particular note should be made of the fact that suits attempting to hold teachers financially liable for injuries to students have never been more numerous. Moreover, the damages sought by such suits are in most cases staggering. The teacher who is sued and eventually found negligent could conceivably spend a lifetime stymied by financial remuneration for a negligence incident which, in the vast majority of cases, could have been avoided.

Teachers, in essence, assume the role of a parent while students are under their jurisdiction. The teacher is legally and morally expected to protect and care for each youngster in the classroom. Taking into consideration the fact that the average American family has only two children to care for and the elementary teacher is expected to effectively supervise some 35 or 40 youngsters each school day, it is not difficult to envision the occurrence of emergencies despite the best-laid plans. Children will be children, and any time large numbers of children are assembled, it is inevitable that emergency-care situations will arise.

In a broad sense every teacher should always anticipate foreseeable risks, no matter what activity the students are performing. Therefore, the teacher must take reasonable steps to prevent the foreseeable risks from becoming a reality and must certainly warn the youngsters about those risks that for whatever reason cannot be reduced or averted. In addition, the teacher also has the legal responsibility and duty to aid any student who might become injured or ill during the school day. This responsibility also implies that by rendering first aid, the teacher will not increase the severity of the injury or illness.

In the event that a child should be injured or stricken with illness while in school, the teacher should always report the incident in writing. Most school systems have, or surely should have, a standard form to be completed by the attending teacher should an emergency situation occur. An example of such a form is the "Standard Student Accident Report Form" (Fig. 7.1), which is suggested as a model accident report form by the National Safety Council.

Understanding and insight of this nature will be most beneficial should the new teacher ever be a defendant in a liability suit. The accused teacher who is found negligent in one or all aspects of liability stands an excellent chance of being found remiss in terms of his or her responsibilities and will surely be forced to endure some rather unpleasant and embarrassing consequences.

Theoretically, then, it would appear that every prospective teacher should be skilled in the basic procedures of emergency care. Unfortunately, this is not at all the case in many teacher-education programs. Because the consequences can be so devastating, the failure to provide adequate training does seem paradoxical.

EMERGENCY-CARE PROCEDURES

Every school has, or certainly should have, a written set of procedures for handling both major and minor emergency-care situations. Again, the new teacher has the responsibility to become familiar with these procedures. The following portion of "Suggested School Health Policies and Procedures for Emergency Care," prepared by Brennan and

(check one)	RECOMMENDED	(check one)

RECOMMENDED
STANDARD STUDENT ACCIDENT REPORT
(See instructions on reverse side)

(check one)
☐ School Jurisdictional
☐ Non-School Jurisdictional

(check one)
Recordable ☐
Reportable Only ☐

School District:
City, State:

General

1. Name

2. Address

3. School

4. Sex   Male ☐
         Female ☐

5. Age

6. Grade/Special Program

7. Time Accident Occurred
   Date: Day of Week: Exact Time: AM ☐
                                                                               PM ☐

Injury

8. Nature of Injury

9. Part of Body Injured

10. Degree of Injury (check one)
    Death ☐   Permanent ☐   Temporary (lost time) ☐   Non-Disabling (no lost time) ☐

11. Days Lost
    From School: From Activities Other Than School: Total:

12. Cause of Injury

Accident

13. Accident Jurisdiction (check one)
    School: Grounds ☐   Building ☐   To and From ☐   Other Activities Not on School Property ☐
    Non-School: Home ☐   Other ☐

14. Location of Accident (be specific)

15. Activity of Person (be specific)

16. Status of Activity

17. Supervision (if yes, give title & name of supervisor)
    Yes ☐
    No ☐

18. Agency Involved

19. Unsafe Act

20. Unsafe Mechanical/Physical Condition

21. Unsafe Personal Factor

22. Corrective Action Taken or Recommended

23. Property Damage
    School $ Non-School $ Total $

24. Description (Give a word picture of the accident, explaining who, what, when, why and how)

Signature

25. Date of Report

26. Report Prepared by (signature & title)

27. Principal's Signature

This form is recommended for securing data for accident prevention and safety education. School districts may reproduce this form adding space for optional data. Reference: *Student Accident Reporting Guidebook*, National Safety Council, 425 N. Michigan Avenue, Chicago, Illinois 60611. 1966. 34 pages.

(over)

Fig. 7.1 Standard student accident report form. (Reprinted by permission of the National Safety Council.)

Ludwig (1971, pp. 143-145), exemplifies the type of written plan that every school should possess regarding the handling of emergency-care situations.

Suggested School Health Policies and Procedures for Emergency Care*

Policies

1. The responsibilities of the school in terms of emergency care are to:

   a) Give *immediate* care.

   b) Notify parents.

   c) See that the child is placed under responsible care, that of either the parents or a physician designated by them.

2. *All* members of the school faculty, school bus drivers, custodians, and lunch room personnel should have training in first aid such that they would be able to carry out the necessary duties in administering emergency care of injuries and sudden illness.

   Training [handwritten annotation]

3. *Every* member of the school faculty, school bus drivers, custodians, and lunch room personnel should have in their possession a first aid manual or guide for quick reference in emergency situations.

   Book on hand [handwritten annotation]

4. *At least one* person in the school should be *skilled* in administering first aid.

   CPR [handwritten annotation]

   a) Principal (in an elementary school is usually called upon to handle serious emergencies).

   b) In high school, a number of persons may be available:

      (1) Coach
      (2) Physical education teacher
      (3) Health coordinator

      (4) Nurse
      (5) Industrial arts teacher
      (6) Those in charge of various laboratories

   At least one person should be designated for this responsibility. This person (or persons) should keep up with the latest advice on emergency care by taking refresher courses and by consulting with medical specialists.

5. In the event of an emergency, the degree of injury or illness or availability of professional help will determine who shall be responsible. The order of preference is:

   a) School physician

   b) School nurse

   c) Trained school personnel assigned first-aid duties. (See item 4 above.)

   d) Individual teachers

   Keep in mind that if *none* of these people listed are available, *you* will have to skillfully attend to the victim at that precise moment until trained assistance arrives.

6. First aid equipment and supplies should be located in strategic areas throughout the school, (i.e., in every classroom, laboratories, home economics room, industrial arts room, lunch room, gym).

   Kit [handwritten annotation]

7. Every school employee should be aware of the location and availability of first aid equipment and supplies.

8. There should be a designated first aid room with equipment and supplies in every school. This room should be unlocked whenever the school is in use.

9. All faculty members and school employees should know the location of the first aid room and the availability of equipment and supplies contained therein.

10. The first aid room will be under the supervision of a designated person, preferably the school nurse.

---

* The material in this section is taken from William T. Brennan and Donald J. Ludwig, *Guide to Problems and Practices in First Aid and Civil Defense*, Dubuque, Iowa: Wm. C. Brown Company. Copyright © 1971 by Wm. C. Brown Company Publishers and reprinted by permission.

11. Every faculty member, employee, and student should have on file, in the first aid room, information relative to notification in case of injury or sudden illness. This information will be filled out at the beginning of the school year on an "Official Notification Card." This information should include:

    a) Parent or relative (and where he or she can be located)

    b) Preferred physician and hospital

    c) Permit signed by parent, allowing the school to call the designated physician or dentist directly in case a parent cannot be reached

12. The phone numbers of the following persons and services should be posted conspicuously near each school telephone:

    a) School physician

    b) School nurse

    c) Substitute physician

    d) Local fire station

    e) Local police station

    f) Hospital or ambulance service

    g) Poison control center

13. Every teacher or employee should be required to fill out a standard sickness and accident report after every reportable incident. This report should be kept on hand in the principal's office. It should include:

    a) Names of persons concerned

    b) Time and date of incident

    c) Location

    d) Nature of accident or illness

    e) Witnesses

    f) Disposition of the case

14. No sick or injured child should ever be sent home unaccompanied by a responsible person or when a responsible person is not at home.

15. Parents or guardians should be notified as calmly and as early as practicable. Every needed assistance should be given them in caring for their children.

16. These policies should be evaluated at the end of each school year and revised in light of the evaluation.

Procedures

1. Care of minor injuries

    a) In elementary grades the classroom teacher stresses the importance of cleanliness of minor wounds, washes the injured areas with soap and water, and applies the sterile dressings.

    b) At other levels the student is referred to one of several places in the building where instructors can apply first aid measures.

    c) Bus drivers, custodians, and lunch room personnel should also be trained in first aid and have supplies handy.

2. Care of major injuries and sudden illness

    a) Immediately summon sufficient help to do the following *simultaneously:*

        (1) Administer first aid.

        (2) Notify school administrator.

        (3) Notify parents.

        (4) Secure physician.

    b) Render immediate care.

        (1) Stop external bleeding (know pressure points). *severe*

        (2) Start artificial respiration in cases of asphyxia (stoppage of breathing).

        (3) Care for shock.

        (4) Do not move a person suspected of neck or back injury.

        (5) Leave the unconscious person alone (no attempt to arouse or give liquids).

c) Be able to render care for common emergencies such as:

   (1) Fainting

   (2) Unconsciousness

   (3) Epileptic seizures

   (4) Insulin shock

   (5) Foreign bodies in eye

   (6) Foreign bodies in air passage

   (7) Foreign bodies in food tube

   (8) Convulsions

   (9) Snake bite — *Special*

  (10) Burns

  (11) Insect bites and bee stings — *Special*

3. Specific care of injuries and sudden illness

  a) For a clean cut:

    (1) Wash around area with soap and water.   *— not usually in schools*

    (2) Apply an antiseptic, preferably hydrogen peroxide. Avoid such substances as alcohol and iodine; they injure tissue.   *why*

    (3) Apply sterile dressing.

  b) Dirty wound:

    (1) Cleanse around wound with soap and water.

    (2) Cleanse with alcohol to remove dirt.

    (3) Apply antiseptic—allow to dry.

    (4) Apply sterile dressing.

  c) Dog bite:

    (1) Wash with water and soap.

    (2) Apply antiseptic (see 3-a-2 above).

    (3) Apply sterile dressing.

    (4) Refer to family doctor.

    (5) Report to police and try to find dog.

d) External bleeding:

    (1) Apply pressure with compress.

    (2) Elevate wound.

    (3) If bleeding persists, apply digital pressure.

    (4) As a last resort, apply tourniquet.

e) Fainting:

    (1) Lay flat on back and elevate the feet.

    (2) Rest, with supervision.

f) Burns:

    (1) First degree—skin reddened but unbroken. Apply cold water. (Seek medical attention.)

    (2) Second and third degree—skin and tissues broken. Apply cold water. (Seek medical attention.)

g) Foreign body in eye:

    (1) Wash with warm boric acid solution.

    (2) Apply loose dressing.

    (3) Refer to family doctor.

h) Epileptic seizure:

    (1) Lay on back and loosen clothing.

    (2) Do *not* restrain patient's movements.

    (3) Do not force a pad into the mouth.

    (4) Allow child to rest following seizure.

    (5) Refer to family doctor.

i) Fractures:

    (1) Do not move the part.

    (2) Immobilize injured part.

    (3) Call parent to take child to family doctor if possible.

In addition to the school's planned emergency-care program, there are also standard first aid measures with which every teacher should absolutely and unequivocally be familiar. The following thoughts and techniques are presented in an effort to provide insight concerning the handling of some of the most serious emergency-care situations that might confront a teacher.

Serious Bleeding

Wounds come in all sizes and shapes. Depending on the type and location of the wound, bleeding may or may not be an extremely important factor in the emergency care of an injured student. If the wound involves a major artery, a child could actually bleed to death in less than a minute. Severe bleeding is truly one of the most urgent conditions requiring emergency care. The loss of a great deal of blood in a short period of time is a tremendous shock to a child's system, not to mention the emotional repercussions of witnessing the sight of blood.

Immediate action is imperative, and the steps to follow should be methodically performed without delay. The basic approach in controlling serious bleeding encompasses one to four measures, depending on the location and severity of the wound. One should always:

1. *Elevate the wound.* Unless there is evidence of a fracture, it is good practice to elevate the bleeding portion of the body as high above the heart as possible. Because it is more difficult for the heart to pump blood up, the blood pressure in the area of the elevated wound is lessened, which enhances further control measures. If at all possible, elevation is the first control measure that should be immediately implemented with any type of bleeding, regardless of severity.

2. *Apply direct pressure.* Direct pressure on a wound is also a very effective method for controlling bleeding. In fact, the combination of elevation and direct pressure will, in the vast majority of cases, effectively control hemorrhage. To apply direct pressure, one simply covers the wound with a sterile compress and steadily applies pressure to the

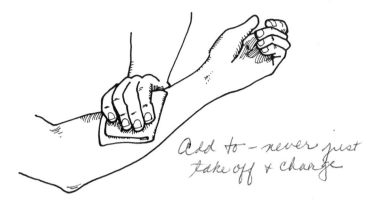

Add to — never just take off & change

Fig. 7.2 Elevating and applying direct pressure to a wound to control bleeding.

injured area. If a sterile gauze compress is unavailable, a clean towel, shirt, pillow case, sweater, or jacket could be used. If there is nothing available that will suffice as a compress, one should apply direct pressure over the bleeding with one's hand. However, any time a compress of a sort is available, it should be used. (See Fig. 7.2.)

3. *Employ arterial pressure points.* If hemorrhaging is so severe that the combination of elevation and direct pressure to the wound does not effectively control the loss of blood, "digital pressure" must be applied. In theory, this approach is relatively simple: One merely applies pressure to a specific point on the arm or leg to temporarily compress the main artery supplying blood to the afflicted portion of the body. There is one recommended pressure point on each arm and leg—where the artery is near the surface of the skin and in close proximity to a bone.

But because pressure-point use tends to stop circulation to the injured limb, this method should be employed only when absolutely necessary, and

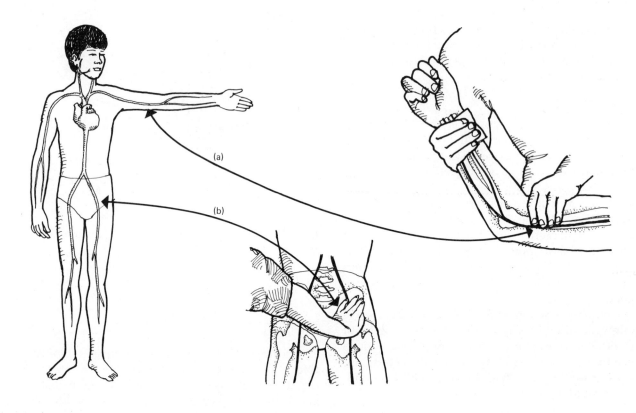

Fig. 7.3 The two major pressure points for controlling hemorrhage.

is best utilized in conjunction with direct pressure and elevation. It is best to have assistance, if possible, when employing all three techniques simultaneously. In addition, pressure-point use should be discontinued as soon as possible; however, one should always be ready to reapply the pressure if profuse, uncontrollable bleeding should recur.

There are two accepted pressure points that can be easily located and employed to control most bleeding (see Fig. 7.3). It is useful to locate these points on oneself or a friend just for practice. A prior knowledge of their location is most advantageous, eliminating indecision and fumbling when and if such action should be needed. A slight pressure with the index finger in each of the areas depicted in Fig. 7.3 will yield a pulse. This pulse signifies that you have located the pressure point.

More specifically, for a severely bleeding arm wound, apply pressure (along with direct pressure and elevation) over the brachial artery, forcing the artery against the arm bone. This pressure point is on the inside of the arm in the groove between the biceps and triceps (the large muscle masses of the upper arm). Pressure is best applied by grasping the victim's upper arm midway between the armpit and the elbow, with your thumb on the outside of the victim's arm and your fingers on the outside. Using the flat side of the fingers (not the fingertips), press toward your thumb, which will create enough force to compress the artery and thus stop the blood flow.

For a severely bleeding leg, pressure is best applied to the femoral artery, in the pelvic area. This pressure point is on the front of the thigh just below the middle of the crease of the groin, where the artery crosses over the pelvic bone on its path to the lower leg. Pressure is best applied by placing the heel of the hand over the pressure point and then leaning forward over your straightened arm to apply pressure against the underlying bone.

It is difficult to conceive of a situation in which the overall combination of direct pressure, elevation, and digital pressure would not effectively control bleeding. However, one additional technique warrants mentioning, especially because of the many misconceptions that have plagued its use for years.

4. *Employ a tourniquet as a last resort*. Only as a last resort would one even entertain the thought of applying a tourniquet. By its very nature, the tourniquet stops all blood flow to an extremity (the only place a tourniquet can be applied), and its use can potentially cause the loss of that limb due to lack of circulation. One would be hard pressed to cite a situation in which use of a tourniquet might be justified. Perhaps if many children were very seriously injured, one might have to quickly apply a tourniquet to an injured child and then move on to another victim. Or, perhaps the complete amputation of a limb might justify the use of a tourniquet. In short, a tourniquet should be applied only when, after a great deal of thought and consideration, there appears to be no other practical approach. Figure 7.4 illustrates the proper application of a tourniquet.

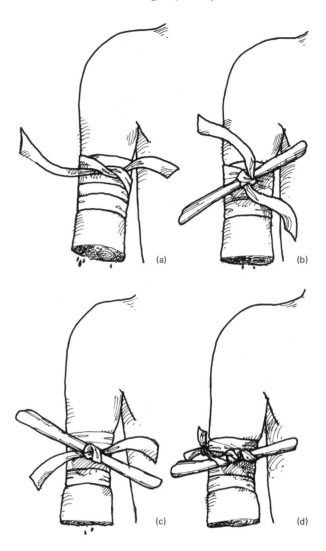

Fig. 7.4 Tourniquet application: (a) wrap twice around arm and tie half-knot; (b) place "windlass" over half-knot; (c) finish knot and turn windlass to tighten; (d) secure windlass with tails of tourniquet.

Stoppage of Breathing

Breathing can cease for many reasons: an overdose of drugs, lack of oxygen, electrical shock, toxic gases, a heart attack, or a blow to the head. In such a situation immediate action is again called for. Without oxygen, the human organism cannot survive. The chances of reviving an individual who has stopped breathing decrease with each passing minute. The person deprived of oxygen for four minutes or longer will undoubtedly suffer irreparable brain damage or death even if artificial respiration is started at that time.

As with serious bleeding, the teacher cannot afford to wait for medical help to arrive on the scene. He or she must have the ability to effectively implement the proper emergency-care procedures immediately if a child's life is to be saved. Oftentimes death may be prevented if the victim's breathing and heartbeat can be restored and maintained until professional medical assistance arrives. A simple procedure known as cardiopulmonary resuscitation (CPR) is designed to do just this, and it can be performed with a minimum of training by anyone. See Fig. 7.5.

Cardiopulmonary resuscitation should be started as soon as possible after breathing stops. Several guidelines should be followed:

1. To determine whether a collapsed victim is conscious, shake the person's shoulders and shout, "Are you all right?" If there is no response and he or she is not breathing, you must then clear and open the airway.

2. Clear the victim's mouth. Always quickly check the victim's mouth and throat region for any foreign debris that might prevent an effective exchange of air between you and the victim. Simply lay the victim down face up, turn his or her head to one side and force the mouth open, and in one sweeping motion wipe the child's mouth and throat clean with your fingers.

3. Next to quick action, the most important key to successful mouth-to-mouth resuscitation is an unobstructed air passage. The jaw of a victim who is not breathing will normally relax, with the tongue dropping back so that it blocks the trachea (windpipe). To correct this situation and to ensure a clear air passageway directly to the lungs, tilt the victim's head back into maximum extension position and pull the jaw upward by hooking your thumb behind the victim's lower teeth.

4. Pinch the victim's nostrils to prevent the air you will blow in from escaping. Then take a deep breath, place your mouth over the victim's, and blow four quick, full breaths in rapid succession into the victim's mouth.

5. Next, check the victim's pulse by locating the carotid artery in the victim's neck. You can find the carotid artery by sliding the tips of your index and middle fingers into the groove beside the voice box. If you cannot detect a pulse, you must provide both the oxygen and the artificial circulation for the victim.

Fig. 7.5 Cardiopulmonary resuscitation: (a) determine ▶ if victim is conscious; (b) quickly clear victim's mouth; (c) tilt victim's head backward and pull up on jaw; (d) first insert thumb into corner of victim's mouth in order to grasp lower jaw and lift it upward and then pinch nostrils closed with free hand; (e) take a deep breath, place your mouth tightly over victim's, and give four quick, full breaths in rapid succession; (f) check for victim's pulse on carotid artery; (g) if no pulse is evident, perform external cardiac compression by applying rhythmic pressure on lower half of victim's sternum.

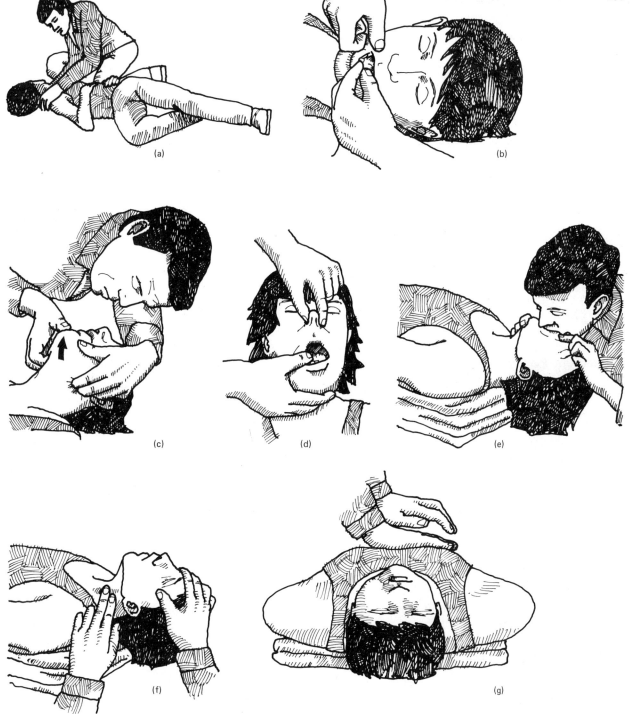

(a)

(b)

(c)

(d)

(e)

(f)

(g)

Table 7.1 CPR with one and two rescuers.

Number of rescuers	Ratio of compressions to breaths	Rate of compression
1	15:2	80 per minute
2	5:1	60 per minute

6. If there is no pulse, you must literally move the oxygenated blood for the victim. This procedure is accomplished by external cardiac compression. By applying rhythmic pressure on the lower half of the victim's breastbone, you actually force the heart to pump blood. Kneel at the victim's side and locate the lowest portion of the sternum, placing the heel of one hand approximately one inch from the tip of the sternum. Place your free hand on top of the one in position. Keep the fingers raised off the chest wall; interlocking the fingers will assist with this matter. Now bring your shoulders directly over the victim's sternum. By keeping your arms straight and by compressing the adult victim's sternum 1½ to 2 inches, you effectively artificially circulate the victim's blood. A period of relaxation must follow compression immediately and be of equal time.

7. A rhythmical, rocking motion helps ensure the proper length of time for both the compression and relaxation cycles. The rescuer's hands are kept in position over the victim's sternum while allowing the victim's chest to return to its normal position between compressions.

Assuming that you are alone in your rescue attempts, you must provide both the artificial respiration and cardiac compression. To effectively restore circulation, you must compress the victim's chest some 80 times per minute and in addition provide two quick mouth-to-mouth breaths every 15 compressions.

If you are fortunate enough to be aided by another trained rescuer, both of you should position yourselves on opposite sides of the victim. One rescuer provides for the breathing, and the other rescuer conducts the cardiac compression. When two rescuers are available, the rate changes to one breath after every fifth compression. The respective ratios and rates with one and two rescuers are given in Table 7.1.

8. The CPR procedure for infants and small children is similar to that used on older children and adults. However, there are a few important differences:

a) When clearing an infant's airway, be careful not to tilt the head too far backwards. An infant's neck is so pliable that a forceful backward tilt might actually block the airway instead of opening it.

b) Rather than trying to pinch shut the nostrils of an infant or small child, cover both the nose and mouth with your mouth and give one small breath every three seconds.

c) When applying cardiac compression for infants and small children, the rescuer should utilize only one hand for compression, placing the other hand under the child to provide firm support for the back.

For infants, only the tips of the index and middle fingers are used to compress the chest at midsternum. The area should be depressed some ½ to ¾ inch at the rate of 80 to 100 times a minute.

For small children, the heel of one hand is used to compress the chest at midsternum. The area should be compressed some ¾ to 1½ inches, depending, of course, on the size of the child. The compression rate should be maintained at 80 to 100 times per minute.

Table 7.2   CPR procedures on infants and small children.

	Part of hand	Hand position	Depress sternum	Rate of compression
Infants	Tips of index and middle fingers	Midsternum	½ to ¾ inch	80 to 100 per minute
Children	Heel of hand	Midsternum	¾ to 1½ inches	80 to 100 per minute

d) For both infants and small children, breaths should be given after every fifth chest compression. Table 7.2 summarizes the procedure employed on infants and small children.

Choking

The most frequent cause of obstruction of the airway is large, poorly chewed foods. The obstruction can be either partial or complete. The emergency-care procedures for the choking victim are relatively simple. If the victim *can* cough, speak, and breathe, it is best not to interfere. However, if the victim is conscious, but *cannot* cough, speak, or breathe, action is required, as follows:

1. Quickly administer four back blows in rapid succession (see Fig. 7.6a);
2. If the back blows prove ineffective, rapidly apply four manual thrusts (see Fig. 7.6b);
3. If the manual thrusts prove ineffective, immediately repeat the sequence of events until they are effective or until the victim lapses into unconsciousness.

Should the victim lapse into unconsciousness, a different series of steps must be taken:

1. Attempt to ventilate the victim, utilizing the same procedures as for stoppage of breathing.

If the victim *can* be ventilated, proceed with mouth-to-mouth resuscitation; if not, undertake cardiopulmonary resuscitation. If at any point the foreign body is seen in the mouth, remove it by finger probes.

2. If the victim *cannot* be ventilated:
   a) Administer four rapid back blows;
   b) Administer four rapid manual thrusts;
   c) Probe the mouth with a finger;
   d) Repeat the entire sequence:
      (1) Attempt to ventilate
      (2) Four back blows
      (3) Four manual thrusts
      (4) Finger probe.

Shock

Shock accompanies all injuries, physiological and/or psychological in nature, and generally is proportional to the severity of the injury. One should always treat for shock in any injury situation.

Shock can be defined simply as a depressed state of many bodily functions due to insufficient blood circulation. A person who develops the condition of shock and is not properly treated will most likely die. Therefore, it is imperative that the proper

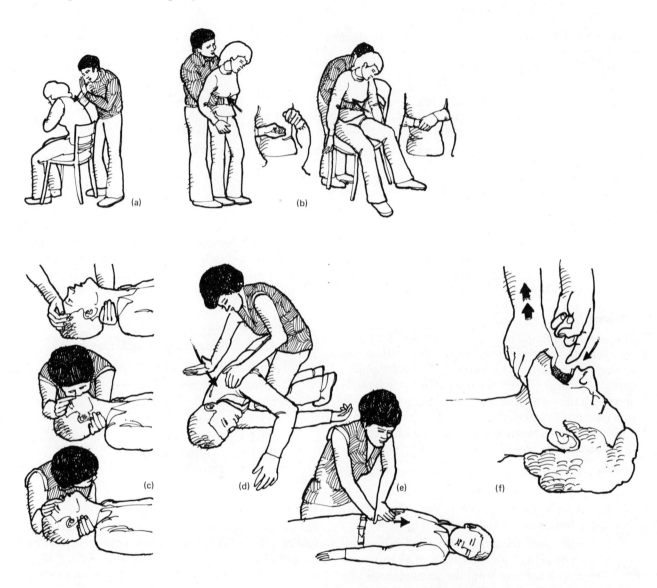

Fig. 7.6 First aid procedures for choking: (a) quickly administer four back blows; (b) if back blows prove ineffective, apply four manual thrusts; (c) ventilate an unconscious victim; (d) if victim cannot be ventilated, administer four back blows; (e) repeat step (b); (f) proceed with a finger probe to remove foreign body, then begin mouth-to-mouth resuscitation or cardiopulmonary resuscitation, if necessary.

emergency-care treatment for shock be administered to the injured.

Telltale signs of shock include:

1. Eyes are vacant and lack luster.
2. Pupils are dilated.
3. Breathing is shallow and irregular, with frequent gasps for air.
4. Pulse is weak or absent.
5. Skin appears pale, cold, and moist.
6. Victim is nauseated.

The treatment procedures for shock are the same for both prevention and care. One should:

1. Keep the victim lying down.
2. If possible, elevate the lower extremities.
3. Maintain normal body temperature, which may require covering the victim with a blanket.
4. Administer fluids if the victim is conscious and not nauseated.
5. Constantly reassure victim and stay with him or her.
6. Keep onlookers away.
7. If possible, attempt to keep the victim from viewing his or her injury.

Common Emergencies

In addition to the more serious types of emergency-care situations, other instances common to the elementary school will also require first aid care.

Diabetic Coma

The diabetic child is a potential emergency-care problem for the elementary teacher. By either not receiving enough insulin or taking in too much insulin on a given day, the diabetic child can exhibit some rather startling signs and symptoms. Diabetic coma occurs when the victim has not received a sufficient amount of insulin to carry on bodily proc-

esses. The victim's face will become flushed, with the lips a brilliant red and the skin quite dry. Ironically, the victim's temperature will be down even though he or she appears to have a fever. Perhaps the most unique characteristic symptom of this condition is the extremely sweet odor on the victim's breath. This condition, acidodis, is a reaction from the body's inability to fully metabolize consumed fats and carbohydrates because of a lack of insulin.

Unfortunately, little can be done for the victim of diabetic coma until a doctor arrives on the scene. The victim needs insulin quickly, and only a person skilled in administering a hypodermic injection of the proper amount of insulin can really be of help to the victim. Obviously a physician should be summoned immediately. Until the doctor arrives, the teachers should make the child feel as comfortable as possible and offer verbal encouragement.

Dr / Mom

Insulin Shock

The opposite of diabetic coma, insulin shock is a case of too much insulin in the blood and far too little sugar. The victim of insulin shock will exhibit all the signs and symptoms of a person who is in deep shock. The skin of the Caucasian becomes quite pallid and moist. The pulse is rapid, but breathing is slow and shallow. Also, there is no sweet smell on the breath of the victim. Because the victim appears to be, and is, in shock, it would be most beneficial for the teacher to have prior knowledge of the student's condition so that there will be no needless waste of time when and if such a condition might present itself.

Again, a physician should be summoned immediately, but because the victim has too much insulin in his or her system and not enough sugar, there are some immediate measures that can be employed. Giving the victim sugar will in many cases cause a rapid recovery. Even if the child lapses into unconsciousness, a teaspoon or so of granular sugar placed under his or her tongue will be absorbed into the bloodstream. Should the child be conscious, a cube or two of raw sugar is again an excellent choice if available, or a candy bar or orange juice, both good sources of carbohydrates, can be substituted. It would be good practice for the teacher who has a diabetic child in class to keep several lumps of sugar in the desk for just such a potentiality.

Epileptic Seizure

The most common cause of convulsions among school children is epilepsy, and an epileptic seizure is not at all an uncommon occurrence among school children. However, due to the nature of the seizure, there is, and probably always will be, a great deal of fear and misconception connected with epilepsy.

The most commonly seen forms of epilepsy are grand mal and petit mal. Of the two, grand mal presents the most difficulty. Oddly enough, the victim of a grand mal seizure has a premonition of what is to come just prior to the seizure. A child who has had previous seizures may quickly move to a more secluded area and lie down, shortly thereafter becoming unconscious. Now the other signs and symptoms of the seizure will be rather apparent— foaming at the mouth, violent convulsions, vomiting, loss of bladder control, defecation, and loud, labored breathing. The seizure normally lasts some three to five minutes, but this may very well seem like an eternity to the attending teacher. Once the seizure subsides, the victim will most likely drop off into a deep sleep for a few minutes and upon awakening may appear to be confused, which is indeed understandable.

To deal effectively with the grand mal seizure requires little skill. Above all, one should *never* restrain a victim during a seizure. The seizure should be allowed to run its course. It is good practice to clear the area of furniture, etc., so as to ensure that the victim will not be hurt. A pillow gently slid under the victim's head is also a help, especially on a hard floor. Do not concern yourself with the victim's biting his or her tongue; it has been found that such action by an epileptic is an exception to the rule. But if the child is biting his or her tongue, try to slip a hard object between the victim's teeth in an effort to prevent further injury. A wooden ruler, a pencil wrapped with a handkerchief, or the corner of a wallet are readily available items that might suffice on the spur of the moment.

When the victim regains consciousness, it is good practice to make him or her feel as comfortable as possible both mentally and physically. The youngster will also benefit from a rest in an undisturbed environment, so as to regain strength and stamina. Should the child lapse from one seizure into another, trained medical help should be summoned at once. In rare instances, a general anesthetic is required to control some seizures.

Petit mal presents far less of a problem. Actually, a petit mal seizure may very well occur with a child and you would not even be aware that such an event was taking place. The victim is perfectly normal just prior to and immediately after the seizure, receiving no premonition of an impending seizure. The seizure lasts for only a very short period of time and consists of little more than minor convulsive movements of the extremities or eyes. At no time does the child lose consciousness during the seizure.

Fainting

Fainting is not rare among young children. It can be caused by many things, but perhaps the most common is an unpleasant sight or situation, e.g., the sight of blood. Fainting occurs when the brain is deprived of a sufficient supply of oxygen, which in turn prompts a condition of immediate unconsciousness.

Without reservation, the best technique for treating someone who has fainted is to lay the victim flat, with the head lower than the legs if possible. If for some reason the victim cannot be stretched out on the floor, the next best alternative is to sit the victim down and bend his or her head between the knees. This technique may help, but is not nearly as effective as laying the victim down flat on his or her back. Once in a supine position, the victim will most likely regain consciousness very quickly. A glass of water with salt is helpful once the victim is fully conscious.

Nosebleed

Nasal bleeding is most common among elementary children. A blow to the nose and excessive nose picking are the most common causes of such a disorder. Rupture of the veins very near the surface of the membrane inside the nose is the source of nasal bleeding.

To treat nasal bleeding, keep the victim in an upright position—sitting, preferably—to elevate the source of bleeding. Insert a wad of sterile cotton in each nostril and then ask the child to compress his or her nostrils with the thumb and forefinger for *no less* than six minutes. Then have the child gently release the nostrils and check for further bleeding. If bleeding is still present, repeat the process. Once bleeding is controlled, leave the cotton wads in place for as long as possible. When they must be removed, do so gently so as not to remove clots and thus restore the hemorrhage.

REVIEW QUESTIONS

1. Define emergency care and state how, when, and why this definition might apply to the elementary teacher.

2. What are the specific guidelines for the responsibilities and liability for school accidents in your state? In light of these guidelines, what steps would you consider to be important (relative to emergency-care techniques) in preparing yourself for a teaching appointment?

3. Defend the statement: "Every prospective teacher should be skilled in the basic procedures of emergency care."

4. Outline an acceptable approach for dealing with an emergency-care situation that involves serious bleeding, or stoppage of breathing, shock, etc.

5. Define diabetic coma (or insulin shock, epileptic seizure, fainting), including the signs and symptoms, and present an acceptable emergency-care approach for dealing with such a situation.

REFERENCES AND BIBLIOGRAPHY

American National Red Cross. *Advanced First Aid and Emergency Care* (Garden City, N.Y.: Doubleday, 1973).

Brennan, William T., and Donald J. Ludwig. *Guide to Problems and Practices in First Aid and Civil Defense* (Dubuque, Iowa: Wm. C. Brown, 1971).

Chayet, Neil L. *Legal Implications of Emergency Care* (New York: Appleton-Century-Crofts, 1969).

Cole, Warren H., and Charles B. Puestow. *First Aid Diagnosis and Management* (New York: Appleton-Century-Crofts, 1965).

Henderson, John. *Emergency Medical Guide* (New York: McGraw-Hill, 1969).

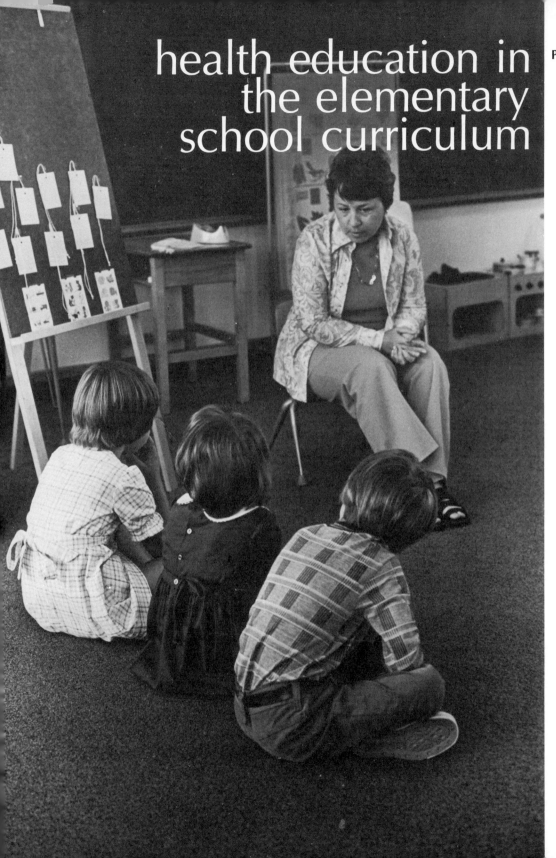

health education in the elementary school curriculum

 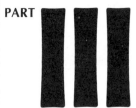

CHAPTER 8

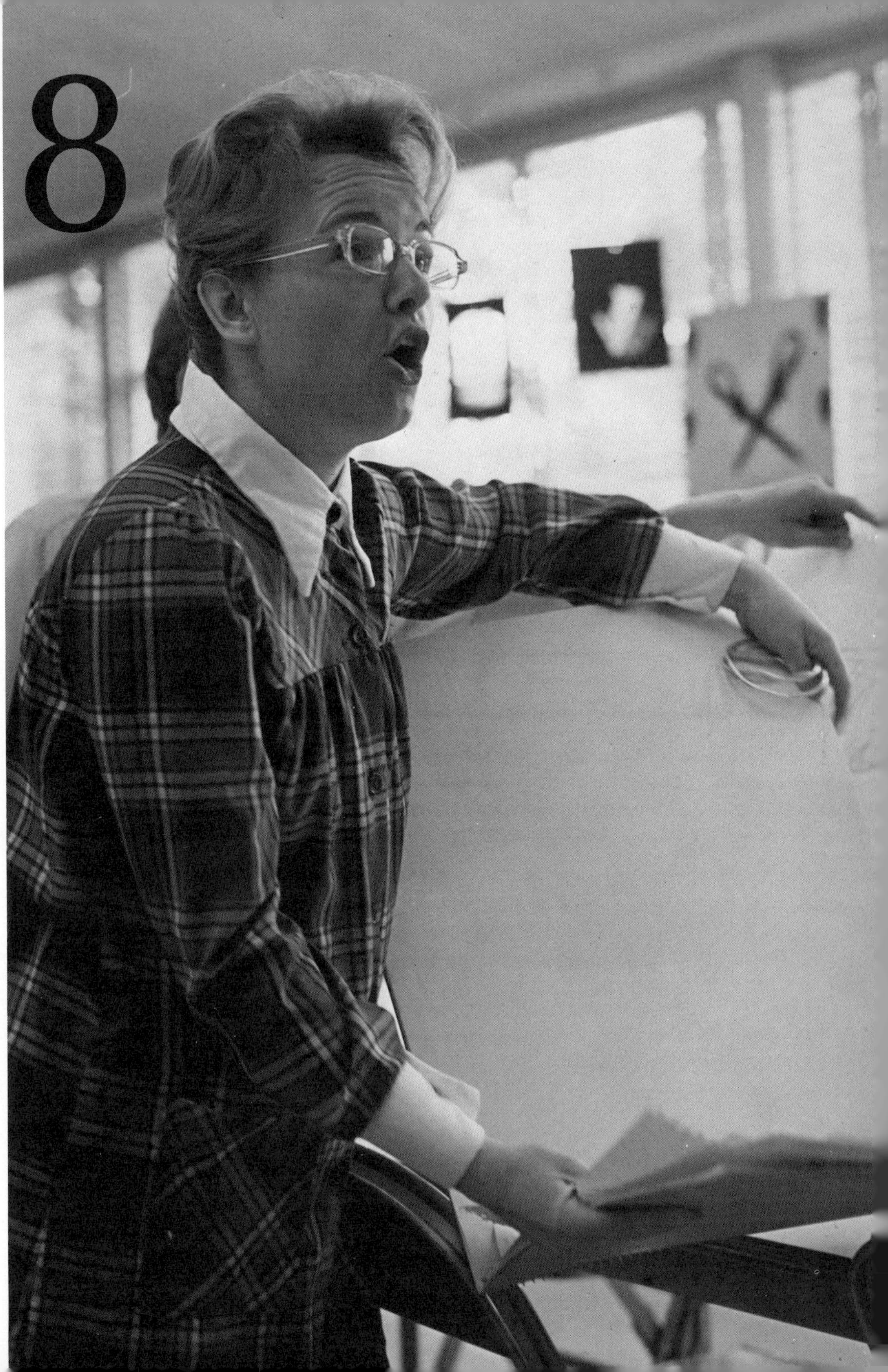

the role of the teacher in the elementary school health program

Teaching at the elementary level is by no means an easy task. The skills required of the elementary teacher are both complex and demanding. In fact, the elementary teacher will have as much, if not a greater, impact on the overall development of the youngster as any of the other immediate forces within the child's environment. Unfortunately, many elementary teachers do not realize the profound influence they can have on the youngsters with whom they come in contact.

This premise has implications for elementary health science. The primary responsibility for the health of the elementary child surely rests with the parents, and the school's role becomes one of supplementation. However, in all too many instances the supplementary role of the school becomes primary. The child may be receiving very little or perhaps no direct health instruction at home. If this is the case and if the child is further deprived of quality health instruction in the school, it is not difficult to forecast the ultimate outcome. The unhealthy child's efficiency level is drastically impaired, and in the long run his or her accomplishment will be altered. Failure in itself can be devastating for a child. Failure of a child at any level for unattended health reasons is inexcusable.

The elementary years are particularly important from a health standpoint. First and foremost is the fact that much of the learned behavior and attitudes about health that will prevail throughout a lifetime are established during the elementary years. If these habits and attitudes are positive in nature, the child will most likely continue through life exhibiting healthy practices and attitudes.

Such theory contributes to the goal of modern health education. In essence, the fundamental concept underlying all health education is the attainment of "intelligent self-direction" on the part of the student in health matters. Essentially, elementary health instruction can, and will, prepare the youngster to do what is necessary for the protection, preservation, and promotion of his or her health.

The vehicle for conveying such an approach is the teacher, who must possess the insight and understanding necessary to effect health education. In terms of elementary health science, this necessitates a precise blending of experiences and informa-

119

tion that will complement the student's immediate health needs and interests.

THE HEALTH EDUCATION PROCESS

The teaching of elementary health education can be thought of as a process whereby health information and experiences are disseminated and implemented in order to influence youngsters' health practices, attitudes, and understandings. In theory, the concept of health education is developed in much the same manner as any of the other traditional subject areas found in the elementary education curriculum. Perhaps the key difference between elementary health instruction and other subject areas is in the realm of expected outcomes. The teaching of elementary health education is specifically aimed at assisting the youngster to develop a sense of intelligent self-direction in health matters. However, what is often so easily said is not as easily accomplished. The process of elementary health education is a complex art requiring the consideration of the many factors which will ultimately have a bearing on the quantity, quality, and effectiveness of the instruction.

For example, before bona fide health instruction is undertaken, the teacher should ponder the following questions:

- Why should I teach health? What can I really hope to accomplish by providing health instruction for my students?
- Just exactly which health topics should I teach about?
- What would be the most effective way for me to teach health?
- When should I teach health?
- What materials would enhance my health instruction?
- How far can I go with the "difficult" areas of health education?
- How can I evaluate my health instruction?

Education that is motivating, relevant, timely, and meaningful and that provides for student/teacher involvement requires careful planning and systematic organization. Health education is no exception to this rule. The quantity and quality of the health education that may or may not take place in your classroom are direct reflections of your motivation, preplanning, and organizational skills.

Haphazard education is more often than not misguided and lacks the continuity of effectively planned educational experiences. A teacher who sincerely desires to be effective with health instruction should make a conscious effort to fulfill several prerequisites. A thorough understanding of the concept of developmental tasks and their relationship to needs, interests, and maturational stages of youngsters (see Chapter 4) is indispensable to curriculum planning. Gaining insight about the basis of health behavior is helpful when planning and implementing the instructional program. The skill and ability to develop concepts (see Chapter 10) is most helpful. Determining sound and attainable expected outcomes is also essential. Teacher qualifications, motivating learning experiences (see Chapter 12), and ultimately evaluation (see Chapter 13) are all additional considerations that should be carefully contemplated before formal instruction is undertaken.

As expressed above, the topic of elementary health instruction is most complicated. It should be approached with a great deal of forethought and planning if one expects to be effective in contributing to the development of positive health behavior on the part of students.

THE TOTAL SCHOOL HEALTH PROGRAM

In an effort to clarify the terminology repeatedly utilized throughout the remainder of the text, the following discussion of the school health program is essential. To this point we have referred to elementary health education as purely a process by which elementary children are exposed to classroom expe-

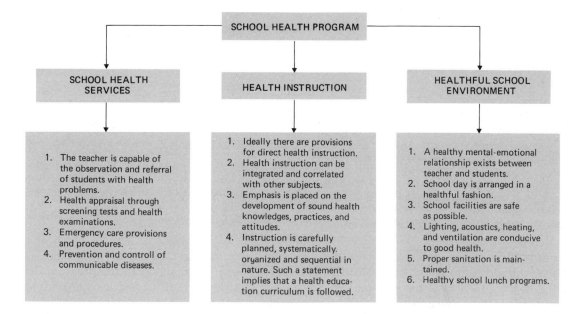

SCHOOL HEALTH PROGRAM

SCHOOL HEALTH SERVICES	HEALTH INSTRUCTION	HEALTHFUL SCHOOL ENVIRONMENT
1. The teacher is capable of the observation and referral of students with health problems. 2. Health appraisal through screening tests and health examinations. 3. Emergency care provisions and procedures. 4. Prevention and controll of communicable diseases.	1. Ideally there are provisions for direct health instruction. 2. Health instruction can be integrated and correlated with other subjects. 3. Emphasis is placed on the development of sound health knowledges, practices, and attitudes. 4. Instruction is carefully planned, systematically. organized and sequential in nature. Such a statement implies that a health education curriculum is followed.	1. A healthy mental-emotional relationship exists between teacher and students. 2. School day is arranged in a healthful fashion. 3. School facilities are safe as possible. 4. Lighting, acoustics, heating, and ventilation are conducive to good health. 5. Proper sanitation is maintained. 6. Healthy school lunch programs.

Fig. 8.1 The school health program.

riences of a health nature. Surely such an approach is an integral part of the school health program, but it is only one aspect of the total elementary health picture.

We can begin by defining the total *school health program* as a combination of the many activities provided by the school in an effort to preserve and promote the health of the school child. It encompasses all of the school functions directed at affecting the health of the child, and it includes *health services, health instruction,* and *healthful school environment* (see Fig. 8.1). None of these activities is mutually exclusive. For the school health program to operate effectively, the interrelationship among these three traditional aspects of the school health program should be carefully outlined.

The *health services* aspect of the total school health program is specifically designed to appraise, promote, protect, and maintain the health of students. Health services are carried out through a wide variety of activities and procedures and re-

quire the cooperative efforts of teachers, physicians, nurses, students, parents, and others. School health services are generally considered to include:

1. health appraisal;

2. counseling relative to appraisal findings;

3. encouragement of and assistance with the rectification of remediable defects;

4. assisting in the planning of educational experiences for the handicapped;

5. pupil observation;

6. referral to the proper medical authorities of any student with a suspected medical problem;

7. assistance in the control and prevention of communicable diseases;

8. provisions for emergency care should a member of the school community become injured or sick.

The *health instruction,* or health education, component of the total school health program is the planned pattern of sequential learning activities designed to favorably influence students' health knowledge, attitudes, and practices. Cognitive input pertains to those learning experiences that emphasize such skills as knowing, analyzing, evaluating, synthesizing, comprehending, and applying gained insight. Attitudes and practices imply affective and action behavior that will in some way influence the youngster's health. Obviously, the health practices of the student while at school are easily observable and offer an opportune situation for evaluation. But just as important are those practices and attitudes the student exhibits outside the school. To effectively influence the health attitudes and practices that will come to govern the student outside the school is indeed a formidable challenge for the elementary teacher.

Rounding out the school health program is the area of *healthful school environment.* The school has a specific responsibility to provide an environment conducive to the students' good physical, social, and emotional health. This aspect includes provisions for a safe and healthful school site; thus such factors as the water supply, sewage and refuse disposal, and grounds free from unnecessary safety hazards must be considered. Heating, lighting, and ventilation are also most important. The food service program is an integral aspect of healthful school environment.

The criteria discussed above are physical in nature. They are essential to the optimal operation of a healthful school environment, but perhaps the most important aspect of a healthful school environment is the people. The establishment of healthy interpersonal relationships among teachers, students, staff, and administrators is paramount if the school is to operate at a truly effective level from a health standpoint.

SPECIFIC RESPONSIBILITIES OF THE ELEMENTARY TEACHER

Within the realm of the school health program, the elementary teacher has many specific responsibilities. Indeed, the elementary teacher has a responsibility to contribute to *all* aspects of the school health program. We have already established the fact that the elementary teacher is in a unique position of authority. For all practical purposes, the elementary teacher occupies the key role in the elementary school health program. The student will surely benefit from a teacher who is interested in and motivated to teach health science. If, on the other hand, the teacher cannot find time for health education, the school health program never really has a chance to play an influential role.

Health Services

The precise role of the elementary teacher in the health services aspect of the school health program is one of *observation* and *referral.* The elementary teacher sees a child every day over an extended period. Such characteristics as appearance, behavior, and emotions are easily compared from one day to the next. If and when abnormalities do appear, the elementary teacher has an obligation to refer the youngster to the proper authorities.

However, responsibility does not stop there. It is imperative that a serious health deviation in the youngster be alleviated. The dedicated and empathic teacher not only refers the afflicted child, but also follows up the case to ensure that the situation is remedied to the fullest extent possible. The fledgling teacher is encouraged to follow all of the proper channels of authority in referring a youngster. Failure to follow the proper procedures may involve you, the child, and the child's parents in an embarrassing legal entanglement. One may have to persevere longer with such an approach, but if the child is ultimately helped, the time and effort will have been well spent.

It is safe to assume that rarely will a year pass without the elementary teacher's being confronted with at least one, if not more, health abnormalities among the students. When such an occasion occurs, the teacher has an expressed responsiblity to obtain help for the child. Chapters 4 and 6 are devoted entirely to a discussion of the observation and referral process.

Healthful School Environment

The elementary teacher has direct control over the immediate environment of the classroom. The physical characteristics of the classroom can do much to either enhance or hinder the learning process. A student who is in a cheery, bright, and comfortable room can't help but feel good about her or his surroundings. Such an atmosphere created in the classroom will have a bearing on the behavior patterns of students.

The classroom environment can also contribute to social betterment on a long-range basis. Children in whose homes the basic practices of good hygiene are not followed can gain valuable insight and experience from a classroom situation that adheres to a higher standard of healthful living. Ideally, through such an experience the deprived student will develop the incentive to establish a higher level of healthful living at home. Obviously, the student who comes from a home that already has a high standard of healthful living will receive reinforcement for his or her present practices.

Needless to say, there is little the elementary teacher can do about the architectural surroundings the school provides. However, the teacher can, in very subtle ways, contribute tremendously to the efficiency of the structure. For example, it is most important that the teacher have burned-out lights replaced in the classroom. An improperly lighted classroom will contribute greatly to eye fatigue.

Room temperature is another flagrantly disregarded aspect of the classroom environment. The room that is either too hot or too cold is a strong deterrent to the learning process. Teachers should be careful not to impose their wishes on students. Because of their activity level, youngsters generally like a cooler room than adults do. The teacher who has difficulty adjusting to the temperature preferred by the students should make a special effort to offset such a discrepancy, perhaps keeping a sweater at school for use when the need arises.

In addition to the temperature of the room, ventilation is also a most important consideration. Whenever possible in the room lacking air conditioning, the windows should be adjusted so as to provide sufficient air transference. When ventilation is poor and the heat is raised beyond a normal level, the students are likely to react with drowsiness, headaches, depression, and a general loss of vigor.

For all practical purposes, the elementary teacher should strive for a classroom temperature of between 66° and 71°F. Humidity can also affect the comfortableness of a classroom. A humidity rating of 50 percent is ideal combined with a temperature of approximately 70°F. However, without a central air conditioning unit in the school, the teacher stands little chance of having any control over the humidity of a classroom.

When we analyze the total concept of a healthful school environment, it becomes apparent that perhaps the most important component is the people themselves. Even if all of the considerations above were the epitome, the social environment would still be totally dependent on the people who occupy it. Certainly, the teacher is the most important of these people. Without his or her skillful guidance, empathy, and love for children, the physical structure of the school lacks life itself. Students will only be as enthusiastic, vibrant, and full of love for life as is their teacher.

Health Instruction

Unfortunately, ineffective health instructional programs at the elementary level continue to plague our schools. This is especially important when we realize that health problems of a sociological and psychological nature are increasing tremendously in both magnitude and complexity in our society. Without question, the need for the development, promotion, and maintenance of sound health practices and attitudes has never been more important.

The elementary school years are crucial for health education. Some basic health knowledge will be acquired by the child; the very foundation for the attitudes that will guide the youngster throughout life is laid; and many of the habits that will affect his or her health are formed. The implications for elementary health education become obvious when one critically perceives the many public health problems that we as citizens and prospective teachers are faced with today.

The point to be made is that formal, planned classroom health education is essential if we are to attempt to prepare young people to make informed decisions about matters concerning their health. The elementary level promises the greatest return from direct health instruction in terms of immediate and long-range positive health behavior.

Elementary health instruction is best directed toward the development of sound health habits and attitudes on the part of the students. Although some health knowledge is essential, it is best implemented so that additional information further enhances positive health attitudes and practices. Actually, health knowledge is considered secondary to the fostering of sound attitudes and practices at the elementary level. The development of a wealth of health knowledge is more appropriate at the junior high and high school levels.

Essentially, the elementary teacher as a facilitator of health education should:

1. Encourage good health and safety practices at all times when the students are at school. Such an approach can be considered as meeting many of the students' immediate health and safety needs.

2. Make an effort to determine the students' interests relative to health and safety matters. Then the teacher can actively pursue activities and experiences that will, in effect, capture the enthusiasm which normally accompanies an interest.

3. Provide those activities and experiences that most creatively develop the health and safety concepts selected for that year at the particular grade level.

4. Take full advantage of "teachable moment" situations if and when they do arise. Many times the lesson learned through such situations is the very information that will be retained throughout a lifetime.

5. Always keep in mind that teaching by example is a most effective form of education. Elementary youngsters are far more aware of hypocritical attitudes and practices than the neophyte teacher might ever believe. The "do as I say, not as I do" philosophy lost its appeal a generation ago. If as an elementary teacher you do intend to influence youngsters' health practices, attitudes, and knowledge, be certain that you exhibit all the characteristics of a healthy, mature adult.

6. Continually evaluate the relevance of the health instruction taking place. Education that does not provide for meaningful tasks and constructive alternatives is education that wastes the time and energy of everyone involved. Motivation is the key to effective instruction. Relevance, in turn, is essential to motivation. Tautologically, then, the task becomes one of confronting youngsters with relevant health- and/or safety-related tasks that will moti-

vate them to act responsibly relative to their health attitudes and practices.

In summary, health education should receive as much attention as any of the other traditional content areas normally associated with elementary school. Anything less than systematic, planned direct health instruction is an injustice.

Teacher-Student Involvement

Dr. William Glasser, the author of *Schools Without Failure* (1969), has much to say about the concept of teacher-student involvement. His premise is that when students become involved at an affective level with responsible teachers, they are better able to make responsible choices and to behave constructively.

All too often, teachers stand aloof from their students and do not become emotionally involved. They avoid being warm, personal, and sincerely interested in their students. Such an approach is indeed unfortunate, especially for the youngster who is lonely and desperately in need of the warmth and recognition an adult can give.

The involvement concept deals directly with the students' mental health. There is perhaps no other aspect of the elementary education program more important than the development and maintenance of the students' emotional well-being. The intriguing feature of such a premise is that so much can be done for the child with such little effort by the teacher. However, a disappointing facet is that "involvement" is difficult to teach. Prospective teachers can be told to empathically involve themselves with their students, but unless they have literally lived such an approach to life, it is indeed difficult to change and adopt such a philosophy. The process of involvement is important at every level of education, but perhaps most so at the elementary level.

Many young students miss an opportunity to identify with an adult who can be considered responsible and successful in the task of coming to grips with life itself. Some youngsters are actually thwarted in their attempts to fulfill their basic needs, as opposed to being afforded an opportunity to identify with an adult who is capable of constructively and effectively assisting them in this process.

Obviously a youngster can, and ideally will, establish a meaningful relationship with an adult other than the teacher. Opportunities for exemplary adult models are numerous: parents, older brothers and sisters, clergy, responsible peers, and a close relative. Unfortunately, however, many children are never given the opportunity to get personally involved with a responsible person. Unlikely as it may sound to the prospective teacher, many young persons will readily admit that their existence as functioning human beings can be attributed to the fact that an understanding teacher took an interest in them as individuals.

As a teacher, it is facetious to think that you can please, and meet the needs of, every student with whom you come in contact. This does not mean that one cannot strive to meet every student's needs. Indeed, you should make a pronounced effort, but be cognizant of the fact that there will invariably be some students with whom you will have difficulty establishing rapport. However, just as there are a few students with whom you will have difficulty communicating, there will be many others who will benefit tremendously from your concern and interest in them as individuals.

Several simple techniques can be implemented to foster the concept of involvement. Some helpful guidelines include the following:

1. Get to know the youngsters' first names as soon as possible. A youngster who is called by name in and out of school knows that you have an interest in him or her as an integral member of the class.

2. Make an effort to know the student's background—home life, interests, hobbies, anxieties, etc. Such a suggestion is not meant to imply

that you should pry such personal information from the student. Just by being a good listener, you can gather a wealth of insight into the child's personal life. Such insight is most helpful when you are attempting to relate to a particular youngster. Having the uncanny ability to empathically identify on a child's level and in his or her present sociological environment is extremely helpful to both you and the student.

Becoming a good listener is, unfortunately, one of the more difficult capacities to develop for most prospective teachers. All too often, the teacher wants to do the talking, give advice, and offer constructive alternatives. Such a procedure is more than likely just what the student does not need. The youngster may actually need little more than a responsible adult who will acknowledge him or her by doing something as simple as listening.

3. Deal with misconduct in a caring way. A child misbehaves in any of a number of ways for a reason. The teacher must adopt the attitude that students are, in fact, responsible for their behavior. By expecting or demanding anything less than responsible behavior, the teacher merely adds to the dilemma that the deviant child is already experiencing. Glasser (1969) would say that behavior is directed by emotion. Successful behavior produces pleasant emotion, and the converse holds true for unsuccessful or unacceptable behavior. Ideally, then, the teacher should make an effort to deal with the deviant child's behavior if any success is expected in the area of dealing with the child's emotional well-being.

By developing a warm, positive, personal involvement with students and working with their present behavior, the teacher stands a good chance of affecting their emotions in a positive manner. Keep in mind that emotion is a result of behavior, but it is the behavior, and the behavior alone, that can be improved. When, and if, we can affect the child's behavior, he or she will automatically begin

to experience feelings of worth. Such a happening can literally snowball into better behavior in every aspect of the child's life.

Assuming that as a teacher, you are willing to become personally involved with a child who has a behavior problem, you must assist that child in changing his or her present behavior if you are really to help. Essentially, the youngster must be induced to make a value judgment about the present behavior. As fatalistic as it may sound, if the child sincerely doesn't believe that there is anything wrong with the behavior, there is little you can do to positively help the child. The child must suffer the consequences of refusing to change the behavior.

However, you should never give up on the child. No matter how many times a child misbehaves or fails, he or she should again and again be asked to make an honest value judgment about the situation. Sooner or later, the youngster will doubt that what he or she has been defending is best for him or her.

If and when such an event should occur, then and only then should the teacher and student together actively pursue a more reasonable and constructive course of behavior. If the child doesn't know a better course, the teacher must suggest some alternatives and actually help the child plan a better approach. Once the child does make a value judgment about his or her behavior and eventually becomes committed to a new course of action, no excuse becomes acceptable for not following through. The teacher who really cares accepts no excuses. In effect, such an approach is discipline at its best. Every child needs discipline and guidance.

In another respect, Glasser's approach to dealing with pupil behavior also accentuates the concept of commitment. It is not enough to just get the child to make a value judgment about his or her behavior. First, the child must be persuaded to choose a better way to behave and then make a commitment to that choice. Commitment of this nature develops a maturity and feeling of worth in a youngster that ideally will carry through a lifetime.

Glasser is also careful to differentiate between discipline and punishment. Schools and society use punishment mainly to deal with misbehavior. The overall positive effects of punishment are questionable. The discipline approach discussed above allows the child to suffer the painful consequences of misbehavior, but no attempt is made to induce excess pain or to be punitive. The child can and should be excluded from the class activities, or school if necessary, for blatant misbehavior. However, the child is excused for an arbitrary time which is completely up to him or her. After proposing an acceptable behavior plan and making a commitment to that plan, the child should be allowed to return to class as an integral member.

If such a system of involvement is to succeed, the teacher cannot accept any excuse for a commitment going unfulfilled. If a teacher does accept an excuse for the breakdown of a commitment by the student, involvement too begins to break down. The sensitive student knows that the teacher who really cares will not let him or her get hurt. Involvement ceases when the person who makes the commitment is then allowed to excuse himself or herself for breaking the commitment.

There is no question but that the concepts of involvement and commitment are well within the province of mental health. Properly employed, such an approach to classroom management can do much to ensure a healthy classroom environment.

The information cited from Glasser's *Schools Without Failure* is only a small portion of Dr. Glasser's philosophy. His comments about memorization, relevance, eliminating failure, classroom meetings, and morality are just as thought-provoking. The interested student is highly encouraged to peruse Dr. Glasser's entire text.

HEALTH BEHAVIOR AS IT RELATES TO HEALTH INSTRUCTION

Basic to a discussion of health education is an understanding of health behavior and those factors most likely affecting it. Insight into the variables that influence health behavior is helpful when attempting to plan learning experiences for pupils. By carefully analyzing the key factors influencing health behavior, we develop greater insight into the reasons why people behave the way they do in health matters.

Hochbaum (1970) has developed an easily interpreted theory concerning health behavior. This theory provides an excellent framework from which to develop several basic behavioral concepts. Hochbaum addresses himself to the fundamental question of why people behave the way they do in matters that have a direct bearing on their health. What makes them do some things but not others? What plays the largest role in influencing individual decisions in health matters?

You'll remember that in Chapter 2, we said that such authorities as Maslow, Erikson, Havighurst, and Glasser perceive the fulfillment of the basic fundamental needs as indispensable to positive and socially acceptable behavior. It is when one of these basic fundamental needs goes unfulfilled that we can expect an alteration in behavior. Obviously such a situation can have a gross effect on health behavior, and very often the results can be catastrophic for both the individual and society.

Hochbaum builds on this premise and introduces further variables which help in answering his basic questions relative to the "whys" of health behavior. His theory begins with early childhood and involves parental influence. He feels that the initial health behavior of the child (from birth through approximately five years) is almost entirely dependent on what the parents consider desirable and undesirable health practices. Through rewards and punishments, the youngster acquires certain health practices which in many cases are continued throughout the individual's life. Keep in mind that in the vast majority of these initial health behaviors, the child is not at all cognizant of why she or he is performing them, except, of course, for the intrinsic or extrinsic motivation he or she receives from parents. When we further realize that the better part of a youngster's personality is developed by age six, we can begin to realize how extremely important these initial health behaviors become. The young child who is reared in an environment not supportive of positive health practices will, unfortunately, more than likely go through life exhibiting poor health behavior.

Such a theory has implications for elementary health instruction. Without question, the typical elementary class is comprised of youngsters from families that are highly supportive of positive health behavior, as well as those that could literally care less. For children from supportive families, health instruction will more than likely add further support to their behavior and supplement the direction provided by the parents. The child from the nonsupportive family presents the immediate challenge. The health instruction provided in school may very well be the only health guidance such a child receives. Therefore, it is imperative that the health instruction be motivating, timely, and relevant.

Hochbaum further believes that much initial, as well as later, health behavior is greatly influenced by incidental happenings. Chance events, overhearing conversations, observation (especially television), playful imitation, etc., all lead to a form of health behavior. Again, such input has implications for elementary health instruction. The teacher can use such incidental happenings to decided advantage. There is perhaps no more meaningful opportunity for health instruction than the "teachable moment." When a chance event occurs that has health implications, it becomes most meaningful to take time at that moment to discuss the health ramifications of such an event. For example, a child suffering a minor cut in the classroom or on the school playground provides an excellent opportunity for presenting the entire class with the proper first aid for a minor wound. Such an approach takes on an entirely different aura because of its obvious relevance.

This segment of Hochbaum's theory also supports the inclusion of role playing of meaningful health situations at the appropriate level. The teacher can always prompt a discussion about the many health-related events taking place on television. Commercials dealing with health products alone could be discussed endlessly as to their relative merits and impact on society. A simple show-and-tell session devoted to health might also provide some interesting incidental learning experiences. In any event, many of the most meaningful learning situations are those that require little, if any, preparation, and they just seem to happen. The skillful teacher takes advantage of just such a situation.

It is interesting to note that many of the youngsters' initially strong attitudes about particular kinds of health behavior are developed long before the health reasons for such attitudes. Ideally, these attitudes and practices will be positive in nature and continually supported at home. By the same token, the school can be an influential factor in promoting and reinforcing proper health behavior. Eliciting and encouraging proper health practices by providing appropriate health learning experiences at the primary level should provide the foundation for the development of sound health attitudes and knowledge. Such an approach becomes particularly important for the youngster who is receiving no, or poor, health guidance at home.

As the child continues to mature, there is a gradual change in the influential factors affecting his or her health behavior. As the child begins the intermediate years, his or her peers begin to become the catalytic force behind health behavior. Now the child may suffer through some value conflicts. He or she may very well be tempted to indulge in behavior that is completely contrary to his or her present beliefs and practices. The child is quickly entering the stage of life that encourages experimentation. By the time the child enters junior high school, peer influence has become one of the most motivating factors in his or her life.

The intermediate grades and early junior high years are highly attitudinal in nature. The child is now actively searching and exploring and is most in need of strong, exemplary models and positive direction. In keeping with our earlier discussion in Chapter 2, it is most important at this stage that the child become involved in learning experiences that deal with the prominent sociological health problems that are likely to touch him or her. We cannot, and must not, bury our heads and deny the possibility of youngsters at this level becoming involved in health behavior that can conceivably have a drastic and irreversible effect on the rest of their lives.

Hochbaum also discusses three other factors he considers to be influential in determining one's health behavior. He feels that pleasure plays an important part in whether or not a youngster will deliberately participate in a poor health behavior. A person may gladly accept the risks involved in poor health behavior in exchange for the pleasure it may promise. It becomes a coping behavior. The challenge for the educator is to provide young people with constructive alternatives to poor health behavior. Many positive and constructive health activities can be substituted for poor health practices which provide pleasure for the individual. Can you think of some of the alternatives?

Many people rationalize particular kinds of health behavior simply because they feel that the potential threat to their health is far removed, so why not indulge in the activity for now. A classic example is the young person's rationalizing that cigarette smoking is safe for a few years because it normally takes some 20 years for the ill effects of smoking to become chronic. Such a rationale is often faulty because the person may have an extremely difficult time breaking a firmly acquired habit or addiction. It is relatively easy to become habituated or possibly even addicted, as many a smoker will attest. Young people need to be made aware of such consequences.

Fear can also have an effect on health behavior. Fear of potential emotional and/or physical agony can lead to behavior designed to remove or ameliorate such a situation. Therefore, fear can be a powerful incentive to involve oneself in rational health behavior.

A discussion of fear as it relates to health behavior should not be construed as a plea for scare tactics in the classroom. There is no place in education for morbid, abnormal, or fearful subject matter. Research has proved that such approaches to education are of little value. They may be shocking and motivating for the moment, but have little carryover value. However, students surely should be made aware of the possible consequences of poor health behavior. An honest and sincere approach is by far the preferred approach.

DEVELOPING HEALTH ATTITUDES, PRACTICES, AND KNOWLEDGE

The relative emphasis placed on the development of health attitudes, practices, and knowledge varies at different educational levels (see Fig. 8.2). Research suggests that at certain developmental stages, children are more inclined to readily establish health practices, at other stages are more likely to develop attitudes, and at still other periods in their lives will seek to procure knowledge.

Piaget (1971) has described the process by which children develop the capacity for grasping concepts. His theory, when applied to elementary health science, is helpful in evolving a pattern of instructional emphasis. Thus the best results will be attained by assigning primary emphasis to the development of health practices during the early years of school life. Theoretically, health attitudes will also be developed as by-products through installation of sound health habits at the primary level.

The middle elementary grades provide the most opportune time for the development of health attitudes. Such a statement should not be construed as meaning that practices and knowledge are disregarded during the intermediate grades. It simply means that the development of attitudes is given

Percent
emphasis

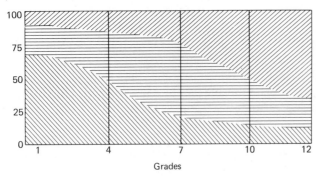

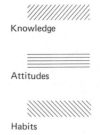

Knowledge

Attitudes

Habits

Fig. 8.2 Changing emphasis to be placed on imparting health knowledge, evolving attitudes, or developing habits at various grade levels.

top priority at that time, due to the fact that the child is most ready for the cultivation of sound and positive attitudes in this period of his or her life. This is the age when the youngster is highly impressionable and easily and readily acquires attitudes. Through the acquisition of desirable health attitudes, health practices already established will be further reinforced.

Knowledge to sustain, support, and reinforce practices and attitudes then becomes important. The upper elementary grades or junior high school should be thought of as the level at which health knowledge becomes increasingly important. Such knowledge is necessary to reinforce previously procured practices and attitudes. Junior high youngsters rapidly become interested in the how and why of health matters. Furthermore, they are now capable of digesting and assimilating such cognitive information. They have reached the maturational level at which factual information is meaningful and relevant to their world.

Keep in mind that the junior high years are highly experimental in nature for the youngster. Peer pressure is intense, and for many youngsters their first real value conflicts are occurring. Young people are in dire need of objective health information at this time. Ideally, such information, combined with previously established practices and attitudes, will assist the child in making an informed decision regarding his or her health behavior.

"DO NOTS" OF HEALTH INSTRUCTION

Anderson (1968) discusses some "do nots" of elementary health instruction. Certain practices that may perhaps outwardly appear appealing have been found to be more injurious than helpful as aspects of health instruction. All too often in the search for motivating devices, the elementary teacher may be inclined to employ questionable materials and/or activities. For example, the elementary teacher should steadfastly avoid employing the following approaches to health instruction:

1. Extrinsic (artificial) rewards for proper or acceptable behavior (e.g., stars, ranking charts, movies, etc.);

2. Unrealistic or unattainable standards;

3. Healthiest-child contests;

4. Health competition among students (e.g., height, weight, grooming, dental caries, etc.);

5. Scare tactics through the use of morbid, abnormal, or fearful subject matter;

6. Ridiculing or humiliating a student;
7. Using a student in class or school as an example of a health defect;
8. Allowing personal prejudices to drastically influence health instruction;
9. Confusing health instruction with physical education;
10. Imposing one's personal values on students.

Perhaps a true-life incident will serve to clarify the point. A fifth-grade teacher permitted his students—both girls and boys—to play softball during their physical education period. It was standard procedure on each occasion for any youngster who hit a home run to receive a candy bar (purchased by the teacher) as a reward. Few girls ever received a candy bar, and personal observation led us to conclude that very few of the girls really enjoyed the activity. How do you react to this situation? Do you perceive any fallacies in such an approach? Undoubtedly, many of these girls were left with mixed emotions about physical activity and baseball in particular. The situation above is a classic example of poor extrinsic motivation on the part of the teacher.

REVIEW QUESTIONS

1. Define the responsiblities of both the home and the school in terms of the health of the elementary child. Allude to the fallacy frequently associated with this approach.
2. Explain the instructional decisions that should be considered prior to implementing health instruction.
3. Discuss the goals of the school health program.
4. Outline the school health program.
5. Explain Hochbaum's theory of health behavior. Cite the rationale surrounding the "relative emphasis" concept of teaching for attitudes, practices, and knowledge at the different educational levels.
6. List the so-called do nots of health instruction.
7. Discuss the merits of teacher-student involvement at the elementary level.
8. Cite and explain several techniques that can be employed by the elementary teacher in an effort to become involved with students.

REFERENCES AND BIBLIOGRAPHY

Anderson, C. L. *School Health Practice* (St. Louis: C. V. Mosby, 1968).

Bruner, Jerome S. *The Process of Education* (New York: Vintage House, 1960).

Cornacchia, Harold J. "Teaching in Difficult Areas in Health," *Journal of School Health* **41** (April 1971): 193-196.

Cornacchia, Harold J., Wesley M. Staton, and Leslie W. Irwin. *Health in Elementary Schools* (St. Louis: C. V. Mosby, 1970).

Crary, Ryland W. *Humanizing the School: Curriculum Development and Theory* (New York: Knopf, 1969).

Foster, Julia C. *The Teaching of Health Education* (Columbus, Ohio: Charles Merrill, 1969).

Glasser, William. *Schools Without Failure* (New York: Harper & Row, 1969).

Hochbaum, Godfrey M. *Health Behavior* (Belmont, Calif.: Wadsworth, 1970).

Holt, John. *The Underachieving School* (New York: Pitman, 1969).

Mead, Margaret. *Culture and Commitment: A Study of the Generation Gap* (New York: Doubleday, 1970).

Pulaski, Mary, and Spencer Pulaski. *Understanding Piaget* (New York: Harper & Row, 1971).

Rash, J. Keogh. *The Health Education Curriculum* (Bloomington: Indiana University Press, 1966).

Read, Donald A., and Walter H. Greene. *Creative Teaching in Health* (New York: Macmillan, 1971).

9

the elementary health education curriculum

WHY INCLUDE HEALTH IN THE ELEMENTARY CURRICULUM?

Never before have children been more acutely aware of what is taking place around them. They are the television generation, and this fact is more responsible than any other for their being exposed to more spectacles in a year that their parents could have been expected to perceive in a decade. Without question, today's elementary youngsters are brighter, more sensitive, and certainly more provocative than their counterparts in any preceding generation. Attitudinally, the child of today matures quite quickly and very often exhibits as much insight as a young person twice as old. Such a phenomenon has implications for elementary health science.

It is generally agreed that there is a strong relationship between one's values and attitudes and one's emotional, physical, social, and spiritual well-being. The earlier in life that one develops a positive outlook relative to health behavior, the greater the chances of living a wholesome, happy, and productive life. It follows that the logical point at which to initiate health education is the elementary classroom. Ideally the health education that takes place in the classroom will supplement the health education the child receives at home and in the community.

It would seem logical that if our socially aware elementary youngsters were exposed to a formal health education program, they would be more inclined to develop a healthy and wholesome outlook toward optimal well-being. Unfortunately, many children are never exposed to formal health education during their developmental years. It is indeed regrettable when a youngster acquires poor health knowledge, attitudes, and practices simply because he or she was never exposed to sound health principles. If we expect young people to avidly seek a meaningful and rewarding life, we must help them to establish a firm foundation of health knowledge, attitudes, and practices early in life. Failure on our part to assist the child with such developmental tasks may very well deprive him or her of the ability to reach maximum potential and enjoy a truly wholesome life.

The responsible and sensitive elementary teacher is concerned about the health and welfare of students. Actually, the elementary teacher has a legal as well as moral responsibility for the promotion and development of positive pupil health behavior. Such an accomplishment is no easy task. The development of optimal well-being is without question one of the most challenging undertakings in life. The informed and concerned elementary teacher can significantly contribute to such a worthy goal.

In addition to this philosophical rationale in support of the inclusion of health education at the elementary level, there are also other, more objective reasons:

1. It is common knowledge that Americans possess poor health practices. Our diet, activity level, dental habits, weight control, and techniques for dealing with stress border on being atrocious at times. For many of us, such poor health practices are a direct reflection of our failure to develop proper health habits at an early age.

2. Undoubtedly, many Americans have difficulty in establishing proper health practices simply because they lack the basic information necessary to make intelligent decisions about health matters. A well-planned and coordinated elementary health science program can contribute immensely to solving such a dilemma.

3. The general attitude of the average American toward well-being is not good and unfortunately appears to be getting worse. Perhaps "future shock" is the best term to describe the state of affairs that confronts most of us. "Obsolete" has become a household word. Change is so rapid that only the heartiest can adjust and keep his or her wits. Technology has done many wonderful things for us, but not without built-in traumas. Reality can become too much to bear, and all too often the occasional escape to a world of illusion becomes

habitual. The drug problem, divorce rate, incidence of venereal disease, and ecological problems are just a few of the indicators of "future shock" in the United States. If we are literally to survive, we must effectively deal with the way of life we have created. Health education at an early age can assist young people as they strive to adjust successfully and cope with a complex and demanding way of life.

4. The most pressing health issues that we as a nation face today are in most instances sociological in nature. Such timely, relevant, and surely significant health topics as mental health, mood-modifying substances, family life and sex education, and ecology are all monumental in terms of present-day social health issues. In addition, they are all highly attitudinal in nature. Education pertaining to these topics will be helpful in developing a socially aware young adult who will be more likely to contribute significantly to the solution of these problems.

5. Health is one of the cardinal objectives of education. Every national policy-forming body in the United States for the past five generations has indicated that one of the major objectives of education is the achieving of good physical and mental health. In addition, most state laws require a teacher to accept certain health obligations and teaching opportunities "for health" in the school. Teachers are also legally bound to do certain health teaching, to recognize illnesses in pupils, and to prevent school accidents. The recommendations in the *School Health Education Study* (1964) not only included health instruction among priorities for the school, but also recognized it as a distinctive responsibility of the school. Implicit in this recommendation was the belief that the content of health instruction belongs to the school curriculum because such knowledge is necessary to direct self-behavior, is most effectively learned in school, and is not available from other public agencies.

APPROACHES TO TEACHING ELEMENTARY HEALTH SCIENCE

Most often when one speaks of approaches to health instruction, one is referring to three distinctly different theories of health education. Health science as a discipline can be developed through correlation, integration, and/or direct instruction. As you might imagine, many authorities disagree as to which one of those approaches is best suited for providing learning experiences of a health nature for elementary school children. The following discussion is provided in an effort to help you form your own opinion.

Correlation

Correlation can be thought of as the incorporation of health education into another appropriate subject area. Such an approach requires as a prerequisite a strong relationship between health and the area with which it is being correlated. Proponents argue that such an approach actually allows the teacher more latitude. It helps remove the traditional barriers of the curriculum and offers a refreshingly new avenue for developing the same old topics. In addition, correlation is purported to actually enrich content information because such a technique broadens and adds relevance to subject-matter areas.

Actually, health science at the elementary level can be incorporated into any of the subjects normally taught in elementary school. Language arts, reading, mathematics, art, geography, music, science, history, and physical education all provide opportunities for learning experiences of a health nature. For example, by having the students chart their height and weight for the year, math principles can be implemented, and a discussion of the relationship among growth, development, and health can be prompted.

Needless to say, the teaching for health through correlation requires a great deal of exper-

tise on the part of the teacher. Assuming that health objectives are established for the year, the teacher is faced with the dilemma of determining which activities are most applicable to developing the health concepts selected for dissemination.

The pitfalls to such an approach are obvious. It would be relatively easy to force the correlation of health education. When sound preplanning is lacking, it is not at all difficult to become irrelevant, waste the students' time, and duplicate someone else's efforts. When a significant relationship does not exist among the ideas being correlated, students can easily miss the point or be totally unaffected by what unfortunately may be very important information. On the other hand, correlation properly implemented can and will do much to help children see the relationship between health and the many and varied aspects of everyday living.

Integration

Integration implies that learning experiences are organized around a central objective, theme, or area of living. Such an approach best lends itself to elementary school because the units taught usually transcend subject-matter lines and are centered on life's activities. The concept of integration can be thought of as a core, broad-fields approach to curriculum organization. For such an approach to be effective, the teacher must skillfully draw on the content of the various school subjects and programs which can best contribute to the concept being developed.

It is easy to understand why correlation and integration are often confused and many times used synonymously. One thing is certain: Where there is an integrated plan, there must be correlation taking place in each of the subject areas involved in the integration process. On the other hand, there certainly can be correlation of health education into another subject or two without such instruction being literally integrated into some overall instructional plan.

Should you still be grappling with the main difference between correlation and integration, the following discussion by Rash should help clarify the issue:

As has been suggested, integration is sometimes erroneously confused with correlation. The confusion results from the complete misuse of the word integration, not from any close similarity in meaning. In reality integration has two meanings. The first, and original, meaning is related to integrate, "to make whole." In this connotation integration is the process of making whole. *The second meaning, resulting from attempts to describe a plan of organization of a school curriculum is defined in the* Dictionary of Education *as: "a curriculum in which subject matter boundaries are ignored, all offerings of the school being taught in relation to broad areas of study and in relation to one another as mutually associated in some genuine life relation."*

*The concept of correlation in which one subject field is related to another subject field is in direct conflict with the concept of integration, in which subject matter boundaries are ignored. Correlation relates to method while integration relates to plan of organization.**

In summary, the elementary classroom does lend itself to such approaches to education. The fact that the classroom is self-contained offers flexibility which the teacher can use to decided advantage. The skillful elementary teacher is afforded the opportunity of moving through a correlation teaching situation to direct instruction or vice versa. When the same teacher is responsible for providing all of the students' curricular learning experiences, there evolves a state of freedom for the teacher that can be found only in the self-contained classroom. However, such freedom is not without its inherent pit-

---

* Reprinted by permission from J. Keogh Rash, *The Health Education Curriculum*, 2nd ed. (Bloomington: Indiana University Bookstore, 1974), pp. 134-135. Reprinted by permission of the author.

falls. For example, it would be easy for the elementary teacher to slight health instruction through sheer laxity because he or she felt that students' health needs were being met entirely through correlation.

The most important point is that we make our overt attempt to meet the students' health needs. Correlation can be most effective in contributing to the accomplishment of such a task. Combined with direct instruction, it becomes even more effective.

Direct Instruction

Direct health instruction simply implies that time is set aside during the school day for health education. Such instruction is planned and directed toward the fulfillment of pupils' health needs and interests.

We have already established the fact that the primary school youngster is held responsible for very little in terms of specific knowledge in regard to health. However, children's natural curiosity will demand more specific information as their capacity for understanding advances. It is especially desirable to provide more and more cognitive information of a health nature from the third grade on. Surely there is no single perfect approach, but one can be reasonably sure that the primary grades best lend themselves to development of sound health practices; the intermediate grades to the establishment of positive health attitudes; and the junior high level to the building of new positive attitudes and in-depth health knowledge. Direct health instruction becomes the vehicle for such an approach.

Perhaps you have now developed your own opinion as to what is the best approach to health education. Keep in mind that no matter what the choice, the teacher is the main aspect on which the responsibility of success rests. We feel that perhaps the most logical approach to health instruction centers on direct instruction implementing correlation where and whenever possible. That way, health instruction is afforded the same amount of emphasis as the other traditional subjects taught at the elementary level.

Combination of Approaches

An example of how the three approaches may be combined to provide health instruction is the Berkeley Project, which encompasses a core curriculum and a specific body system as a control theme in each grade. The core material varies with grade level. For example, the digestive system is studied in grade 4, the respiratory in grade 5, and the cardiovascular system in grade 6. In every grade level the model is composed of five basic phases: awareness, appreciation, structure and function, disease and disorders, and prevention. The underlying philosophy is to first orient the student to discover, as from dissection of a body organ, how it works and then how that body system works together with other body systems. Rather than having the teacher lecture about each of the body systems, a series of learning stations is set up in the classroom, each focusing on one aspect of the body system, with a different set of reference materials and work sheets. Students use multimedia learning aids, such as books, models, filmstrips, slides, and overhead transparencies. After mastering the topic at the station, a student teaches other students in his or her group. Students go from station to station, studying the structure and function of a body system, as well as the risk factors associated with the diseases, disorders of the body system, and ways of preventing these in the body.

One of the outstanding features of this approach is that the elementary teachers are pre-trained in in-service workshops. Teachers are acquainted with the five phases of the health unit for each grade, as well as key concepts, content, and learning experiences to be used in the classroom. The Berkeley Smoking and Health Project is one of the most effective health instructional approaches being used in the United States. Further information about this approach is available from:

Community Program Development Division
Bureau of Health Education
Center for Disease Control
Atlanta, Georgia 30333

THE ELEMENTARY HEALTH CURRICULUM

To speak of the elementary health education curriculum is a much more difficult task than one might imagine. First and foremost, it is the aspect of health education that you, the prospective elementary teacher, will probably be able to affect the least. Should you be asking yourself "why," perhaps Fenton's discussion of textbook writing and course of study development might help in clarifying the statements above:

In the past, university professors and public school teachers wrote the textbooks used in the schools. Usually the most qualified experts, busy at research, refused to turn their hands to writing. Moreover, publishers feared to risk their stockholders' money on radical new approaches which might fail on the market. As a result, one text looked pretty much like another, and almost all lagged behind the latest research.

Typically, a board of education, accepting the recommendations of a small committee of teachers, authorized the use of one text in preference to others. Starting with the text, a committee of teachers developed a course of study during summer vacation. It often turned out to be an expanded table of contents followed by an extensive bibliography. No teacher can develop an imaginative curriculum in a month. Then the textbooks, along with the course of study, passed into the hands of classroom teachers. The curriculum reformers recognized that conventional texts and courses of study were built-in obstacles to chance.*

Curriculum can be thought of as the "what" to teach. In most school districts, the elementary

---

* Reprinted with permission from Edwin Fenton, *The New Social Studies*, p. 2. Copyright © 1967 by Holt, Rinehart and Winston.

health education curriculum has been established by a group of so-called experts supposedly well qualified and willing to extend themselves in a more imaginative manner than those cited by Fenton. Ideally, the elementary health curriculum should be designed to meet the health needs and interests of the students and should be flexible enough to provide for individual differences from school to school and class to class. Needless to say, such an undertaking, if it is properly approached, is a monumental project and requires much time, skill, and insight from its designers.

In recent years all disciplines have undergone some rather radical curricular changes. Some have enjoyed more success than others. Just over a decade ago, for example, the new mathematics created a fever among students, teachers, and parents alike. The repercussions of the new math are still being felt today. About the same time came the increased emphasis on science. Spurred by Sputnik and financed generously by private foundations and the government, these new reforms have spread throughout American schools. However, the rash of books and articles written since then in an attempt to explain the new math and science to bewildered parents who are diligently trying to understand so they can help their children testifies in a negative fashion to the success of many of these curricular reforms. Perhaps even more interesting is the fact that already a newer math, designed to consolidate and improve on the work of the original group of reformers, is on the drawing boards. The dilemma in health science—that of identifying a new and relevant curriculum, initiating it, and having it accepted by the teachers and public at large—is similar to that of mathematics and science. Obviously, radical curriculum revision is not without many innate problems.

THE SCHOOL HEALTH EDUCATION STUDY

The discipline of health education has not been immune to curricular investigation and eventual revision. At about the same time that most other content areas were receiving critical evaluation, so was health education. It was rather obvious around 1960 that the health education curriculum was out of date when compared to any of the other subjects in the school curriculum. Following Sputnik I's appearance in orbit, many schools quickly moved to bolster their math and science curriculums, often at the expense of health instruction.

Such action prompted one of the most important national status and curricular studies in the field of education. The School Health Education Study (SHES) was born in the fall of 1960. Financed by the Samuel Bronfman Foundation, the study was initially designed to determine the national status of health education and to provide the data necessary for the creation of a sound school health instruction program. Initially, the study was funded for only one year. Later the scope of the study was expanded, and the Bronfman Foundation continued its support through 1965. Approximately one-third of a million dollars was allocated for the completion of the study.

In its early stages, the study consisted of two surveys. One survey was designed to determine the actual status of, and practices common to, health instruction in the nation's public schools. Particular attention was paid to: the time devoted to such instruction; whether it was required or not; the course content by grade level; organizational patterns; student groups; course titles; by whom taught; teacher qualifications; credit value, if any; special facilities; textbooks; in-service teacher training; problems peculiar to health instruction; and any recommendations. The second survey was designed to determine the actual health behavior of the students in terms of knowledge, attitudes, and practices.

In 1961 the SHES team selected a valid statistical sample of the approximately 35,000 public school systems in the United States. More specifically, they randomly selected 135 school systems in 38 states for surveying purposes. The survey forms dealing with the status of instruction were completed by the chief administrative office of each participating school system. The student health behavior instrument was administered to students in one sixth, one ninth, and one twelfth grade in each of the cooperating school systems. The gathering of data continued through 1962. After a great deal of analyzing and refining, the SHES staff published a summary report of its findings (1964).

The report essentially confirmed the worst suspicions of the SHES staff. Health education at all levels was in dire difficulty. The subsequent publication, *School Health Education: A Call for Action*, more vividly depicted the status and quality of health education in the nation's schools. Among the most important conclusions were:

*The response by school administrators and teachers . . . revealed a marked deficiency in the quantity and quality of health education in both the elementary and secondary schools. The problems confronting school personnel included: failure of parents to encourage health habits learned at school; ineffectiveness of instruction methods; parental and community resistance to discussions of sex, venereal disease and other controversial topics; insufficient time in the school day for health instruction; inadequate professional preparation of the staff; indifference toward and lack of support for health education on the part of some teachers, parents, administrators, health officers and other members of the community; inadequate facilities and instructional materials; student indifference to health education; lack of specialized supervisory and consultative services. . . . ***

Regarding the health behavior, knowledge, attitudes, and practices of the surveyed students, there were equally appalling findings. For example:

The health behavior—knowledge, attitudes and practices—of students was likewise appalling. The sixth graders surveyed could answer correctly—on the average—just over 20 of their 40 test questions. Ninth and 12th graders, on the average, could answer about 50 of 75 questions correctly. Girls, consistently, did somewhat better than boys. Consistently, too the students were not practicing many of the things they did know—but one sixth grader in five regularly brushed his or her teeth after meals; three out of four ninth grade boys (and half the girls) said a parent or counselor would be their last resort on a question concerning sex.

*Equally appalling were the misconceptions held by a great many students. Up to 70 percent of the seniors surveyed, for example, firmly believed that: fluoridation purifies drinking water, legislation guarantees the reliability of all advertised medicines, popular toothpastes kill germs in the mouth and prevent cavities, chronic diseases are contagious, pedestrians are safe under all circumstances in marked crosswalks, venereal diseases can be inherited, venereal diseases have never been a social problem, public funds support the voluntary health agencies, the best man to see for a persistent cough is a pharmacist.***

As appalling as the findings above may appear, it is not at all surprising that such conditions and beliefs existed, in view of the general quality and quantity of health instruction in 1962.

After the summary report was published in 1964, the SHES Advisory Committee charted a course of action designed to combat the poor status of health education. The original scope of the project was expanded to include the designing of a school health education curriculum for grades K-12. Eight health education specialists from five states were selected to develop the curriculum, and four sites were selected to implement the curriculum for testing purposes once it was completed. The four tryout centers represented the major geographical subdivisions of the United States.

The writing team began work in 1964 and quickly moved to explore the possible approaches to the development of a school health education curriculum. After a great deal of research and discussion, it was determined that a concept approach to health education appeared to be the most realis-

---

* From School Health Education Study, *Education Age,* St. Paul, Minn.: 3M Education Press, 1967, pp. 6-7.

tic, potentially effective, and economical way to develop a functional and sound school health education curriculum. The rationale behind such an approach was based on the premise that health is not a fact, but a comprehensive, generalized, and unified concept. Health is physical, mental, social, and spiritual in nature. It is also inherently a matter of knowledge, attitudes, and practices into which must be incorporated the interaction among the individual, his or her family, and the total community. Hence there are many component dimensions which are interdependent and combine to influence one's health status. Helping young people to recognize and understand this dynamic interaction became the challenge for the SHES writing team.

PHILOSOPHY OF ELEMENTARY HEALTH SCIENCE

In summary, elementary health science should be considered an integral aspect of the elementary education curriculum. After all, what is more important than our young people's health? Without health, life can never offer the true zest which accompanies optimal well-being.

Through elementary health education, we can actively assist young people in becoming self-actualizing human beings who are capable of making intelligent and informed decisions about their health behavior. Behavior is the most influential factor in determining the health of the student. Heredity and environment are also important factors in determining one's health status, but behavior is generally the most crucial constituent.

Based on the premise above, we attempt to influence youngsters' behavior by dealing with their health knowledge, attitudes, and practices. Health as a concept is highly value-oriented and attitudinal in nature. The school health program, with its interrelated components, should provide the example and guidance necessary to influence and assist young people in attaining optimum health.

CONTENT AREAS OF HEALTH EDUCATION: WHAT SHOULD WE BE TEACHING?

Haag (1965, p. 246) lists 13 content areas of health education; Kilander (1968, p. 278) cites 11; Willgoose (1974, pp. 407-413) discussses 12; Cornacchia, Staton, and Irwin (1970, p. 158) mention 20; Fodor and Dalis (1966, p. 41) list 11. At first glance, there would appear to be little agreement among the authorities as to just what content areas should be taught under the auspices of elementary health education. Further analysis, however, reveals much more agreement than might initially be anticipated. Some authors combine particular content areas into larger ones; others prefer to subdivide larger areas into more concise topic areas.

In an effort to help clarify the matter of health content areas, we have selected the California State Department of Education publication entitled *Framework for Health Instruction in California Public Schools* (1970) as a working example of an elementary health education curriculum. California's curriculum guide is an excellent exemplary model for our purposes, because it is up to date, developed by a highly competent team of experts, well field-tested, and utilizes the conceptual approach. The overall emphasis of the framework is placed on behavioral objectives. Attitudes and behaviors are stressed rather than merely health knowledge.

Development of the Framework

It is interesting to note how the California framework was developed. Two major steps were undertaken in its preparation: (1) the determination of the health needs of California school-age children; and (2) the development of the framework on the basis of these needs.

The needs of California school-age children were determined by reviewing the literature and asking for the opinions of authorities asked to sit on an ad hoc committee. The committee was composed of representatives from the fields of medicine, dentistry, public health, allied health professions representing health content areas, and education. Once the health needs of the children had been determined, a document listing the needs was prepared and was sent to the project consultants for use in preparing the framework.

After much careful deliberation and analysis, the final draft of the framework was developed. It organized material into ten content areas, with an overview, major concepts, grade-level concepts, suggested behavioral objectives, and suggested examples of content for each of these areas. The ten content areas identified were: consumer health; mental-emotional health; drug use and misuse; family health; oral health, vision, and hearing; nutrition; exercise, rest, and posture; disease and disorders; environmental health hazards; and community health resources. The California health instruction curriculum follows.

California
health
instruction
curriculum ▶

Consumer Health[1]

Major concept	Primary level	Intermediate level	Junior high level
I To maintain health requires effort, time, and money, but failure to maintain health is detrimental and more costly.		**Grade-level concept: Prevention and early treatment are less costly than results of neglecting one's health.** *Objective:* Discusses why prevention and early treatment are economical. *Content:* (1) immunization reduces illness; (2) preventing or treating dental caries early saves teeth and money; (3) precautionary measures prevent permanent damage; (4) precautionary measures promote more effective use of one's talents.	**Grade-level concept: Disease and premature death are detrimental and costly.** *Objective:* Illustrates how disease and premature death are detrimental and costly. *Content:* (1) personal costs; (2) loss of productivity; (3) rising costs of facilities and personnel for health care; (4) pain or discomfort.
II Scientific knowledge and understanding are bases for effective evaluation, selection, and utilization of health information, products, and services.	**Grade-level concept: Adults can help children solve health problems.** *Objective:* Names appropriate sources of help in various situations of injury, illness, and disorders. *Content:* (1) parents; (2) doctors; (3) dentists; (4) nurses. *Objective:* Tells how physicians, dentists, and nurses protect our health. *Content:* (1) early detection; (2) treatment before extensive damage occurs; (3) health counseling.	**Grade-level concept: The source of health information influences its accuracy.** *Objective:* Identifies various reliable sources of health information. *Content:* (1) professional personnel; (2) professional associations; (3) public health agencies; (4) approved voluntary health agencies; (5) insurance companies. *Objective:* Explains factors that influence the accuracy of health information. *Content:* (1) who provides the information; (2) why the information is provided (motives); (3) date of information.	**Grade-level concept: Discretion in selection and utilization of health products can both enhance health and save money.** *Objective:* Summarizes factors to consider when evaluating, selecting, and using health products. *Content:* (1) labels; (2) cost; (3) generic versus brand names; (4) prescription versus nonprescription drugs. *Objective:* Discusses the effects on health when products are not used wisely. *Content:* (1) may cause direct harm; (2) may cover up symptoms of disease.

III Self-diagnosis and self-treatment may be dangerous to an individual.

Grade-level concept: Mass media may be misleading sources of health information.

Objective: Names health products that are commonly misrepresented.

Content: (1) cosmetics; (2) nonprescription drugs; (3) tobacco; (4) dentifrices.

Objective: Identifies types of mass media that may include misleading sources of information.

Content: (1) radio and television commercials; (2) advertising in periodicals; (3) articles in periodicals; (4) books on health topics.

Grade-level concept: Advertising may mislead individuals in their selection and use of health information, products, and services.

Objectives: Cites examples of appeals that are used by advertisers.

Content: (1) plays upon emotions; (2) appeals to the sexes; (3) makes unstated assumptions; (4) appeals to the good life; (5) utilizes hero worship.

Objective: Describes the impact of advertising techniques on individuals.

Content: (1) buying products that are not needed; (2) buying products that may be harmful to the consumer; (3) selecting personnel not qualified to care for the consumer's health problem.

IV Quackery and faddism raise false hopes, delay proper medical attention, and cause financial waste.

Grade-level concept: Superstitions and misconceptions about health may be dangerous.

Objective: Describes the origin of health superstitions and misconceptions.

Content: (1) old wives' tales; (2) folk medicine; (3) quacks; (4) faddists.

Objective: Cites ways in which health superstitions and misconceptions may be dangerous.

Content: (1) delay in seeking treatment; (2) likelihood of acquiring poor eating habits; (3) raising of false hopes; (4) creation of anxieties.

Grade-level concept: Quackery and faddism are dangerous to health.

Objective: Identifies examples of health quackery and faddism.

Content: (1) false cures for cancer; (2) ineffective treatment for arthritis; (3) food faddism.

Objective: Predicts potential hazards of faddism and quackery.

Content: (1) raising false hopes; (2) delaying proper medical treatment; (3) incurring damage because of improper treatment.

¹ NOTE: Descriptions of *objectives* and *content* throughout the ten content areas of this document are intended as EXAMPLES ONLY. *Framework for Health Instruction in California Public Schools.* Sacramento, Calif.: California State Department of Education, 1970.

Mental-Emotional Health

Major concept	Primary level	Intermediate level	Junior high level
I Mental health is influenced by the interrelationship of biological and environmental and cultural, factors.	**Grade-level concept: Health practices influence and are influenced by one's emotions.** *Objective:* Describes personal health practices which influence and are influenced by one's emotions. *Content:* (1) sleep and rest; (2) eating; (3) physical activity; (4) posture.	**Grade-level concept: Biographical factors influence one's mental health.** *Objective:* Discusses biological factors that influence mental health. *Content:* (1) nervous system; (2) endocrine glands; (3) heredity; (4) physical appearance. **Grade-level concept: One's environment helps to determine one's mental health.** *Objective:* Summarizes environmental factors affecting mental health. *Content:* (1) physical factors (housing, climate); (2) social factors; (3) ethnic factors.	**Grade-level concept: No one factor is solely responsible for one's mental health.** *Objective:* Describes the interrelationship of biological and environmental influences on one's mental health. *Content:* (1) heredity sets limits, and environment determines levels of attainment; (2) stress situations in one's environment cause biological reactions, which in turn may cause anxiety; (3) a pleasant environment may bring about feelings of calm and tranquility.
II Developing and maintaining optimal mental health include understanding oneself and others.	**Grade-level concept: Making friends and getting along with others make life more satisfying.** *Objective:* Lists ways of making and keeping friends. *Content:* (1) being friendly; (2) being fair; (3) respecting the rights of others. *Objective:* Tells how one can gain satisfaction through family and friends. *Content:* (1) companionship; (2) someone to confide in; (3) security.	**Grade-level concept: People are similar in many ways, but each individual is a unique person.** *Objective:* Explains the importance of setting realistic goals within the limits of one's strengths and weaknesses. *Content:* (1) goals can be achieved; (2) undue pressure and frustration can be limited; (3) satisfaction from achieving goals can be realized. *Objective:* Illustrates ways in which individuals are similar. *Content:* (1) physical needs (shelter, food, safety); (2) emotional needs (love, security, companionship). *Objective:* Provides examples to show how individuals are unique. *Content:* (1) size and shape; (2) rate of growth; (3) skills and abilities; (4) feelings and thoughts; (5) interests.	**Grade-level concept: Individuals who have good mental health exhibit some common characteristics.** *Objective:* States the characteristics of the mentally healthy individual. *Content:* (1) understanding and liking oneself; (2) understanding and getting along with others; (3) meeting the daily demands of living in an effective way. **Grade-level concept: Individuals are basically worthy and make contributions to society.** *Objective:* Discusses the importance of recognizing and accepting the contributions of others. *Content:* (1) encourages individuals to make contributions; (2) helps individuals to feel worthwhile; (3) helps in the rehabilitation of individuals.

III Stress, an unavoidable product of our culture, can be either productive or detrimental.

Grade-level concept: Young children, as well as adults, have responsibilities.

Objective: Indicates how assuming responsibility helps to reduce stress.

Content: (1) obtains personal satisfaction; (2) gains the respect of others; (3) eliminates source of stress.

Objective: Identifies achievable responsibilities at home and at school.

Content: (1) helps with family chores; (2) maintains own room; (3) does assigned school work to best of ability.

Objective: Tells how stress may result from undue concern about responsibilities.

Content: (1) worrying about not carrying out responsibilities satisfactorily; (2) being overly concerned about trying to please; (3) failing to carry out responsibilities.

Grade-level concept: Individuals react differently to stressful situations.

Objective: Compares and contrasts the values and limitations of stress.

Content: (1) stress may be a motivating factor; (2) some individuals work better when under mild stress; (3) stress may cause undue concern and may interfere with normal response.

Objective: Identifies typical situations in which stress occurs.

Content: (1) competition (baseball); (2) sibling rivalry; (3) parental expectations; (4) pressure of school curriculum.

Objective: Explains ways that individuals reduce stress.

Content: (1) modify goals; (2) change activity; (3) balance work and play.

Grade-level concept: Peer pressures produce stress which individuals can learn to handle.

Objective: Interprets how peer pressures can affect an individual's behavior.

Content: (1) may become a blind follower; (2) may desert his peer group; (3) may have conflict with parents owing to difference in expectation of peer group and parents.

Objective: Summarizes factors that determine when it is appropriate to make one's own decision and when one should follow the advice of others.

Content: (1) individual maturity; (2) personal understanding of the situation; (3) importance of the decision; (4) ability of others to help.

Objective: Indicates ways of handling stress produced by peer pressures.

Content: (1) talking it out; (2) working off anger; (3) taking one thing at a time; (4) assuming leadership responsibilities.

IV Maladjustive behavior varies in its impact on the individual and society.

Grade-level concept: Emotions, when not controlled, can be harmful.

Objective: Identifies basic emotions and discusses how they may be helpful or harmful.

Content: (1) anger—motivation or carelessness; (2) fear—caution or panic; (3) love—security or overdependence.

Objective: Tells positive ways of relieving emotions.

Content: (1) talking with someone; (2) playing; (3) working; (4) enjoying a hobby.

Grade-level concept: Individuals vary in their ability to adjust to the demands of living.

Objective: Identifies ways in which individuals adjust to the demands of daily living (adjustment mechanisms).

Content: (1) rationalization; (2) projection; (3) identification; (4) other adjustment mechanisms.

Objective: Discusses how maladjustive behavior may result from misuse of adjustment mechanisms.

Content: (1) explaining away problems instead of solving them; (2) consistently blaming others; (3) indulging in excessive day dreaming.

Grade-level concept: Maladjusted individuals can be helped.

Objective: Identifies types of maladjustive behavior.

Content: (1) phobias; (2) obsessions; (3) anxieties; (4) depression; (5) delusions of grandeur.

Objective: Discusses the importance of early detection.

Content: (1) treatment more effective; (2) shorter hospitalization period; (3) efforts less costly.

Objective: Categorizes the types of services available.

Content: (1) medical and psychiatric; (2) recreational; (3) vocational.

V Qualified help is available for those with maladjustive behavior.

Drug Use and Misuse

Major concept	Primary level	Intermediate level	Junior high level
I When used properly, drugs are beneficial to humanity.	**Grade-level concept: Medicines are helpful for maintaining health.** *Objective:* Tells how medicines may be beneficial. *Content:* (1) prevent infection; (2) relieve pain; (3) control coughs; (4) ease upset stomach. *Objective:* Discusses why medicine should be taken under supervision of parent as prescribed or recommended by a physician or a dentist. *Content:* (1) the correct drug for illness; (2) proper dosage; (3) proper frequency of use.	**Grade-level concept: Drugs with different properties are prescribed for medical use.** *Objective:* Gives examples of different forms in which common medicines may be taken. *Content:* (1) pill—aspirin; (2) injection—penicillin; (3) liquid—cough medicine; (4) capsule—antihistamine. *Objective:* Tells differences between prescription and nonprescription drugs. *Content:* (1) prescription drugs are prescribed by a doctor or a dentist; (2) nonprescription drugs are sold over the counter; (3) more rigid controls are needed for the manufacture and sale of prescription drugs; (4) prescription drugs are generally more potent; (5) nonprescription drugs are intended usually for minor ailments of short duration.	**Grade-level concept: Medicines can help the individual to function more effectively.** *Objective:* Describes ways in which medicines can be used to benefit the individual. *Content:* (1) to control communicable diseases; (2) to control chronic disorders; (3) to aid in surgery and to relieve pain; (4) to aid in the treatment of mental disorders.
II Many factors influence the misuse of drugs.	**Grade-level concept: A variety of conditions contribute to the misuse of medicines.** *Objective:* Discuss conditions under which a person might take the wrong medicine. *Content:* (1) not reading the label; (2) taking medicines in the dark; (3) accepting substances from strangers; (4) using another person's medicine; (5) taking more than the prescribed dose; (6) taking medicine from an unlabeled bottle.	**Grade-level concept: Misuse of drugs often starts early in life.** *Objective:* Explains why misuse of drugs often starts early in life. *Content:* (1) being motivated by curiosity; (2) imitating adults; (3) using accidentally; (4) being influenced by other users; (5) acting on a dare; (6) experimenting. *Objective:* Summarizes examples of the misuse of drugs. *Content:* (1) uses medicines prescribed for another person; (2) takes more than the prescribed or recommended amount; (3) does not follow a prescribed or recommended time schedule; (4) uses nonprescription drugs indiscriminately; (5) takes drugs for "kicks."	**Grade-level concept: Physical, emotional, and social factors influence the misuse of drugs.** *Objective:* Identifies physical and emotional factors that lead to the misuse of drugs. *Content:* (1) self-medication (relieving pain); (2) escape from reality; (3) compensation; (4) medically induced drug dependency; (5) attempts to overcome fatigue. *Objective:* Explains how social pressures can lead to the misuse of drugs. *Content:* (1) experiencing the influence of peer groups; (2) seeking false status; (3) rebelling against authority; (4) engaging in individual and group experimentation.

III Tobacco is harmful, and alcohol and other drugs, if misused, are harmful to the individual and to society.	**Grade-level concept: Some substances that are commonly used can be harmful if misused.** *Objective:* Identifies substances that can be harmful if misused. *Content:* (1) cola drinks; (2) tea and coffee; (3) alcohol; (4) medicines (aspirin, vitamins, diet pills, antibiotics, antihistamine).	**Grade-level concept: Individuals react differently to the chemicals contained in tobacco, alcohol, and other drugs.** *Objective:* Cites individual differences that cause people to react differently to drugs. *Content:* (1) bodily size; (2) sensitivity; (3) metabolism. *Objective:* Describes individual reactions to drugs. *Content:* (1) may become psychologically dependent; (2) may become physiologically dependent; (3) may have drug reaction-sensitivity; (4) may lose control of behavior.	**Grade-level concept: Tobacco, alcohol, and other drugs may cause harmful effects that are immediate and long-range.** *Objective:* Identifies potential harmful effects of drugs. *Content:* (1) *effects from tobacco:* (a) immediate (cardiovascular, mucous membrane, human performance, blood chemistry); (b) long-range (heart disease, lung cancer, emphysema, other circulatory disorders); (2) *effects from alcohol:* (a) immediate (intoxication, reaction time, sense organs, blood chemistry, neuromuscular coordination); (b) long-range (alcoholism, liver malfunction, brain damage); (3) *effects from other stimulants, depressants, or hallucinogens:* (a) immediate (stimulation or depression of nervous or circulatory system, hallucinations, distortion of senses, death caused by overdose); (b) long-range (dependence, chromosomal change, mental disorder, shortening of life expectancy); (4) *synergistic effects* (result of combination of drugs): death, masked symptoms.
IV The individual and society need to accept responsibility for preventing the misuse of tobacco, alcohol, and other drugs.	**Grade-level concept: Each person must treat medicine and other substances with respect.** *Objective:* Cites ways in which the individual shows respect for drugs. *Content:* (1) uses only when necessary; (2) takes only in recommended amounts and at recommended times; (3) takes only under supervision.	**Grade-level concept: Personal goals and practices established early in life can help one to avoid the misuse of drugs.** *Objective:* Discusses the values of personal goals and practices in avoiding the misuse of drugs. *Content:* (1) self-respect; (2) respect for one's body; (3) healthy standards of behavior; (4) sound personal decisions.	**Grade-level concept: One can live a normal, full, and happy life without misusing drugs.** *Objective:* Illustrates ways to cope with social pressures other than through use of drugs. *Content:* (1) having realistic goals; (2) participating in productive leisure-time activities; (3) achieving social relationships; (4) making one's own decisions.

Family Health[2]

Major concept	Primary level	Intermediate level	Junior high level
I The family and its members exert a significant influence on one another.	**Grade-level concept: Children can become responsible family members.** *Objective:* Discusses one's contributions and responsibilities as a family member. *Content:* (1) cooperates with others; (2) performs assigned duties; (3) considers rights of other family members.	**Grade-level concept: Family living provides opportunities for learning and practicing ways of achieving health.** *Objective:* Predicts favorable health outcomes of family living. *Content:* (1) good interpersonal relationships; (2) proper nourishment; (3) precautions against disease; (4) care for those with diseases or disorders. *Objective:* Indicates personal responsibility that contributes to the health of the family. *Content:* (1) personal health practices; (2) caring for others when they are ill; (3) getting along with other members.	**Grade-level concept: The family influences the ability of its members to make adjustments in society.** *Objective:* Describes factors that influence the family members. *Content:* (1) cultural backgrounds of parents; (2) family dwelling; (3) health practices of family members; (4) economic position of family; (5) different family structures (one-parent family, mother-dominant family, grandparents in home, others); (6) family value system.
II Human masculinity and femininity are determined by biological, emotional, and social factors.	**Grade-level concept: One's role as a boy or girl starts early in life.** *Objective:* Explains similarities and differences between boys and girls. *Content:* (1) growth; (2) physical skills; (3) expected behavior.	**Grade-level concept: Differences between boys and girls become greater as they grow and mature.** *Objective:* Compares and contrasts changes that occur in boys and girls as they grow and develop. *Content:* (1) individual rates of growth and maturity; (2) effect of hormones on secondary sex characteristics; (3) differences in interest. **Grade-level concept: Attitudes that one develops about sex influence behavior.** *Objective:* Discusses how one shows attitude about sex. *Content:* (1) vocabulary; (2) choice of personal reading material; (3) treatment of the opposite sex.	**Grade-level concept: The sex drive is a normal component of growth and development.** *Objective:* Discusses reasons why the sex drive is important. *Content:* (1) perpetuates humanity; (2) influences human behavior. *Objective:* Identifies factors that influence one's sex drive. *Content:* (1) biological makeup of the individual; (2) early childhood experiences in the home; (3) parental attitudes; (4) nature and extent of influences in the environment.

III Effective preparation, the ability to adjust, and respect for and understanding of one's marriage partner tend to produce successful marriages.	**Grade-level concept: Many attitudes about marriage develop early in life.** *Objective:* Describes influences that affect one's attitudes about marriage. *Content:* (1) social relationships; (2) types of home life; (3) family relationships; (4) environmental factors; (5) value systems.	**Grade-level concept: Dating plays an important role in preparation for marriage.** *Objective:* Identifies the functions of dating. *Content:* (1) sense of belonging; (2) learning to get along with the opposite sex; (3) learning social behavior; (4) enjoyment. *Objective:* Describes the various aspects of dating behavior. *Content:* (1) responsibilities to dating partner, self, and family; (2) standards of behavior; (3) implications of "going steady."	
IV Persons may function more effectively in their roles as males or females when they understand each other and understand that reproduction is a normal process.	**Grade-level concept: The ability to grow and reproduce is characteristic of living things.[3]** *Objective:* Indicates that all living things come from other living things. *Content:* (1) plants and animals grow and reproduce; (2) human beings grow; (3) newborn babies have special needs.	**Grade-level concept: Human reproduction is a normal function of living.[3]** *Objective:* Describes the normal reproductive system. *Content:* (1) reproductive systems; (2) physical development and bodily changes; (3) influences of heredity.	**Grade-level concept: Problems associated with the maturing process can be controlled.** *Objective:* Draws conclusions regarding ways in which the individual, the family, and society can reduce problems related to the maturing process. *Content:* (1) recognizing physical and social problems that can be prevented by sound knowledge and education; (2) accepting responsibility for individual behavior; (3) showing respect for others.
V Family planning may help to improve the health of family members.			

[2] The philosophy under which the five concepts in this content area should be developed is that adopted by the State Board of Education in its Resolution dated April 10, 1969. The Board recognized that the California Constitution prescribes "moral improvement" as one of the principal purposes of the public schools and resolved that "a Family Life and Health Education program be included as a necessary part of our over-all educational system (grades K-12) in order to aid in the carrying out of the full intent of the Constitution."

[3] Guidelines in the Resolution adopted by the State Board of Education April 10, 1969, include the following: "Earliest instruction relative to human reproduction not to be introduced prior to age of 9." Provisions of Education Code Section 8506 should also be kept in mind when planning instruction relating to human reproduction.

Oral Health, Vision, and Hearing

Major concept	Primary level	Intermediate level	Junior high level
I Neglect of oral health affects individuals of all ages.	**Grade-level concept: Oral neglect reduces the effectiveness of baby teeth as well as that of permanent teeth.** *Objective:* Describes the purposes of baby teeth and permanent teeth. *Content:* (1) maintain shape of face; (2) aid in eating; (3) assist in speech; (4) baby teeth maintain space for permanent teeth.	**Grade-level concept: Oral neglect affects appearance and social relationships.** *Objective:* Identifies ways in which oral health influences appearance and social relationships. *Content:* (1) unpleasant breath; (2) unsightly teeth; (3) rejection by peers. **Grade-level concept: Neglect of teeth interferes with their function.** *Objective:* Classifies teeth according to type and function. *Content:* (1) incisors—cutting; (2) canine—tearing; (3) molars—grinding.	**Grade-level concept: Oral neglect may result in oral disorders, which in turn may affect other organs and systems.** *Objective:* Identifies oral disorders that may result from neglect. *Content:* (1) dental caries; (2) abscesses; (3) periodontitis. *Objective:* Describes possible systemic effects that may result from oral disorders. *Content:* (1) infections in adjacent body parts (mouth and neck); (2) connective tissue damage to heart, kidney, and joints.
II Most oral disorders can be prevented.	**Grade-level concept: Tooth decay can be prevented or controlled.** *Objective:* Indicates parts of a tooth affected by tooth decay. *Content:* (1) crown; (2) root; (3) nerve. *Objective:* Lists ways of preventing tooth decay. *Content:* (1) brushes teeth properly or rinses mouth after eating; (2) chooses proper foods; (3) visits dentist regularly.	**Grade-level concept: Many factors contribute to tooth decay and its prevention.** *Objective:* Identifies factors that contribute to tooth decay. *Content:* (1) heredity; (2) tooth structure; (3) the nature of saliva; (4) bacteria in the mouth; (5) sugar in the mouth. *Objective:* Summarizes ways in which tooth decay can be prevented. *Content:* (1) by eating properly; (2) fluoridation of drinking water; (3) proper oral hygiene; (4) regular visits to the dentist.	**Grade-level concept: Personal decisions are important in preventing and treating oral disorders.** *Objective:* Describes personal decisions that are important in preventing or treating oral disorders. *Content:* (1) choice of foods; (2) choice and use of toothbrush and dentifrice; (3) utilization of qualified dental personnel. **Grade-level concept: Use of fluorides is an effective way of preventing tooth decay.** *Objective:* Describes the means of providing fluorides. *Content:* (1) public water supply; (2) topical application by dentist; (3) prescribed tablets; (4) bottled water. *Objective:* Compares claims made for and against fluoridation. *Content:* (1) claims made in favor of fluoridation: it is an inexpensive process, reduces tooth decay significantly, is safe, reaches all people, reduces cost of dental repair; (2) claims made against fluoridation: it forces people to drink fluoridated water against their will, is dangerous to health, is a type of socialized medicine.
III Oral disorders can be treated.	*Objective:* Tells why one should go to a dentist. *Content:* (1) early detection of tooth decay; (2) treatment of decayed teeth. **Grade-level concept: Practices harmful to oral health can be avoided.** *Objective:* Discusses practices that can be harmful to oral health. *Content:* (1) thumb sucking; (2) pencil chewing; (3) nail biting; (4) careless behavior; (5) excessive eating of sweets.		

IV Most disorders of vision and hearing, which may occur at any age, can be prevented or treated and corrected.

Grade-level concept: One's vision and hearing can be protected.

Objective: Tells why vision and hearing should be protected.

Content: (1) one can enjoy one's environment more; (2) learning is enhanced; (3) work tasks can be carried out more effectively; (4) recreation and play can be better enjoyed; (5) communication is improved.

Objective: Identifies practices that protect one's vision and hearing.

Content: (1) vision—seeking proper and sufficient light, using safety glasses when needed, protecting eyes from irritation or injury by foreign substances, avoiding direct visual contact with sun or bright lights, taking vision tests; (2) hearing—blowing nose gently, using care in diving, keeping foreign objects out of the ear, avoiding excessive noise, taking hearing tests.

Grade-level concept: Vision and hearing disorders are caused by many factors.

Objective: Identifies factors that contribute to vision and hearing disorders.

Content: (1) heredity; (2) structure; (3) growth changes; (4) infections; (5) accidents.

Objective: Explains why early detection and early treatment of vision and hearing disorders are important.

Content: (1) to avoid complications; (2) to alleviate academic, social, and personal problems.

Grade-level concept: Persons of all ages can be afflicted with vision and hearing defects.

Objective: Describes common defects of vision and hearing.

Content: (1) vision—refractive errors, muscle imbalance, color deficiency, glaucoma; (2) hearing—conduction defects, nerve damage, brain damage.

Grade-level concept: Most vision and hearing disorders can be treated or corrected.

Objective: Lists treatment and corrective procedures for vision and hearing disorders.

Content: (1) vision—corrective lenses, eye exercises, treatment of infections, surgery; (2) hearing—removal of obstructions from outer ear canal, use of hearing aids, treatment of infections, surgery.

Nutrition

Major concept	Primary level	Intermediate level	Junior high level
I Nutrition is important in the everyday functioning of an individual.	**Grade-level concept: Food has a variety of important functions.** *Objective:* Identifies purposes of food. *Content:* (1) for energy; (2) for growth and repair; (3) for enjoyment.	**Grade-level concept: Good dietary practices can help prevent personal health problems.** *Objective:* Summarizes personal health problems that may result from poor dietary practices. *Content:* (1) skin problems; (2) dental problems; (3) fatigue; (4) impaired growth and development; (5) constipation; (6) overweight and underweight.	**Grade-level concept: Nutritional practices contribute to the development of diseases and disorders.** *Objective:* Describes chronic diseases and disorders which may be associated with nutritional practices. *Content:* (1) obesity; (2) underweight; (3) diabetes; (4) cardiovascular disease; (5) acne; (6) allergies; (7) central nervous system disorders; (8) vitamin deficiency disease; (9) dental disorders. *Objective:* Identifies common disorders of the digestive system. *Content:* (1) indigestion; (2) constipation; (3) ulcers; (4) appendicitis; (5) colitis; (6) hemorrhoids. *Objective:* Discusses how nutritional choices and eating habits contribute to diseases and disorders. *Content:* (1) overeating; (2) eating too many sweets; (3) eating too much fat; (4) omitting necessary nutrients.
II Individuals throughout life require the same nutrients but in varying amounts.	**Grade-level concept: Developing a liking for a variety of foods at each meal helps to ensure that needed nutrients are provided.** *Objective:* Classifies foods into four basic food groups. *Content:* (1) milk group; (2) meat group; (3) grain and cereal group; (4) fruits and vegetables. **Grade-level concept: Good breakfasts are as important as any other meal in providing required nutrients.** *Objective:* Tells why good breakfasts are important. *Content:* (1) length of time since evening meal; (2) provides energy for morning activity; (3) contributes to total daily needs. **Grade-level concept: Snacks can contribute to good nutrition.** *Objective:* Identifies nutritious snacks that can supplement regular meals. *Content:* (1) fruits; (2) vegetables; (3) protein foods.	**Grade-level concept: The "four food groups" provide all nutrients needed by the body.** *Objective:* Lists nutrients provided by the four basic food groups. *Content:* (1) carbohydrates; (2) fats; (3) proteins; (4) vitamins; (5) minerals; (6) water. *Objective:* Explains the primary contributions of different nutrients to normal body functioning. *Content:* (1) carbohydrates and fats—supply energy; (2) protein—promoting growth and repair; (3) vitamins and minerals—regulating body functions. **Grade-level concept: The digestive process enables one to utilize food.** *Objective:* Specifies the function of digestion in the utilization of foods. *Content:* (1) converts ingested food to nutrients the body can use; (2) provides for absorption of nutrients from the digestive tract; (3) provides for elimination of body wastes.	**Grade-level concept: Lack of sufficient nutrients can lead to nutritional deficiency diseases.** *Objective:* Relates specific nutritional deficiencies to the diseases they cause. *Content:* (1) vitamin D—rickets; (2) vitamin C—scurvy; (3) iron—anemia; (4) protein—kwashiorkor; (5) iodine—goiter; (6) vitamin A—night blindness.

Main concept	Grade-level concept	
III Food processing and preparation influence the nutritional value and safety of foods.	**Grade-level concept: Foods come from a variety of sources.** *Objective:* Names sources of foods. *Content:* (1) plants; (2) animals; (3) synthetic substances. *Objective:* Tells where food is processed. *Content:* (1) dairy; (2) cannery; (3) bakery; (4) meat-packing plant; (5) frozen food–processing plant; (6) home.	**Grade-level concept: Food values are conserved and enhanced by proper processing and preparation.** *Objective:* Indicates how processing and preparation conserve and enhance food values. *Content:* (1) destroys pathogenic organisms—pasteurization; (2) preserves foods—canning, quick freezing, dry freezing, and dehydrating; (3) restores lost nutrients—using additives. **Grade-level concept: Control of commercial preparation and commercial processing of foods helps to protect consumers.** *Objective:* Specifies federal and state agencies that impose controls on purity and quality of foods. *Content:* (1) the federal Food and Drug Administration; (2) U.S. Department of Agriculture; (3) California State Department of Public Health. *Objective:* Describes control measures to protect consumers. *Content:* (1) setting standards; (2) inspections; (3) testing.
IV Nutrition is a significant factor in weight control.	**Grade-level concept: Eating practices influence one's weight.** *Objective:* Identifies eating practices that can contribute to overweight or underweight. *Content:* (1) eating too much or too little; (2) making poor choices of foods.	**Grade-level concept: Energy balance determines an individual's weight.** *Objective:* Indicates factors that influence energy balance and help to control one's weight. *Content:* (1) caloric values derived from food; (2) calories expended through activities; (3) calories required for normal body processes; (4) illness; (5) body type, or build. **Grade-level concept: Obesity is a social problem as well as an individual problem.** *Objective:* Presents examples of how individual weight problems can affect the individual and society. *Content:* (1) affects self-image; (2) affects relationships with other individuals; (3) contributes to onset of chronic disease; (4) shortens life expectancy.
V Dietary fads and misconceptions can be detrimental to health.	**Grade-level concept: Special foods or supplements are not usually required to meet normal nutritional needs.** *Objective:* Lists reasons why special foods or supplements are not usually required to meet normal nutritional needs. *Content:* (1) regular foods contain essential nutrients; (2) excess of supplements may be harmful; (3) special foods are more expensive.	**Grade-level concept: Individuals who follow the advice of food quacks and food faddists can endanger their health.** *Objective:* Summarizes food fads and misconceptions, particularly the ones listed as follows. *Content:* (1) those concerning the processing of foods; (2) those about soil depletion; (3) those concerning the values of specific foods; (4) those having to do with organic versus inorganic growing practices. *Objective:* Concludes, by identifying some of the resulting problems, that food faddism and food quackery may threaten optimal health. *Content:* (1) individuals may fail to obtain a balanced diet; (2) following a quack's advice may delay necessary treatment of specific disorders.

Exercise, Rest, and Posture

Major concept	Primary level	Intermediate level	Junior high level
I Physical fitness is one important component of total health.	**Grade-level concept: Play that includes physical activity is healthful as well as fun.** *Objective:* Lists the benefits of play and physical activity. *Content:* (1) helps one to get along with others; (2) helps one to feel better; (3) helps one to grow in strength and agility; (4) helps one to sleep more soundly.	**Grade-level concept: Regular physical activity is beneficial to one's body.** *Objective:* Identifies benefits of physical activity to one's body. *Content:* (1) aids in personal appearance; (2) helps to develop strength and coordination; (3) helps to maintain weight control; (4) improves circulation and respiration; (5) improves muscle tone; (6) improves appetite.	**Grade-level concept: Regular physical activity can help reduce the risk of chronic disorders.** *Objective:* Describes ways in which physical activity helps to delay or prevent chronic disorders. *Content:* (1) improved circulation and increased heart strength—against cardiovascular diseases; (2) increased vital capacity—against respiratory diseases; (3) weight control—against obesity.
II A balanced program of exercise and rest contributes to fitness.	**Grade-level concept: Individuals do better in physical activities when they have enough rest and sleep.** *Objective:* Tells how rest and sleep help one to perform physical activity more effectively. *Content:* (1) permits recovery from fatigue; (2) improves alertness; (3) restores vitality; (4) improves efficiency.	**Grade-level concept: A variety of physical activities, along with adequate rest and sleep, contribute to one's fitness.** *Objective:* Summarizes the contributions of a variety of physical activities to physical fitness. *Content:* (1) running—endurance; (2) tumbling—agility; (3) lifting, pushing, pulling—strength; (4) stretching—flexibility. *Objective:* Discusses the effect of physical activity on the need for rest and sleep. *Content:* (1) energy is expended; (2) muscles tire; (3) fatigue products accumulate.	**Grade-level concept: Different degrees of fitness are needed for various activities.** *Objective:* Compares caloric demands for different types of activity. *Content:* (1) running—3.7 cal/lb/hour; (2) ping pong—2.5 cal/lb/hour; (3) walking—1.1 cal/lb/hour. *Objective:* Discusses factors that influence the degree of fitness required for different types of activities. *Content:* (1) amount of physical contact called for; (2) energy demanded; (3) endurance required; (4) agility and coordination needed. **Grade-level concept: Fatigue is influenced by physical, emotional, and environmental conditions.** *Objective:* Summarizes factors that contribute to fatigue. *Content:* (1) physical activity; (2) tension; (3) noise; (4) heat, humidity; (5) disease; (6) inadequate rest and relaxation. *Objective:* Discusses means of preventing and treating fatigue. *Content:* (1) adequate rest periods; (2) adequate caloric intake; (3) change of activity; (4) length of work periods; (5) level of enjoyment of activity; (6) prevention, early detection, and care of disease; (7) control of the environment—noise, heat, humidity.

III Posture affects appearance and body function.	**Grade-level concept: Good posture helps one look and feel better.** *Objective:* Identifies the values of good posture. *Content:* (1) makes one feel better; (2) makes one look better; (3) helps one carry out daily tasks. *Objective:* Demonstrates good posture in a variety of situations. *Content:* (1) standing; (2) sitting; (3) walking; (4) lifting; (5) reclining. **Grade-level concept: A variety of poor health practices contributes to postural defects.** *Objective:* Lists practices that contribute to poor posture. *Content:* (1) improper nutrition; (2) lack of activity; (3) ill-fitting clothing and shoes; (4) poor walking, standing, sitting, and reclining habits.	**Grade-level concept: The development of the skeletal and muscular systems plays a major role in establishing good posture.** *Objective:* Describes how the skeletal and muscular systems affect one's posture. *Content:* (1) the skeleton provides the framework for supporting the soft tissues of the body; (2) the muscles provide strength for support and movement. **Grade-level concept: Correction of postural defects can best be accomplished before one completes one's growth.** *Objective:* Provides reasons for correcting postural defects during the growth period. *Content:* (1) defects are more difficult to correct when growth is completed; (2) early correction prevents complications; (3) early correction helps a person develop a better self-image.	**Grade-level concept: Good body posture contributes to effective functioning.** *Objective:* Describes how good posture contributes to effective functioning. *Content:* (1) increases efficiency of movement; (2) lessens fatigue; (3) improves circulation and respiration; (4) assists the functioning of internal organs; (5) decreases the danger of later chronic disorders; (6) affects mental outlook and vice versa.

Diseases and Disorders

Major concept	Primary level	Intermediate level	Junior high level
I The occurrence and distribution of diseases and disorders are affected by one's heredity and environment.	**Grade-level concept: Children are susceptible to a variety of diseases and disorders.** *Objective:* Describes common childhood diseases and disorders. *Content:* (1) communicable disease; (2) vision and hearing disorders; (3) orthopedic problems. *Objective:* Identifies factors contributing to diseases and disorders. *Content:* (1) lack of sanitation; (2) individual susceptibility; (3) heredity; (4) exposure; (5) poor nutrition.	**Grade-level concept: Through the years people have been faced with a variety of diseases and disorders.** *Objective:* Interprets how diseases affecting humans have changed over the years. *Content:* (1) prevalence of various diseases and disorders over the years; (2) changing emphasis from communicable disease to chronic disease; (3) increase of mental and emotional disorders. **Grade-level concept: Communicable diseases are caused by microorganisms.** *Objective:* Identifies the role of microorganisms as the cause of communicable disease. *Content:* (1) nature of microorganisms; (2) factors influencing their growth; (3) how they cause disease. *Objective:* Traces the process of infectious disease. *Content:* (1) source; (2) transmission; (3) susceptible host. **Grade-level concept: Many factors contribute to chronic disorders.** *Objective:* Summarizes factors contributing to chronic disorders. *Content:* (1) hereditary factors and predisposition to disease; (2) environmental factors (contamination of environment, overexposure); (3) health status of individual (physical and mental); (4) communicable disease; (5) accidents.	**Grade-level concept: Even though most communicable disease rates have been decreasing, infectious diseases are still serious threats.** *Objective:* Portrays graphically changes in the incidence of selected communicable diseases. *Content:* (1) measles; (2) poliomyelitis; (3) diphtheria; (4) smallpox; (5) venereal disease. *Objective:* Describes the causes and effects of certain major communicable diseases that are still threats. *Content:* (1) bacterial (venereal disease, tuberculosis, streptococcus infection); (2) viral (influenza, hepatitis, colds); (3) fungi (athlete's foot, ringworm); (4) protozoa (dysenteries, malaria); (5) parasitic (worm infestations). *Objective:* States reasons why communicable diseases are still threats. *Content:* (1) increased international travel; (2) increased population; (3) disregard for sanitary procedures; (4) failure to be immunized. **Grade-level concept: Chronic disorders are increasing as threats.** *Objective:* Identifies the major chronic disorders and their incidence among various age groups. *Content:* (1) cardiac and circulatory diseases; (2) cancer; (3) diabetes; (4) mental illness; (5) allergies; (6) orthopedic defects; (7) vision and hearing impairment; (8) neurological disorders; (9) dental disorders.
II Diseases and disorders have both a personal and an economic effect on individuals and society.	**Grade-level concept: Diseases and disorders influence the way one feels and acts.** *Objective:* Lists ways in which diseases influence one's feelings and actions. *Content:* (1) getting along with others; (2) missing school; (3) restricting play activities; (4) leading to additional and future health problems; (5) disrupting family routine.	**Grade-level concept: Diseases and disorders can have immediate and long-range effects on individuals.** *Objective:* Identifies immediate and long-range effects of disease and disorders. *Content:* (1) immediate (effects on body system and ability to perform academically and physically); (2) long-range (longevity and productivity as parent and as worker).	**Grade-level concept: Communicable diseases affect both the individual and society.** *Objective:* Summarizes effects of venereal diseases on the individual and on the community. *Content:* (1) interpersonal relations; (2) family relationships; (3) cost of diagnosis and treatment; (4) loss of work hours; (5) possibility of chronic disease.

Grade-level concept: Children can help handicapped individuals to feel accepted.

Objective: Tells how a child can help a child who is handicapped to feel accepted.

Content: (1) being friendly; (2) inviting child to play; (3) avoiding making fun of anyone who is handicapped.

Grade-level concept: The course of history has been changed by disease.

Objective: Reports how diseases have influenced history.

Content: (1) effects of epidemics (outcomes of wars, of population growth, of the productivity of people); (2) delay of progress (yellow fever in Panama Canal region, malaria in tropical countries, premature deaths of leaders as a result of chronic disease).

Objective: Identifies prevalent communicable diseases that affect the individual and society.

Content: (1) tuberculosis; (2) common cold; (3) influenza; (4) skin diseases; (5) infectious hepatitis; (6) mononucleosis; (7) venereal diseases.

Grade-level concept: Chronic disorders affect individuals of all age groups.

Objective: Describes chronic disorders that affect the school-age child.

Content: (1) allergies; (2) congenital disorders; (3) skin disorders (acne); (4) epilepsy; (5) emotional disorders; (6) dental caries.

Grade-level concept: Individuals can adjust to handicaps and contribute to society.

Objective: Cites examples of individuals who contribute to society despite their handicaps.

Content: (1) Helen Keller—blind, deaf, dumb; (2) Beethoven—deaf; (3) Franklin D. Roosevelt—crippled by poliomyelitis.

III There is variation in the extent to which diseases and disorders can be prevented and controlled.

Grade-level concept: Children can take personal action to prevent or control diseases and disorders.

Objective: Describes how one prevents or controls diseases and disorders through individual actions.

Content: (1) maintaining personal cleanliness; (2) keeping the environment clean; (3) staying home when ill; (4) receiving protective immunization; (5) following the advice of parents and doctors; (6) following the health practices of proper nutrition, exercise, and rest; (7) wearing corrective devices when needed.

Grade-level concept: The control of diseases and disorders depends on a combination of medical advances and individual action.

Objective: Discusses contributions that have been made to protect individuals from diseases and disorders.

Content: (1) immunizations; (2) modern sanitation; (3) chemotherapy; (4) radiation; (5) surgery; (6) prosthetics.

Objective: Identifies actions that should be taken by an individual to support medical advances that help protect people from diseases and disorders.

Content: (1) reporting illness; (2) improving health practices; (3) understanding risk factors.

Grade-level concept: Many diseases and disorders that are primary threats to youth can be effectively prevented and controlled.

Objective: Illustrates how specific diseases and disorders can be effectively prevented and controlled.

Content: (1) diagnosis; (2) case finding; (3) early detection; (4) prompt medical treatment; (5) sanitation and environmental controls; (6) immunizations.

Objective: Discusses the importance of early diagnosis and treatment.

Content: (1) remove the abnormal tissue before it spreads; (2) destroy microorganisms; (3) restore normal function of vital organs; (4) restore chemical balance in the body (e.g., insulin).

Environmental Health Hazards

Major concept	Primary level	Intermediate level	Junior high level
I An individual's environment, including aesthetic characteristics, influences his or her total health.	**Grade-level concept: One's surroundings affect one's total health.** *Objective:* Discusses factors in one's surroundings that influence human health. *Content:* (1) cleanliness; (2) orderliness; (3) attractiveness; (4) climate.	**Grade-level concept: A clean, safe environment is healthful and can be enjoyed.** *Objective:* Describes the value of a clean, healthful environment. *Content:* (1) provides clean air and water; (2) prevents accidents; (3) helps to develop pride in the environment. *Objective:* Discusses the relationship between the environment and how one feels. *Content:* (1) the peacefulness that is characteristic of a natural setting; (2) contentment with a well-kept home and neighborhood.	**Grade-level concept: Conservation of the nation's resources protects the total health of its citizens.** *Objective:* Identifies resources which should be conserved to protect health. *Content:* (1) recreational areas; (2) sources of food and water; (3) air.
II There are ever-changing health hazards in one's environment.		**Grade-level concept: New discoveries and inventions create hazards in the environment.** *Objective:* Summarizes the results of new discoveries and inventions. *Content:* (1) air pollution and the automobile; (2) water and soil pollution and burgeoning technology; (3) noise and industry; (4) ionizing radiation and nuclear advances; (5) contamination and space exploration.	**Grade-level concept: The environment can detract from one's health.** *Objective:* Summarizes selected hazards that detract from a healthy environment. *Content:* (1) polluted air, water, and soil; (2) excessive noise; (3) pesticides; (4) misuse of antibiotics; (5) other chemicals and radiation. *Objective:* Reports on the physiological effects of environmental health hazards. *Content:* (1) cardiovascular; (2) respiratory; (3) intestinal; (4) neurological; (5) genetic.
III The potential for accidents exists everywhere in the environment.	**Grade-level concept: Hazards may be reduced but not always completely eliminated.** *Objective:* Identifies potential hazards in the environment and lists possible ways of reducing these hazards. *Content:* (1) at home; (2) at school; (3) going to and from school; (4) at play; (5) in handling animals; (6) using tools and appliances.	**Grade-level concept: Environmental conditions in the community can be safe or unsafe.** *Objective:* Explains practices that reduce the potential for accidents. *Content:* (1) pedestrian safety; (2) bicycle safety; (3) fire safety; (4) home safety; (5) recreational safety, such as camping, hunting, boating, and swimming.	**Grade-level concept: Accidents are caused—they don't just happen.** *Objective:* Lists those accidents most likely to occur to the junior high school student and how they can be prevented. *Content:* (1) while riding bikes or motorbikes; (2) while using shop equipment; (3) while participating in recreational activities. *Objective:* Interprets the interrelationships of factors that cause accidents. *Content:* (1) human behavior; (2) equipment; (3) physical environment.

Concept	Grade-level concepts		
IV Individuals should be prepared to act effectively in case of accidents.	**Grade-level concept: All injuries should be cared for immediately.** *Objective:* Explains why immediate care of injuries is important. *Content:* (1) prevents infection; (2) prevents further infection; (3) saves lives. *Objective:* Tells about the care that should be provided for simple injuries. *Content:* (1) washing minor wounds; (2) applying band-aids to protect minor wounds; (3) giving support to injured joints. *Objective:* Indicates those persons who should provide care for the injured. *Content:* (1) physicians; (2) nurses; (3) qualified first aid personnel.	**Grade-level concept: Understanding first aid procedures helps one to act quickly and correctly in emergencies.** *Objective:* Traces sequence of steps in providing first aid for the injured. *Content:* (1) administer urgently needed first aid; (2) keep injured persons comfortable; (3) call or send for help.	**Grade-level concept: Prompt care that is given in emergencies can save lives and prevent further injury.** *Objective:* Demonstrates the basic skills of emergency first aid care. *Content:* (1) controlling bleeding; (2) restoring breathing; (3) administering first aid in the case of poisoning. *Objective:* Discusses methods of avoiding further injury. *Content:* (1) securing proper transportation; (2) obtaining competent medical care.
V Maintaining a healthful, safe environment is the responsibility of the individual, the family, and society.	**Grade-level concept: Children, as well as adults, have responsibilities for maintaining a healthful, safe environment.** *Objective:* Describes an individual's responsibility for maintaining a healthful, safe environment. *Content:* (1) keeping the premises clean and free from litter; (2) keeping belongings out of the way to prevent injuries; (3) refraining from playing with matches, medicines, and poisons; (4) reporting unsafe conditions at home and at school.	**Grade-level concept: Healthful, safe recreational areas enhance the enjoyment of the environment.** *Objective:* Presents examples that show how recreation areas can be made safe and enjoyable. *Content:* (1) keeping lakes and streams pure; (2) preventing forest fires; (3) protecting natural resources; (4) maintaining campsites.	**Grade-level concept: Community control activities protect the health and safety of individuals.** *Objective:* Describes the responsibilities of the individual and those of governmental agencies regarding their roles in health and safety. *Content:* (1) control of air, water, and soil pollution; (2) reduction of noise; (3) control of the use of pesticides and other chemicals; (4) fluoridation of water supplies. **Grade-level concept: Safety procedures are valuable only if they are used.** *Objective:* Explains the responsible use of safety equipment and the sound application of safety procedures. *Content:* (1) motor vehicle (using seat belts and auto accessories; observing traffic laws); (2) industry (using safety goggles, protective devices, safety guards; following safety regulations); (3) recreation (knowing correct firearm usage); (4) home (using power equipment, storing inflammable materials and poisons, handling garden supplies).

Community Health Resources

Major concept	Primary level	Intermediate level	Junior high level
I Utilization of community health resources benefits the health of the individual and the community.	**Grade-level concept: Children, as well as adults, can use community health services.** *Objective:* Identifies and describes community health resources that affect health. *Content:* (1) fire department; (2) police department; (3) school nurse; (4) physician; (5) dentist; (6) hospital; (7) health department. *Objective:* Tells how to obtain help from selected community resources. *Content:* (1) telephoning for help; (2) asking school personnel; (3) asking parents and other adults.	**Grade-level concept: Utilizing the services of the health department promotes good health.** *Objective:* Identifies services offered by the health department. *Content:* (1) immunization; (2) maternal and child health; (3) morbidity and mortality statistics; (4) environmental inspections; (5) health education. *Objective:* Explains how using services offered by the health department can be beneficial. *Content:* (1) preventing disease; (2) protecting the health of parent and child; (3) protecting food and water; (4) providing health information.	**Grade-level concept: Community health agencies make their greatest contribution when citizens take advantage of available services.** *Objective:* Identifies various community health agencies and their sources of financial support. *Content:* (1) governmental—taxes; (2) voluntary—contributions; (3) professional—dues; (4) commercial—profits. *Objective:* Classifies services offered by community health agencies and the value of these services when utilized. *Content:* (1) education—offering the help of resource persons and materials; (2) research—solving community health problems; (3) service—preventing disease.
II The health of the community is a shared responsibility of the individual and the community.	**Grade-level concept: Cooperating with local health helpers protects an individual and his or her family.** *Objective:* Tells how one can cooperate with police officers, fire fighters, the school nurse, physicians, and dentists. *Content:* (1) obeys laws; (2) reports fires and fire hazards; (3) follows instructions. *Objective:* Explains how cooperation affects the individual and the community. *Content:* (1) being immunized and staying home when sick are ways of protecting oneself and others; (2) keeping the home and the community clean helps to prevent disease; (3) following rules and regulations helps to prevent accidents.	**Grade-level concept: Supporting health department regulations is one way of promoting individual and community health.** *Objective:* Cites examples of laws and regulations affecting the health of the community (local, state, national). *Content:* (1) pet control laws; (2) sanitation regulations; (3) insect control laws; (4) restaurant inspections. *Objective:* Summarizes factors that influence the effectiveness of health regulations. *Content:* (1) knowing health regulations; (2) following health regulations; (3) encouraging others to follow health regulations; (4) reporting violations of laws and regulations involving health and sanitation.	**Grade-level concept: Maintaining community health depends on each citizen's cooperating with and supporting local and state health agencies.** *Objective:* Cites ways in which the student can serve agencies, hospitals, schools, and other health organizations. *Content:* (1) engaging in volunteer service as nursing and clerical aides; (2) serving on school safety committees; (3) helping to conduct health surveys.

III Nations need to cooperate with one another to identify and solve international health problems.	**Grade-level concept: Cooperative efforts within the World Health Organization help to improve international health.** *Objective:* States examples of services offered by the World Health Organization to individual nations. *Content:* (1) provides publications; (2) reports on communicable diseases; (3) provides direct services to control disease. *Objective:* Explains why cooperative efforts to solve world health problems are necessary. *Content:* (1) communicable diseases can spread from country to country; (2) developing countries need outside assistance; (3) health problems of one country can affect other countries.	**Grade-level concept: United States agencies extend help to other countries in solving their health problems.** *Objective:* Identifies specific agencies and the help they provide to other countries. *Content:* (1) U.S. Public Health Service—medical care and information; (2) CARE—food and clothing; (3) AID—communicable disease control and education; (4) Peace Corps—improvement of environmental conditions.
IV A variety of opportunities exist for careers in the health sciences.	**Grade-level concept: Through careers in health science, individuals have contributed to humanity for many years.** *Objective:* Identifies health workers who have made major contributions to society. *Content:* (1) Pasteur—germ theory; (2) Reed—pioneering efforts against yellow fever; (3) Lister—antiseptic conditions; (4) Curie—radium; (5) Roentgen—X ray; (6) Fleming—penicillin; (7) Salk—polio immunization; (8) Nightingale—nursing.	**Grade-level concept: Health science personnel are required to meet the needs of a growing population.** *Objective:* Compares and contrasts career opportunities in health sciences. *Content:* (1) medicine; (2) dentistry; (3) nursing; (4) public health; (5) health education; (6) other paramedical and paradental fields.

REVIEW QUESTIONS

1. Cite several reasons why health education should be included in the elementary education curriculum. Substantiate your support with documentation.

2. Differentiate among correlation, integration, and direct instruction. Cite the strengths and weaknesses of each.

3. Outline the history of the School Health Education Study and discuss the relevant findings of the study.

4. Discuss the formulation and implementation of the Framework for Health Instruction in California Public Schools. Cite the ten content areas included in the curriculum.

REFERENCES AND BIBLIOGRAPHY

Anderson, C. L. *School Health Practice* (St. Louis: C. V. Mosby, 1968).

Cornacchia, Harold J., Wesley M. Staton, and Leslie W. Irwin. *Health in Elementary Schools* (St. Louis: C. V. Mosby, 1970).

Fenton, Edwin. *The New Social Studies* (New York: Holt, Rinehart and Winston, 1967).

Fodor, John T., and Gus T. Dalis. *Health Instruction: Theory and Application* (Philadelphia: Lea and Febiger, 1966).

Framework for Health Instruction in California Public Schools (Sacramento: California State Department of Education, 1970).

Haag, Jessie Helen. *School Health Program* (New York: Holt, Rinehart and Winston, 1965).

Kilander, H. Frederick. *School Health Education* (New York: Macmillan, 1968).

Michaelis, John U., Ruth H. Grossman, and Floyd F. Scott. *New Designs for the Elementary School Curriculum* (New York: McGraw-Hill, 1967).

NEA-AMA. *Healthful School Living* (Washington, D.C.: National Education Association of the United States, 1957).

_____. *Health Education* (Washington, D.C.: National Education Association of the United States, 1961).

_____. *School Health Services* (Washington, D.C.: National Education Association of the United States, 1964).

Oberteuffer, Delbert, Orvis A. Harrelson, and Marion B. Pollock. *School Health Education* (New York: Harper & Row, 1972).

Rash, J. Keogh. *The Health Education Curriculum* (Bloomington: Indiana University Press, 1966).

School Health Education Study: A Summary Report. (Washington, D.C.: School Health Education Study, 1964).

School Health Education Study. *Health Education: A Conceptual Approach to Curriculum Design* (St. Paul, Minn.: 3M Education Press, 1967).

School Health Education Study: Education Age (St. Paul, Minn.: 3M Education Press, January-February, 1968).

Sorochan, Walter D. "Health Instruction—Why Do We Need It in the 70's?" *Journal of School Health* (April 1971): 209-214.

Willgoose, Carl E. *Health Education in the Elementary School* (Philadelphia: Saunders, 1974).

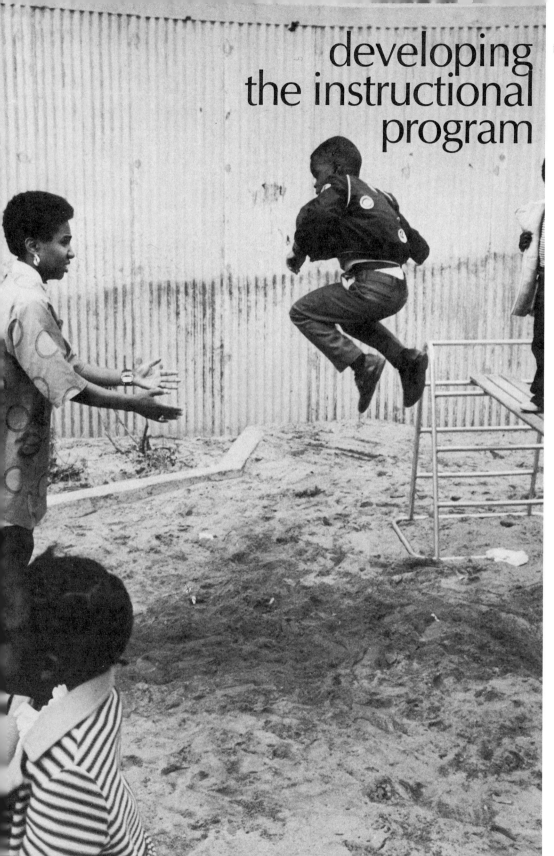

developing
the instructional
program

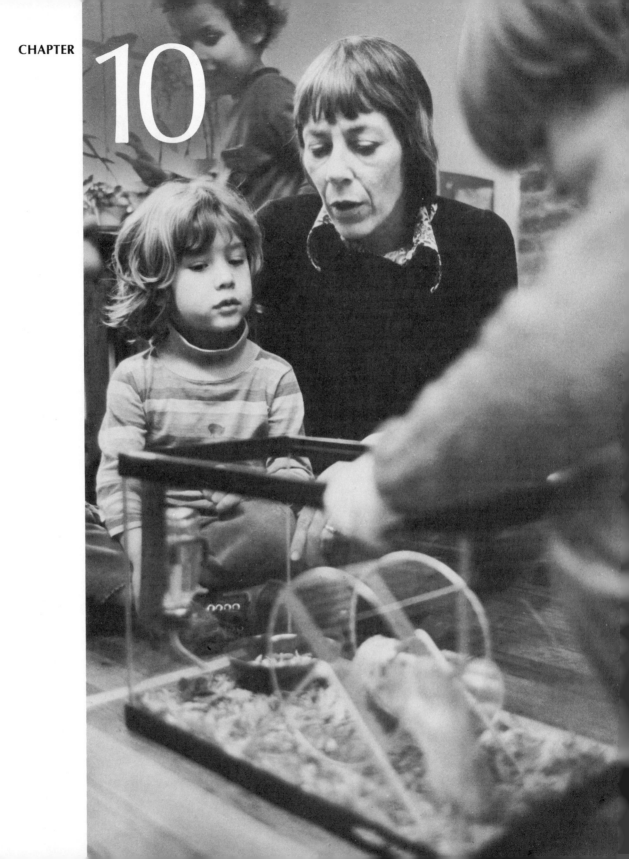

a conceptual approach to elementary health instruction

INTRODUCTION

Like the gills of a trout, the sensory organs extract from the flow of daily experience the mental "oxygen" from which the brain can make its concepts and create the intellectual life. The brain, however, cannot think without sensory data. Conversely, the senses cannot receive preconstructed concepts; they can only accept sensory impressions from the actual referent of our concepts. There is no way into the brain except through the senses. Hence, the teacher must feed sensory impressions to the students, and then coach them through discussion as the students (not the teacher) turn the sensory data into concepts through their own mental processes. *

Traditional teaching of the past has often consisted of the implementing and memorizing of facts by passive children. Often these facts were unrelated to one another or to the child's personal well-being. Teachers emphasized the provision of health information, assuming that once in possession of the necessary facts, children would take intelligent action. Unfortunately, the assumption is not very

---

* Asahel D. Woodruff, *The Psychology of Teaching*, New York: Longmans, Green, 1951, p. 69. Reprinted by permission of the David McKay Company, Inc.

valid today. One has only to reflect on the misuse of drugs by teenagers and adults or the nutritional malpractices by both groups to realize that the mere provision of facts has not resulted in the application of these facts and the accompanying establishment of better health.

It has only been since 1960 that health educators have turned to the concept approach in an attempt to structure or modify personal health habits and public health practices. Among such approaches have been the School Health Education Study-3M project entitled *Health Education: A Conceptual Approach to Curriculum Design* (1967), the American Association for Health, Physical Education and Recreation publication *Health Concepts: Guides for Health Instruction* (1967), the National Dairy Council's *Big Ideas in Nutrition Education and How to Teach Them—Grades K-6* (1970), the American Home Economics Association's national project *Concepts and Generalizations* (1970), and numerous state curriculum guides, such as the *Framework for Health Instruction in California Public Schools* (1970).

Under such an approach, the child should arrive at his or her own health concepts through an active thinking process. The concepts become internalized; hence they become meaningful, and the child restructures his or her thinking, feelings and values, and habits, thereby modifying or changing his or her behavior(s). The foundation for the conceptual approach to health instruction has been devised in part from the content and the beliefs of the preceding chapters. The concept of well-being presented in Chapter 1 structures the basic values and meanings that health can have for the child today as well as when she or he matures into an adult. Chapter 4 makes us aware that maturation provides a state of readiness to understand. Before understanding can develop, the child's brain and nervous system must develop, and the sense organs—used for perceiving—must become functionally mature. Physical growth and development set the pace for socioemotional maturity, which in turn paces the intellectual and conceptual development of the whole child.

Definition of Concept

Just what is a concept? There is little agreement as to what a concept really is, although there is general agreement that concept formation is desirable in transmitting health information to children and also in providing the means for understanding such information. More important, concepts may even be used to mediate and/or reinforce desirable habits and behaviors.

One of the problems stifling such educational approaches is the confusion surrounding use of the term "concept." In literature dealing with teaching in general, one can find the terms concept, conceptual scheme, theme, organizational thread, major generalization, major concept, minor concepts, subconcepts, fundamental or key idea, big ideas, and major principles used synonymously. "Concept" provokes further anguish when the elementary teacher discovers that each learner evolves his or her own concepts. It is with these ambiguities in mind that we move toward further clarification.

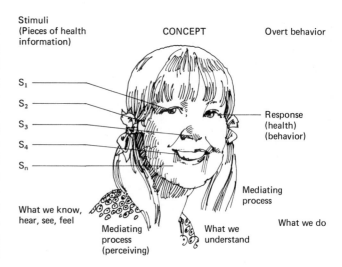

Fig. 10.1 A simple behavioral process, showing the mediating linkage among stimuli, concept, and behavior.

A concept is a person's mental image of an object or event. Woodruff (1951, p. 84) defines concept as "some amount of meaning more or less organized in an individual mind as a result of sensory perception of external objects or events and the cognitive interpretation of the perceived data. *It is a relatively complete and meaningful idea in the mind of a person.* It is an understanding of something. It is his own subjective product of his way of making meaning of things he has seen or otherwise perceived in his experience." The School Health Education Study (1967, p. 6) reinforces this definition by viewing concepts as "the summarizers of experience; they are inventions of the mind to explain or group certain categories of perception. Concepts are mental configurations invented to impose order on an endlessly variable environment and to make adequate responses to events a possibility." Concepts result when the learner relates the facts and information to himself or herself and makes them meaningful. An effort to illustrate such a process is presented in Figs. 10.1 and 10.2. This implies that

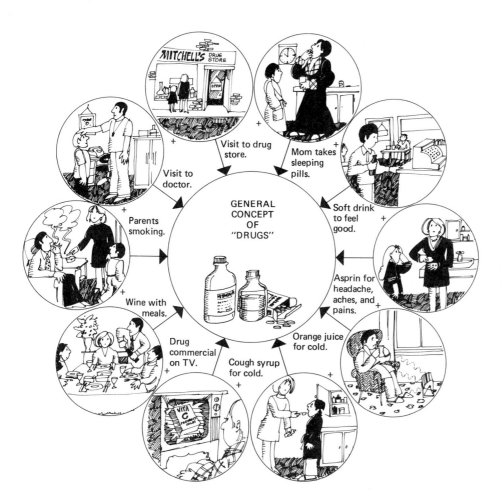

Fig. 10.2 A big idea, or concept, evolves from perceived stimuli.

there are different levels of concepts, with each level relevant to a specific maturational (age) stage. The meaning of ''concept'' will become clearer by understanding the process of concept formation.

Value of Concepts

Concepts result when a child understands. Health behavior, in turn, is influenced by the child's con-cepts of well-being. The type of adjustment the child makes to life is greatly influenced by his or her understanding of the environment, other people, and self. For example, the child who understands the danger of automobiles will be more cautious and careful in crossing a street than a child who lacks such an understanding. One of the greatest values of understanding well-being is that it enables a child to adapt to changes, both personal and environmental. Managing and controlling a developing and changing body is another such example. The child who understands these changes and why they occur will react with less fear, anxiety, or resentment than the child who does not understand.

The child's "own" concepts are important because she or he is better able to think positively about self and others, as well as to control his or her feelings. The child's concepts are important because they determine to a large extent what he or she does. The more health concepts a child has, the better developed and the more accurate they will be, and the greater the child's understanding will become.

The conceptual approach to health instruction is based on the premise and hope that it will allow children to better relate health information to themselves and to their environment, thereby making such information more meaningful. Once information becomes meaningful, it may then be used by children to guide them in everyday life experiences.

Concepts as Mediators of Behavior

Concepts are mediators of what we do. Consider Figs. 10.1 and 10.2 as a way of understanding this idea (see Bourne, 1966, p. 31). The child interprets the numerous pieces of health information or stimuli (S_1-S_n) by synthesizing, organizing, and classifying the information. Eventually the commonness of all the stimuli are perceived, and a big idea, or concept, emerges. The sudden revelation, in turn, provides the motivation for a new behavioral response. The concept is the mediator of a subsequent behavior, just as the stimuli were mediators of the concept itself. It is the link between the desired health behavior and the fragmented pieces of health information and observations. Concepts as mediators are building blocks from which higher abstract concepts evolve and which in turn augment behavior.

The teacher's task is to provide learning experiences so that the child will perceive the concept for himself or herself.

FORMING CONCEPTS

Concepts may be formulated from the way human beings behave. Facts, when synthesized, may be grouped to suggest at least three distinguishable ways of forming new concepts: (1) perceiving a common characteristic from numerous variable phenomena; (2) combining old concepts or grafting new ones onto old ones; and (3) inferring underlying states or constructs from observations and experiences (Brookbeck, 1965). Analysis of what is involved in each case may throw some light on the subtle and devious process by which concepts are formed.

When the numerous variable phenomena have similar structures, or interpret similar behavior among individuals, or relate a unique relationship between individuals, or have a similarity of function or organization, a common characteristic may be perceived. The newly derived concept is more abstract than the variable data suggesting it. For example, the various functions of the pituitary gland are summarized by the concept: "The pituitary gland is the master gland in the body" (see Fig. 10.3).

New concepts may also be formed by combining those concepts already at hand. For example, by speculating that two or more variables act jointly, a child therefore forms a new concept out of them. For example, a concept on nutrition: "Eating a balanced diet regularly keeps us healthy," and a concept on stress: "Emotional stress causes many disorders," may be used as cues and synthesized to evolve a new concept: "Well-being is enhanced by right style of living." The new concept is valid, since it operates according to sociocultural and physiological laws, has universal application, and is significant for well-being. However, most children will obviously need more than two concepts, or big ideas, as cues to evolve a new or major concept.

The third way of evolving new concepts is to infer underlying states or constructs. From our observations we frequently make inferences to some-

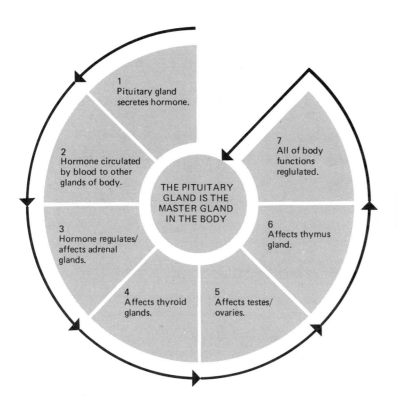

1
Pituitary gland
secretes hormone.

2
Hormone circulated
by blood to other
glands of body.

THE PITUITARY
GLAND IS THE
MASTER GLAND
IN THE BODY

7
All of body
functions
reglulated.

3
Hormone regulates/
affects adrenal
glands.

6
Affects thymus
gland.

4
Affects thyroid
glands.

5
Affects testes/
ovaries.

Fig. 10.3 Illustration showing how a major concept may be evolved from supporting information.

thing not observed (see Fig. 10.4). In order to help explain certain manifest behavior, the teacher or child may formulate concepts that name unobserved states of an organism to which a type of behavior can be associated. For example, children might rush into the classroom from recess, with the teacher forming a concept by remarking: "You behaved like a herd of buffalo." The children's behavior is inferred from an indirect movie or television experience, with which everyone in this culture is familiar, but which no one has directly observed. Such a concept is referred to as a construct.

There are other theories (see Bourne, 1965; Pulaski and Pulaski, 1971; Selberg, Neal, and Vessel, 1970; Woodruff, 1951) of how concepts are formed and categorized. Most of these suggest a developmental sequence, arguing that conceptual behavior is based on a sequential decision-making activity in which later decisions are contingent on earlier ones. The diversity of theories suggests that there is no agreement on how such a process evolves internally. More research is needed in this area.

The internal application of concepts as mediators of behavior seems a rational approach to exploring concept formation. Such an approach has merit for elementary school teachers, in that the main emphasis is to evolve constructive

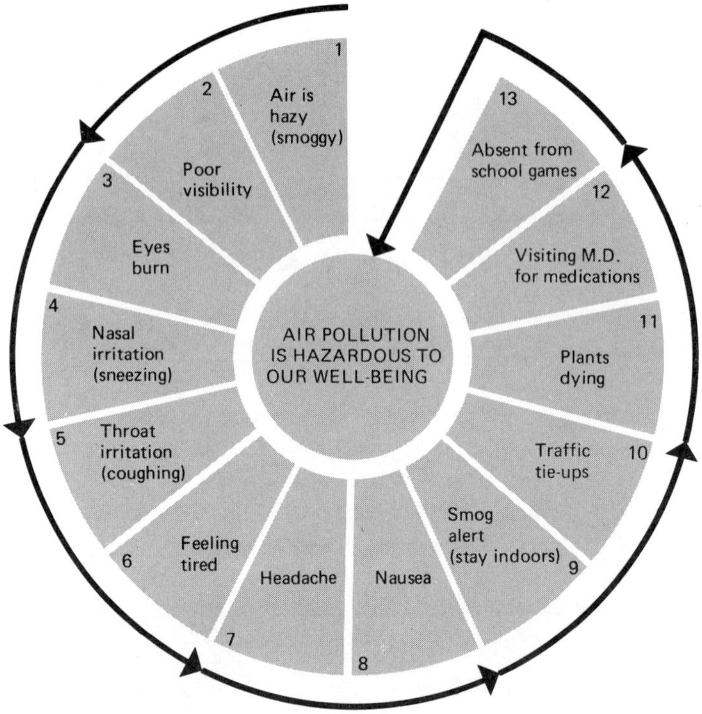

Fig. 10.4 A series of perceptive experiences may contribute to the building of a key concept. At each progressive step of the sensory experiences (planned and incidental), the child evolves emotional responses, which in turn help him or her to generalize more and more about air pollution.

sociohygienic habits. New concepts evolved by teachers and children may be formed by one or more of the suggested ways.

Criteria of Good Concepts

Related to the general definition of concept are criteria for identifying a good concept. Brookbeck (1965), Gage (1965), and Phenix (1964) suggest that a good concept may be identified as:

1. A generalized summary statement about pieces of content or information;

2. An abstract idea of what the detailed and specific content is all about;

3. Representing meanings of an object or an event;

4. Representing a class (body systems), a process (well-being), or a property (height) expressed by a symbol (inches);

5. Reflecting or supporting a basic theory or law (that explains behavior, cause, and effect);

6. Defined in terms of observable individuals;

7. Specifying what is the same in different individuals;

8. Generalizing about time;

9. Valid if it yields successful predictions or outcomes;

10. Implicating desirable behavior, ability, or skill;

11. Reworded or organized at various levels of complexity (complexity of concepts increases with age and experience);

12. Always symbolized and easily evolved from pictorial material;

13. Moving from specific to general, from simple to complex, and from concrete to abstract.

The criteria above are abstract. They help to clarify what good concepts should represent and how such concepts should be structured. Unfortunately, many of the initial concepts evolved by children are too simple and may not meet these criteria. Teachers should keep in mind that children's concepts differ from those of adults more in degree than in kind. For example, children's concepts: are more personalized; change with age; and move from simple to complex, from concrete to abstract, from discrete to organized, from egocentric to more "social" as new meanings are associated with old ones to become part of a system of ideas. Concepts are cumulative for children. In addition to these characteristics, children's concepts are emotionally weighted. Teachers' concepts may have similar characteristics to those of children, but will be on a higher abstract level. Elementary teachers should regard the criteria as general guides to help them in evolving lesson-plan concepts. The application of such guides is presented in the next section.

Steps in Forming Concepts

Prospective teachers are no different from their pupils in evolving concepts. The secret of this process of concept formation lies in understanding the definition of the term "concept." Since a concept is a big idea, or generalization, it may be thought of as a summary about a number of facts. Everyone can form concepts, but not everyone can form good concepts. The basis for this observation lies in the process of development. Children and adults at different stages of development and maturity will vary in the kinds of concepts they evolve about a topic. Teachers should have some expertise in this process if they are going to be able to develop and teach a concept lesson plan.

Teachers need to develop an awareness of the following essentials of forming worthwhile concepts:

1. A basic belief in the fact that optimal well-being is a vehicle to accomplish and therefore is a prerequisite to more abundant living;

2. Familiarity with the criteria for identifying good concepts;

3. Familiarity with the different kinds of concepts;

4. Familiarity with the purpose and function of concepts;

5. Familiarity with the subject matter about which concepts are to be formed;

6. Familiarity with the semantic structural components of a good concept.

The criteria for identifying good concepts, the different kinds of concepts, and the purpose of concepts have already been discussed. Having a rich knowledge of the content is a prerequisite to forming good concepts. A teacher cannot teach something she or he knows nothing about, much less evolve concepts. The more the teacher knows, the easier it will be to evolve concepts. Lack of familiarity with subject matter tends to stifle the formation of teacher-evolved concepts. Often an alert teacher will discover a concept from the readings on the topic. Good writers often begin a paragraph with an introductory statement that provides clues for the reader about the remainder of the paragraph. Likewise, writers will often end the paragraph with a statement summarizing the contents of the paragraph. Teachers should become aware of paragraph structure and be "looking" for potential concepts at the beginning and end of a paragraph. Locating concepts in this manner has limitations, however, because someone else's concept may not be meaningful for the teacher. Therefore, teachers should be receptive to rephrasing, in their own words, someone else's concepts. Only then will someone else's concept have meaning to the prospective teacher. But the secret to evolving relevant concepts is possessing a large body of knowledge as background. Although concepts may be stated by someone else, they need to be discovered by the teacher as a learner. Concepts learned from books tend to be superficial. On the other hand, concepts discovered through enriched learning experiences tend to be more meaningful and self-directing. These observations also hold true for children.

The remaining prerequisite to forming sound concepts is familiarity with the semantic structural components of a concept. A good concept has at least three identifiable parts:

1. A *main theme*, such as air pollution or cigarette smoking.
2. A phrase suggesting, specifying, or implying a certain kind of behavior or *consequence*, e.g., hazardous.
3. A statement of *future ramifications* made by stating the expected outcome and/or by designating persons or things, e.g., to one's well-being.

For example, consider the following concept: Cigarette smoking is hazardous to one's well-being. We can divide this concept into its structural components as follows:

1. *Main theme*—"cigarette smoking";
2. *Consequence*—"is hazardous";
3. *Future ramifications*—to one's well-being.

The three semantic parts of a concept should be stated simply and in as few words as possible. The shorter the "word" length of a concept, the better. As a rule of thumb, a concept sentence should not be longer than 10 to 12 words. Concepts longer than this tend to be splattered and are confusing for the

elementary child. Both a child and a teacher may forget the main theme when they get to the end of a "long-winded" concept. If the concept is to communicate understanding and act as a mediator of health behavior, it must be short, concise, abstract, and simple. Only then do words, as concepts, begin to have power as mediators.

Competence in forming sound, relevant, and worthwhile concepts accrues from practice. The mastery of such a skill may be reinforced in teacher training institutions by college professors providing learning opportunities for prospective teachers to evolve concepts. Such competence is essential to planning lessons.

REVIEW QUESTIONS

1. Define the term "concept."
2. How can concepts be helpful to the instructional process?
3. What criteria make up a good concept?
4. How long should a concept be?
5. How do children's concepts differ from those of a teacher?
6. What are the structural components of a concept?
7. Quote several acceptable health-related concepts.

REFERENCES AND BIBLIOGRAPHY

Big Ideas in Nutrition Education and How to Teach Them: Grades K-6 (Los Angeles: Dairy Council of California, 1970).

Bourne, Lyle E., Jr. *Human Conceptual Behavior* (Boston: Allyn and Bacon, 1966).

Brookbeck, May. "Logic and Scientific Method on Teaching," in *Handbook of Research on Teaching*, ed.

N. L. Gage. (Chicago: Rand McNally, 1965), pp. 44-93.

Concepts and Generalizations: Their Place in High School Home Economics Curriculum Development (Washington, D.C.: American Home Economics Association, 1967).

Framework for Health Instruction in California Public Schools (Sacramento: California State Department of Education, 1970).

Gage, N. L. *Handbook of Research on Teaching* (Chicago: Rand McNally, 1965), pp. 48-72, 884-887.

Health Concepts: Guides for Health Instruction (Washington, D.C.: American Association for Health, Physical Education and Recreation, 1967).

Hurlock, Elizabeth B. *Child Development* (New York: McGraw-Hill, 1964).

Inhelder, Barbel, and Jean Piaget. *The Growth of Logical Thinking* (New York: Basic Books, 1959).

Klausmeier, Herbert J., and Chester W. Harris, eds. *Analyses of Concept Learning* (New York: Academic Press, 1966).

Komisar, Paul B., and C. J. B. MacMillan. *Psychological Concepts in Education* (Chicago: Rand McNally, 1967).

This Is Marshall McLuhan, Part I (film) (New York: McGraw-Hill, 1967).

Phenix, Philip H. *Realms of Meaning* (New York: McGraw-Hill, 1964).

Phillips, John L., Jr. *The Origins of Intellect: Piaget's Theory* (San Francisco: Freeman, 1969).

Pulaski, Mary, and Spencer Pulaski. *Understanding Piaget* (New York: Harper & Row, 1971).

School Health Education Study. *Health Education: A Conceptual Approach to Curriculum Design* (St. Paul, Minn.: 3M Education Press, 1967).

Selberg, Edith M., Louise A. Neal, and Mathew F. Vessel. *Discovering Science in the Elementary School* (Reading, Mass.: Addison-Wesley, 1970).

Woodruff, Asahel D. *The Psychology of Teaching* (New York: Longmans, Green, 1951).

_____. "The Use of Concepts in Teaching and Learning," *Journal of Teacher Education* (March 1964): 81-89.

CHAPTER 11

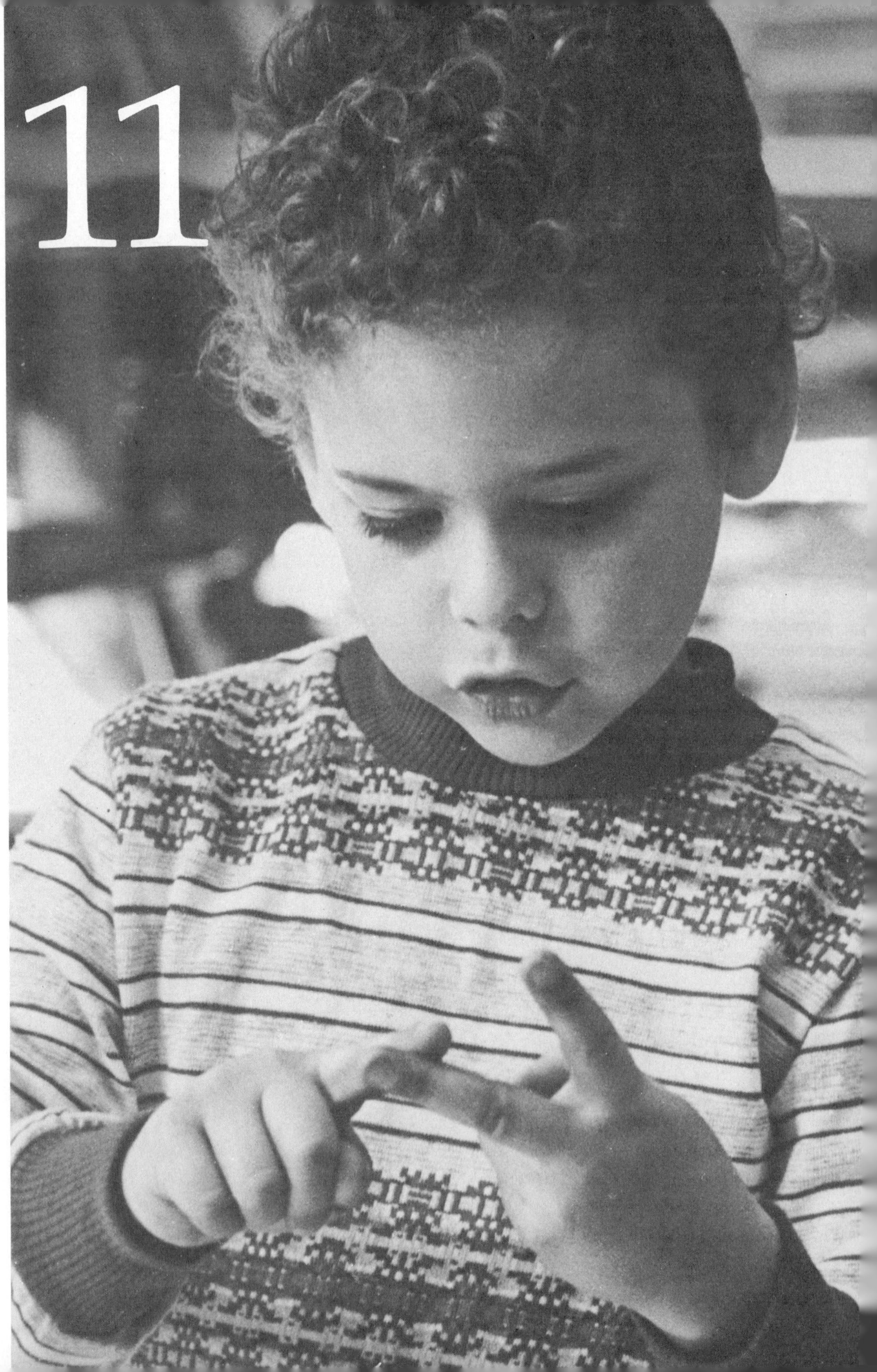

stating behavioral objectives

expected student outcomes

Behavioral objectives are statements that describe what students will be able to do after completing a prescribed unit of instruction (Kibler *et al.*, 1970). Other terms used for behavioral objectives are: objectives, outcomes, goals, or competencies. For the purposes of this text, the term most frequently used will be *"expected student outcomes."*

In essence, these expected student outcomes serve to further the instructional process once concepts for a particular unit of instruction have been developed. Like concepts, they provide direction to both the instructor and the student in terms of what should be taught, how it should be taught, and whether or not that which is taught is attained by the learner.

Properly stated behavioral objectives are not only useful, but also essential to a quality health education program. Failure to prepare behavioral objectives leaves both the instructor and the student with no direction in terms of unit design,

goals, and evaluation procedures. On the other hand, properly stated outcomes serve to communicate the goals of the instructional unit to all interested parties. They identify the specific content to be covered, the expected changes in student behavior, and the form of evaluation necessary to ensure accountability.

LEVELS OF SPECIFICITY

Instructional objectives can be written in degrees of specificity. They can be very general (e.g., "to promote healthful behavior"), or they can be highly specific (e.g., "in a half-hour essay examination at the culmination of the unit, the student will be able to describe the physical effects that transpire in the body from the time tobacco smoke is first inhaled into the respiratory system. The student's response must be complete, sequential, and correspond with the description found in the textbook.") Somewhere in between are objectives that omit some of the more definitive aspects of the specific type of objective cited above, but are more inclusive and pointed than the general objective listed above. For

The material in this chapter is adapted from Walter D. Sorochan and Stephen J. Bender, *Teaching Secondary Health Science*, New York: Wiley, 1978. By permission.

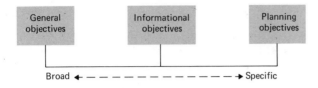

Fig. 11.1   Continuum of objectives.

example, "The student will be able to describe in logical sequence the physiological effects tobacco smoke has on the body once it has been inhaled" is an objective that is somewhere in the middle of the continuum of the behavioral objectives presented. Kibler *et al.* (1970, p. 20) define these categories of objectives as general, informational, and planning, respectively. Figure 11.1 depicts the location of the three different types of objectives on the continuum of objectives. Some objectives, of course, would not fit neatly into any of the three categories. They likely would be found somewhere in between the two extremes. However, to simplify the objectives issue, we have arbitrarily elected to focus on the "informational" and "planning" instructional objectives in this text.

VALUE OF PLANNING AND INFORMATIONAL OBJECTIVES

Planning objectives, which are very specific in nature, are developed specifically for the planning and evaluating of instruction. They are teacher-oriented objectives that are most helpful for guiding the curricular process. Kibler *et al.* (1970, p. 22)

perceive teachers and instructional designers benefiting in several ways from defining planning objectives:

1. Given clearly defined goals to work toward, teachers can design instructional experiences to achieve them and can evaluate the effectiveness of such experiences according to whether the goals are achieved.

2. Students can be examined prior to beginning instruction to determine whether they have already mastered any of the objectives. Information regarding their preparedness for the instruction to follow can also be obtained.

3. Each student can be evaluated on mastery of the unit's objectives. In this way every student can be required to master all objectives. This is in contrast to grading students on how well they performed in comparison with the rest of the class (grading on the curve) or in achievement of a certain percentage of the objectives of the unit. *

Informational objectives, by contrast, are specifically designed to inform others of what the teacher hopes to accomplish in a given instructional unit. Informational objectives are more or less abbreviations of planning objectives, being developed by the teacher after the planning objectives have been established. Kibler *et al.* (1970, pp. 22–23) perceive students, curriculum planners, student advisers, teachers, and administrators as benefiting in the following ways from the use of informational objectives:

1. Several studies have demonstrated that students can be more efficient learners if they are provided with objectives (Mager and McCann, 1961; McNeil, 1966; Miles, Kibler, and Pettigrew, 1967). Perhaps one of the reasons students do better when given copies of the objectives of a unit of instruction is that they are spared the frustrations

---

* From Robert Kibler and others, *Behavioral Objectives and Instruction.* Copyright © 1970 by Allyn and Bacon, Inc., and reprinted with permission.

and time-consuming effort of trying to guess what the teacher expects of them.

2. Given such clearly specified objectives, curriculum planners are better able to arrange sequences of courses or units of instruction. Knowing what students (hopefully, all students) are able to do at the end of courses and what students are able to do at the beginning of courses (prerequisites), it should be possible to eliminate unnecessary overlap of courses and to identify and fill in gaps between courses.

3. Students and their advisers are able to plan their course programs better when they can read course descriptions which include informational objectives.

4. Through clear behavioral objectives, teachers are able to tell other teachers what they teach. Stating that "students learn to name each state and its capital in the United States" tells considerably more than stating "United States geography is taught."

5. Teachers and administrators can determine the level of objectives students will be able to achieve in terms of the three taxonomic classifications to be discussed in Chapter III (in Kibler et al.). For example, in the cognitive domain, objectives can be classified as knowledge, comprehension, application, analysis, synthesis, and evaluation, thereby avoiding undue emphasis on a certain level of objectives.

STATING BEHAVIORAL OBJECTIVES

For the purposes of this text, we will focus on the developmental procedures surrounding planning and informational objectives.

Planning Objectives

As previously stated, planning objectives are most helpful to teachers in preparing a unit of instruction. They are more precise and include more spe-

---

* From Robert Kibler and others, *Behavioral Objectives and Instruction.* Copyright © 1970 by Allyn and Bacon, Inc., and reprinted with permission.

cific details than do informational objectives. Recall that the example of a planning objective on p. 175 describes quite specifically the *behavior* (the student will be able to *describe*) the student will be expected to exhibit to be deemed competent with reference to the objective. In addition, the *content* or result of the student's behavior (*physiological efforts that transpire in the body from the time tobacco smoke is first inhaled into the respiratory system*), plus the *conditions* under which the behavior is to be performed (*half-hour written essay examination at the culmination of the unit*), and the *standard* to be utilized in determining whether or not the performance is satisfactory (*the student's response must be complete, sequential, and correspond with the description found in the textbook*) must all be included for the objective to be termed a planning objective.

In an effort to simplify the foregoing analysis of the component parts of a planning objective, the following list of elements is provided (Kibler *et al.,* 1970, p. 33):

1. WHO is expected to perform the required behavior. For our purposes this will almost always be "the student," "learner," "pupils," etc.

2. The BEHAVIOR to be exhibited by the student to demonstrate his competency. Verbs like "write," "speak," "demonstrate," etc., describe this component. There is a need to use sound action verbs for clarity's sake.

3. The CONTENT or result of the student's behavior which will be evaluated to determine the student's level of competency. With cognitive oriented planning objectives, it is merely what the student will be able to discuss, define, identify, etc.

4. The CONDITIONS under which the student is expected to perform the behavior. Examples might be a "one-hour examination," "in front of class," etc.

5. The STANDARDS which will be employed to determine whether or not the student is minimally competent. Statements such as, "Ninety percent" or *"three out of five satisfactory responses,"* are indicative.*

Now let us view another exemplary planning objective that exhibits all of the elements described above: "In a 15-minute quiz the day following instruction, the student will be able to describe the physiological process by which an individual becomes intoxicated due to alcohol abuse. The student's answer must be in complete agreement with the lecture outline presented in class." Note that all of the previously listed elements are present:

1. *Who*—"the student."
2. *Behavior*—"to describe."
3. *Content*—"physiologic process by which an individual becomes intoxicated due to alcohol abuse."
4. *Conditions*—"15-minute quiz the day following instruction."
5. *Standard*—"the student's answer must be in complete agreement with the lecture outline presented in class."

Informational Objectives

Whereas planning objectives guide the instructor in the instructional process, informational objectives are designed to convey instructional intent to others. The informational objective is less specific than the planning objective, but by no means is it less important.

It is sound educational practice to provide students with a copy of the informational objectives for each unit of instruction. It will help them become more efficient learners by providing direction to their learning activities. It also helps the student to understand better his or her own competency level once the unit of instruction is complete and the evaluation procedures have been inplemented.

---

* From Robert Kibler and others, *Behavioral Objectives and Instruction.* Copyright © 1970 by Allyn and Bacon, Inc., and reprinted with permission.

In that informational objectives are abbreviations of planning objectives, it is wise to develop informational objectives after the planning objectives have been established. This simply means that the informational objective contains all of the elements of a planning objective except the "conditions" and "standards." The "who," "behavior," and "content" aspects still remain intact. For example, "The student will be able to describe the physiological process by which an individual becomes intoxicated due to alcohol abuse" is an example of an informational objective. Note that the "conditions" ("in a 15-minute quiz the day following instruction") and "standard" ("the student's answer must be in complete agreement with the lecture outline presented in class") have been omitted. However, none of the informational impact of the objective is lost. Other teachers, administrators, and students are still well informed as to what is to be taught in a given class and what the students are expected to grasp.

In conclusion, it can be stated that the three key elements of an informational objective are the "who," the desired observable "behavior," and the "content," or result the student is expected to experience. The greater the clarity of these elements, the greater the probability that the objective will clearly communicate to the recipient what he or she is to learn from the given unit of instruction.

A WORD ABOUT PRECISENESS

It is always good practice to make planning and informational objectives as precise as possible. For example, "the student realizes that immunization is one way of controlling communicable disease" and "the student knows about communicable disease" both possess the essential elements (who, behavior, content) of objectives, but they are far too vague. In the first objective, the term "realizes" has many interpretations. One would have to ask what evidence would be required to determine if the pupil does indeed "realize." In the second objective, both the behavioral dimension ("knows") and the content dimension ("communicable diseases") are too broad. Does "knows" mean simple recall, being able to tell in one's own words, or explaining relationships? The words "communicable disease" could conceivably mean anything from the sense of a single communicable disease to a complete understanding of the infectious-disease cycle.

Less precise terms, such as "understand," "know," and "realize," are open to broad interpretation. When utilized in the construction of objectives, they serve only to contribute to ambiguity and confusion. It is much more advantageous to employ other terms that better describe or define the behaviors sought. The use of more precise terms strengthens the educational process by providing better direction to both the student and the teacher. The student will know better what is expected of him or her, the teacher will be better able to provide learning opportunities that will enable the student to attain the objective, and there will be a better opportunity for more precise evaluation. The following list (Fodor and Davis, 1974, p. 46) provides a contrast between behavioral terms that are vague and open to many interpretations and those that are more precise in describing behavior.*

Less precise terms— many interpretations	More precise terms— few interpretations	
Know	Define	Interpret
Realize	Distinguish	Describe
Enjoy	Recall	Name
Believe	Recognize	Construct
Understand	Demonstrate	Compare
Appreciate	Apply	Translate
Value	Organize	State
Comprehend	Discuss	Illustrate
Desire	Identify	Summarize
Feel	List	Classify
Respect	Diagram	Select
	Acquire	Order

* From John T. Fodor and Gus T. Davis, *Health Instruction: Theory and Application.* Copyright © 1974 by Lea & Febiger and reprinted with permission.

CLASSIFYING BEHAVIORAL OBJECTIVES

We have already established the fact that behavioral objectives should be stated in terms of changes in student behavior. These behaviors can be defined as thinking, feeling, and doing. By using such terms, we can begin to determine the classes of behaviors reflected in the objectives we prepare. Classification can be helpful because it can:

1. Assist with avoiding overconcentration in any one area when formulating instructional objectives;
2. Provide insight into the appropriate instruments for evaluation.

For instructional purposes, objectives can be classified into one or more of the following behavioral domains:

1. *Cognitive:* Behavioral objects that range from recall or recognition of knowledge to the development of intellectual skills and abilities.
2. *Affective:* Behavioral objectives that emphasize a feeling tone, an emotion, or a degree of acceptance or rejection. Objectives in this domain are often vaguely described as appreciations, attitudes, interests, or values and are difficult to measure.
3. *Action:* Behavioral objectives that emphasize some muscular or motor skill, manipulation of material and object, or act that requires neuromuscular coordination.

Within each of the behavioral areas, it is possible to classify objectives into progressive labels of development. Bloom *et al.* (1956) and Krathwohl *et al.* (1964) conducted a systematic survey of the educational objectives in the cognitive and affective domains and prepared taxonomies for the two classes of behavior. To date, there has not been any effort to develop a taxonomy for the psychomotor domain.

The following list of Bloom's three domains provides an analysis of the 16 terms that may be used in describing behavior more closely. Note the progressive levels of development for each domain.

1. Cognitive domain (intellectual processes of the learner)
   a) Low level
      (1) Knowledge—recognition and recall of information, terms, classes, procedures, theories, structures
      (2) Comprehension—interpretation of what has been learned
   b) High level
      (1) Application—use of knowledge in *new* situations
      (2) Analysis—breaking whole units into related parts (deduction)
      (3) Synthesis—combining elements into new wholes (induction)
      (4) Evaluation—judging materials and methods, using standards of criteria
2. Affective domain (emphasis on emotional processes, e.g., feelings, interests, values, and adjustments)
   a) Low level
      (1) Receiving—passive attention to stimuli (i.e., sensory inputs)
      (2) Responding—reacting to stimuli (complying, volunteering, and so forth)
   b) High level
      (1) Valuing—actions consistent with a belief or value
      (2) Organization—commitment to a set of values (discussion, formulating values)
      (3) Characterization—total behavior conforming to internalized values (e.g., philosophy)
3. Action domain (emphasis on motor behaviors involving neuromuscular coordination)
   a) Low level
      (1) Perception—sensitivity to stimulus normally leading to action (e.g., cue. sensing, and so on)
      (2) Preparation—involves readiness to perform (e.g., possesses knowledge, bodily stance, willingness)
      (3) Orientation—knowing and/or deciding an appropriate response to be made
   b) High level
      (1) Pattern—a learned response that is habitual, smooth, and confident (e.g., a skill pattern or low error response)
      (2) Performance—response that is a complex motor action involving a high degree of skill (e.g., polished behavior, complicated responses, made with ease and control)

REVIEW QUESTIONS

1. Differentiate between informational and planning objectives.
2. What purpose do objectives or expected outcomes serve?
3. Cite the key components of both a planning and an informational objective.
4. Why is it important to make the action aspect of the expected outcome as precise as possible?
5. How are expected outcomes traditionally classified?

REFERENCES AND BIBLIOGRAPHY

Bloom, B. S., *et al.*, ed. *Taxonomy of Educational Objectives: Domain* (New York: David McKay, 1956).

Fodor, John T., and Gus T. Davis. *Health Instruction: Theory and Application* (Philadelphia: Lea and Febiger, 1974).

Gronhund, Norman E. *Stating Behavioral Objectives for Classroom Instruction* (New York: Macmillan, 1970).

Kibler, Robert J., *et al. Behavioral Objectives and Instruction* (Boston: Allyn and Bacon, 1970).

Krathwohl, D. R., *et al. Taxonomy of Educational Objectives: Affective Domain* (New York: David McKay, 1964).

Mager, R. F. *Preparing Instructional Objectives* (San Francisco: Fearon, 1962).

Sorochan, Walter D., and Stephen J. Bender. *Teaching Secondary Health Science* (New York: Wiley, 1978).

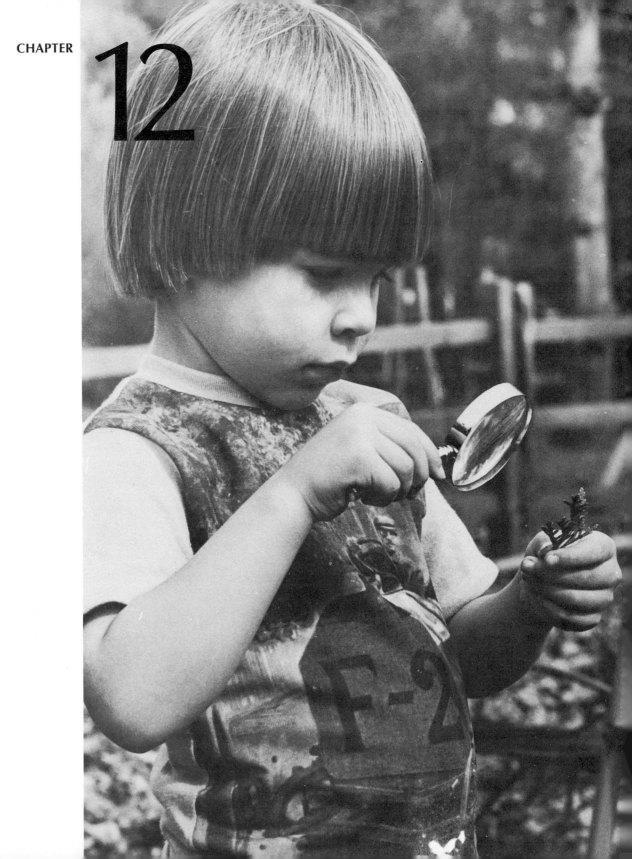

appropriate elementary
health education
learning experiences

To see
To hear
To touch
To feel
To wonder?

  To do
  To discover
  To understand
  To learn . . .

    To be
    To feel good
    To be well
    To live
    To be happy!

The poem above suggests the nature and purpose of this chapter. The first part of the poem has to do with the natural ability of children to learn. You should be able to recognize these as the body senses children use to receive "messages" from the teacher. The middle part of the poem suggests how the message (information) is internalized through learning experiences. What does the latter part suggest? All three are involved in the learning process.

Teaching is both a science and an art. Teachers apply the elements of science and the scientific approach in selecting relevant content, materials, and methods and in projecting expected behavioral objectives. But the effective blending of these into an educational recipe to ensure continuing progress of children toward optimal well-being and more abundant living is an art. This chapter provides suggestions on how elementary teachers may develop greater skill in the art of teaching "for health." The methods suggested are neither bad nor good. Their value, like that of the airplane or the television set, depends on the way in which they are used. Methods should motivate children to discover understandings and feelings and to thereby evolve their own concepts. Obviously some methods do a better job than others. But methods alone are not enough. The message they pass along needs to be reinforced by materials and visual aids. Thus the medium of the method is enriched by the materials and becomes a message. The teacher blends methods and materials to provide essential and

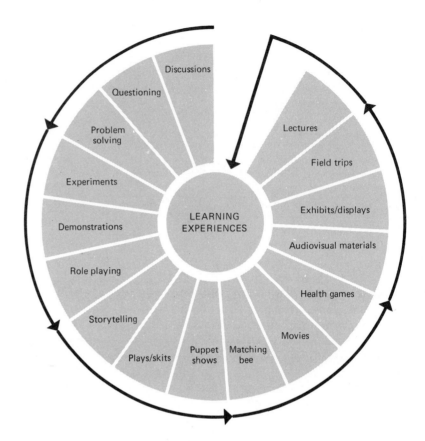

Fig. 12.1 Conceptualization of this chapter.

worthwhile learning experiences so that children may internalize the message. Out of such learning experiences should emerge constructive sociohygienic behaviors.

The first part of this chapter explores the nature of methods and how methods may be used. The second part explores methods relevant to elementary school health science instruction. Teaching aids and materials and their relationship to methods are discussed in the final section. The chapter content is appropriately summarized in Fig. 12.1.

Examples of each of the methods are not included in this chapter. Instead, numerous examples of how methods and materials may be used are included in later chapters dealing with lesson plans.

DEFINITION

There was a time when teaching was accepted as the act of delivering priceless pearls of wisdom to a captive audience of learners. It was also assumed that the mere "telling" of things to be learned fulfilled the obligation of the teacher. Fortunately, today this misconception of teaching is seldom found among elementary teachers. The emphasis in teaching "for health" today is behavioral in nature rather than being placed on the imparting of facts and information.

Teaching has been recognized as a process of stimulating and directing learning (Humphrey, Johnson, and Moore, 1962). Although both teaching and learning take place at the same time, learning is what happens to the pupils, whereas teaching is what the teacher does. Rash (1965, p. 44) defines health teaching as fostering an environment favorable to learning. The word "method" is defined in *Webster's Seventh New Collegiate Dictionary* as "orderly procedure or process . . . orderly arrangement." Obviously this is not an adequate meaning for the word in the teaching context, where it not only covers strategy and tactics of teaching, but also involves what is to be taught at any given time, identification of the expected behavioral objectives or pupil outcomes, the means by which content is to be taught, the order in which the content is to be taught, and evaluative procedures (Broudy and Palmer, 1965; Oberteuffer, Harrelson, and Pollock, 1972). All of these aspects of the teaching act need to be considered when selecting or using a method. Obviously the term "method" covers the "how" of teaching. What we are most concerned with in this chapter is that phase of the teaching act that the teacher chooses and uses in designing teaching/ learning strategies. The teacher reaches into his or her "bag of tools" for the most appropriate technique or activity to help children to discover for themselves the concept, feeling, or habit. Such learning experiences include role playing, plays, demonstrations, experiments, discussions, as well as other activities. Activities of this nature may be referred to as learning experiences, or strategies. The teacher simply manipulates the classroom activity so as to help each child have a specific experience which in turn allows the child to progress toward or achieve proficiency in specific behavioral or sociohygienic skills or tasks.

Beginning teachers are often mesmerized by the various teaching/learning strategies. We have found that prospective teachers are more concerned

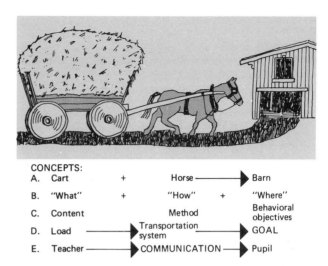

CONCEPTS:

A.	Cart	+	Horse ──────▶		Barn
B.	"What"	+	"How"	+	"Where"
C.	Content		Method		Behavioral objectives
D.	Load ──────▶		Transportation system	──────▶	GOAL
E.	Teacher ──────▶		COMMUNICATION ──▶		Pupil

Fig. 12.2 Conceptualization of the relationships among content, method, and expected pupil outcomes. Which should be considered first in teaching for optimal well-being? Method is simply a way of communicating the ideas and information from teacher to pupil.

about "how" to teach than about the "what" or the "where." This procedure is a good example of putting the horse before the cart. Before the horse is harnessed to the cart, we must have a load for it to pull, and we must also know where the barn is. The analogy between this illustration and teaching is illustrated in Fig. 12.2. The load of hay may be thought of as the subject matter to be taught, the horse as the vehicle or technique of moving the hay, and the barn as expected pupil outcomes. Methods are like the horse; they help the teacher to communicate the information to the pupils. All three—what, how, and where—are interrelated aspects of the teaching/learning process. In health teaching, perhaps how to teach becomes a more critical issue than what and when to teach.

NATURE OF METHOD

Although method consists of many elements, it is more than a collection of tricks, artifices, and ruses; it is a systematic pattern into which are woven knowledge, purpose, skill, respect for others, and a combination of the basic means of communication. The core of content—the facts and knowledge—needs to be presented to the pupils so that they can assimilate, relate to, and internalize the material.

Communication requires sharing and participating. The teacher, as a speaker, only starts the process; the student, as a hearer, must complete or do it. The teacher has information, an idea, an attitude, a feeling, or an undertaking to share with the pupils. The process of transmitting these elements and receiving responses constitutes communication, which may be verbal, nonverbal, or both. The teacher represents only a part of this process, for the process also involves receiving and reacting on the part of the pupils. Thus communication is a two-directional process because the teacher, in addition to transmitting, must also receive and react to the responses of the pupils; thus the teacher is continually adapting the teaching method on the basis of feedback from the pupils.

Selecting the best way or technique to communicate with children is most important. Perhaps the first thing the teacher should be aware of is how children can receive information or communication. Weaver and Cenci (1960, p. 6) point out that we learn through our senses. Table 12.1 summarizes the importance of body senses in learning. Most health and living experiences are sociological in nature, so the feelings we get from the reactions of others play a significant role in how we behave hygienically.

The implications for teaching are many. The nature of the topic and the behavior expected may

Table 12.1 Importance of body senses to learning.

Sense	Importance (in education) (Victor, 1970, p. 6)	Estimated importance in health science instruction
1. Sight	75%	52%
2. Hearing	13	13
3. Touch	6	6
4. Smell	3	3
5. Taste	3	3
6. Balance	-	3
7. Kinesthetic	-	
8. Feeling (emotions)	-	20

call on one of the lesser-rated senses far more than the table indicates. This may be especially true at the primary level, where children are unable to read yet. Teaching through the senses becomes very important at this level. When peer-group pressure to conform in behavior becomes important, especially in the intermediate grades, the sense of feeling becomes important. Educators in general have failed to recognize the potentiality of this sensory area. The teacher must be always conscious to:

1. utilize those senses most important to the child in relation to the specific lesson at hand;

2. stimulate senses as often as possible for retention of learning; and

3. utilize a combination of as many of these senses as possible.

We have all experienced hearing a sentence or word that recalled a song; a phrase that made us recall a poem; a familiar scene, an event; an exercise, our good physical feeling; a smell, a process; a touch, a material; a social occasion, a wonderful feeling of belonging and happiness; or a taste, a good or a poor product. When the teacher stimulates a special sense or more than one sense, he or she is giving the student an additional dimension to learning and recalling. Senses are the receivers of communication.

One may conclude that the goal of all methodology is to facilitate communication so that children internalize the information presented.

FACTORS AFFECTING METHODOLOGY

There is no one best way to teach effectively. "One man's meat is another's poison." However, some approaches may be more appropriate than others. The basis for the first statement should be obvious. There are many variables affecting the selection and use of methods (see Broudy and Palmer, 1965; Gage, 1965; Phenix, 1964; Veneker, 1964). These include:

1. teacher behavior (such as personality, dress, deportment, mannerisms, use of voice and diction, movement and tics, mastery of subject matter, communicative skill, exemplar model, and so on);

2. pupil receptivity and motivational behavior (closed or open mind, desire to learn);

3. media of teaching (methods, materials, instruments, audio-visual aids, etc.);

4. socioemotional environment of the classroom and school;

5. sociocultural traditions and influences of community (we tend to teach how we were taught);

6. pupil maturity (physical, emotional, social, intellectual);

7. expected pupil outcomes (teacher objectives) for the lesson;

8. content or subject matter (what to teach, scope).

All of these variables affect the learning process. Much research has been conducted in an effort to provide evidence that one method is superior or better than another. Because early researchers overlooked these variables in their research designs or ignored controlling them during the research, the conclusions they reached were biased and inconclusive. Gage, in his *Handbook of Research on Teaching* (1965), reviewed all of the educational research on teaching methodology up to 1964. His conclusions are noteworthy:

1. Methods of teaching reflect teacher effectiveness and consistency in communicating and affecting students by providing worthwhile learning experiences.

2. Up until 1950, most research attempted to discuss and describe patterns of teacher behavior or teacher roles. Considerable research was conducted from 1950 to 1964 on the effectiveness of various teaching methods. For example, is the lecture method better than the discussion or TV approaches? Reviewers of such research have found that these studies were all weak in experimental design; did not specify, and hence did not control, learning and teaching variables; and did not specify teacher roles or teacher behaviors. Hence the conclusion about research on effectiveness of teaching, up to 1964, was that different teaching procedures produced little or no difference in the amount of knowledge gained by students. There is little evidence to favor one method over another.

3. Effectiveness of each teaching method and teaching aid depends on the specific instructional objectives or pupil outcomes. There is a need to base methods on educational goals, as stated in terms of behavioral objectives, outcomes, and such attainment. If this is done, any classroom procedure that does the job of achieving the goals or outcomes is a good one.

4. There is a need to base teaching methods and their use on a learning model stemming from psychological research and developmental task theory.

5. Different teaching methods emphasize certain principles and neglect others.

6. There is a great need to design teaching methods that make as much use as possible of a wide range of learning principles.

7. Effective use of teaching methods and the success of those methods are dependent on: (a) teacher personality; (b) teacher motivation and subject interest; (c) teacher interest in pupils; (d) teacher mastery of subject matter; (e) teacher behavior or perception of his or her role as a teacher; (f) teacher aspirations for ideal teaching; (g) teacher acquaintance and exposure to various methods of teaching; and (h) teacher understanding of pupil's developmental tasks and learning processes.

There have been many research studies on the effectiveness of teaching methodology since 1964. Most of these have been unable to incorporate Gage's recommendations for controlling the variables involved in the teaching process. The general conclusions of Gage and his reviewers are still valid today. Thus selecting and using appropriate learning experience becomes an art—a prescriptive judgmental phase of teaching much like the physician's approach to selecting and prescribing a course of treatment for a patient.

APPLICATION OF METHODS

Learning experiences are the means by which children learn both the content and the process of health science. Children acquire understandings, attitudes, and habits that help them to attain, maintain, and conserve their well-being at an optimal level and to also live more abundantly. The teacher should use a wide variety of learning experiences to help children realize these ultimate goals.

Many teachers use many more learning activities than are necessary to ensure satisfactory learning. This excessive use tends to prolong the unit unnecessarily, slow down learning, and dull pupil interest. The experienced teacher employs learning activities wisely and economically, realizing that sometimes one activity is enough for an understanding to be gained. Occasionally one good learning activity will suffice to provide an understanding of more than one concept. Other times, when a concept is difficult or abstract, more than one activity may be necessary to achieve an understanding. Slow learners usually learn better when more than one activity is used.

The grade level may also influence the number of learning experiences needed. In the lower grades, the children's attention span is short, and their ability to think abstractly is not well developed; therefore, more than one activity is often necessary to obtain a satisfactory understanding. To help a child perceive a concept, the teaching/learning strategy may need to be repeated several times, or another strategy may need to be introduced. However, in the upper grades one well-chosen activity is usually sufficient. In all cases the best procedure is for the teacher to use as many— but *only* as many—activities as are necessary to ensure satisfactory learning. Teachers need to exercise their freedom to choose and modify methods in light of specific situations. In practice, no method can or should remain static; all of them yield to the purposes and procedures of particular classes. Method is an inclusive and modifiable process and not a predetermined formula. The effective teacher does not select a method, but instead develops a flexible procedure that is applicable to a particular situation. Effective teaching and learning do not come as a result of merely using the visual method, or a field trip, or a discussion. Progress in social learning is the result of the subtle blending of the varied elements that constitute growth and development. Chapter 4 set the stage for making the elementary teacher sensitive to developmental concepts and learning principles. Chapter 10 suggests that certain methods or learning experiences help children to internalize facts and evolve desirable sociohygienic habits. Chapter 11 suggested the need for the teacher to be concerned about selecting learning experiences that help pupils to attain expected outcomes (behavioral objectives in a lesson plan). Prospective teachers would do well to review these chapters before reading the remainder of this chapter. They should reflect on the major concepts of these earlier chapters when selecting and using learning experiences.

LEARNING EXPERIENCES FOR HEALTH INSTRUCTION

Because of the nature of elementary school children, the subject matter with which they deal, and the educational goals established for them, some learning experiences are more appropriate than others. Some appropriate experiences for primary children may include storytelling, puppet shows, skits and plays, simulation or acting out, demonstrations, problem solving, and discussions. In addition, there are many others that may be used by elementary teachers: exhibits and displays, health fairs, field trips, surveys, guest speakers, debates, panels, lectures, programed instruction, and contract-teaching. Learning experiences at the intermediate level may include all of the primary experiences, as well as education cardboard games, experiments, role playing, and matching bees.

The learning experiences to be discussed appear appropriate for elementary school children in that they have a great potential for helping children to discover concepts and to apply them to everyday living. It is for these reasons that these learning experiences will be explored in some depth.

The following criteria can be used to determine whether a particular learning experience is appropriate:

1. Does the learning experience contribute to pupils' attaining the *expected behavioral objectives* or *outcomes?*

2. Does it help children to evolve and discover the *topic concept* (this discovery occurs only through the learning experience!)?

3. Is it *action-oriented* instead of listening-oriented? That is, learning experiences that contribute to developing affective behaviors should take precedence over those focusing primarily on cognitive behaviors. Likewise, learning experiences that evolve or modify health habits and behaviors (action behavior) should take precedence over those that focus on cognitive and/or affective behaviors.

4. Does it *teach through two or more sense organs?* A learning experience that communicates through two or more body sense organs [eyes, ears, nose (smell), tongue (taste), skin (touch), glands (emotions), muscles (neuromuscular)] is more effective, clearer, and more enduring than one that communicates through just one sensory organ. The information picked up by one sense organ should be reinforced by another. Thus the ears are complemented by the eyes in receiving health information. If a third sensory organ (e.g., nose and smelling) were added, the total learning impact on the student would be stronger and more enduring. More important, it would help the student to more readily discover the health concept. Keep in mind that the only way a person can receive information or messages about the outside the body world is through the sense organs. The more sense organs involved in recording and decoding the information, the more meaningful the information becomes.

5. Is it economical in terms of teacher/pupil time and cost (e.g., the materials and visual aids)?

6. Is it appropriate for the subject matter as well as for the expected pupil outcome?

Discussion and Questioning

These two approaches to effective learning take place in all classroom learning experiences. Both are used as follow-up to most other learning experiences. Questioning the students as a means of treating the topic at hand is the teacher's chief means of directing or channeling discourse. The students, in return, question the teacher and one another about the topic. Questions prompt thinking about specific subjects. In a discussion topics are formulated as questions because a question sets the mind working. According to research, questions constitute about one-third of a classroom discourse, and teachers ask about 86 percent of the questions (Hyman, 1970, p. 217). Because questioning is so essential in the classroom, special attention is given to it here.

A discussion involves the verbal interaction of a number of individuals who perceive one another as participants in a common activity. It is a socializing procedure designed to utilize cooperative participation toward the resolution of a particular problem or question. Discussion usually requires some degree of moderation to guide group thinking effectively. It provides children with an opportunity to review facts and to synthesize them into meaningful generalizations that have practical applications to health problems.

A good classroom discussion requires: (1) an emotionally favorable classroom environment that permits students the appropriate freedom of expression, and (2) that the participants possess sufficient information to discuss the topic or question in a meaningful way. The first condition results from the teacher's general spirit or attitude. He or she should avoid the use of ridicule and generally regard any sincere student response as a useful contribution to the discussion. The second condition, concerning adequate knowledge, is important if one is to avoid the rambling and unproductive "pooling of ignorance" type of discussion. There-

fore, discussions are usually more successful after the students have done some reading or viewed a film, a puppet show, skit, role-play activity, demonstration, or experiment.

Discussion usually centers on the teacher—with the teacher directing the questioning. Often the teacher may want to get more participation from the pupils and can get this from small-group discussions, or *buzz sessions*. Three to five children may be organized into a small group. A leader and a recorder may be appointed. The theme or basic goal of the group is identified in writing on a piece of paper. After 10 to 20 minutes of buzzing—researching for ideas, sharing feelings, suggesting alternative solutions, and so on—the pupil recorder from each group should make a brief oral report. The teacher, as mediator, should entertain questions from the class, allow the pupils to answer, and in the end summarize the discussion. Buzz sessions of this type are effective in sensitizing students to the feelings of their peers as well as to different reactions to critical health issues.

Questioning facilitates a good discussion. Questions should lead students to think, to reason, to clarify, and to classify information. Questions may also be asked in order to:

1. *Get a particular student to participate.*
2. *Check on the student's comprehension.*
3. *Attract a student's attention.*
4. *Test a student's knowledge of the topic.*
5. *Diagnose a student's knowledge of the topic.*
5. *Diagnose a student's weaknesses.*
6. *Break the ice and get a discussion going.*
7. *Allow a student to shine before his classmates.*
8. *Establish an explanation for a problem.*
9. *Review work for yesterday's absentees.*
10. *Build up a student's security when the teacher is quite sure the student will respond correctly.*

11. *Learn about a student's personal activities (which affect his classroom performance).*

12. *Attack issue A rather than B.**

In order to use questions to direct discussion, the teacher must deliberately phrase the questions appropriately to the context of the discourse and the maturational level of the students. The teacher's role as a discussion leader is to facilitate participation. He or she does more than ask questions. The teacher summarizes and also sharpens the responses and reactions by rephrasing them. He or she plays discussion "traffic cop," acknowledging students who wish to speak and requesting others to comment on previous remarks.

The teacher should not expect correct answers to all of his or her questions. To act out the mediator role, the teacher should formulate key questions in advance and include them as part of his or her lesson planning. Formulating written key, pivotal questions will serve as a a basic guide. However, the teacher needs to be flexible to the spontaneity of the classroom discussion.

Perhaps the greatest task facing the teacher in regard to questioning is to encourage the students to question both the teacher and one another. The questions that students ask should arise from a desire to understand both the topic at hand and the position taken by the other participants.

Problem Solving

As a learning experience, problem solving has great relevance for children to everyday living. Its use in this way can help children to develop their thinking, creative expression, critical analysis, and logical reasoning. Perhaps its greatest appeal lies in helping children to learn how to cope with their day-to-day problems. Thus problem solving, like

* Ronald T. Hyman, *Ways of Teaching*, 2d ed., Philadelphia: J. B. Lippincott, 1974, pp. 290-291. Reprinted by permission of the author.

discussion and questioning, has the potential of permeating all learning experiences. Its format and nature change with the topic, the students, and the learning experience.

Problems occur when children are unable to find personal and socially acceptable and worthwhile solutions to sociohygienic situations. Problems, small and big, are an expected everyday occurrence, and meeting them head on and resolving them contributes to successful living. Problem solving is a discovery technique and provides an opportunity for children to apply what they learn in the classroom to the solution of everyday problems. It helps to counter wasteful trial-and-error approaches to solving problems and to avoid the feeling of failure in living.

The process of problem solving is a natural one. The teacher and pupils identify realistic or hypothetical problems and proceed to solve them. There are two basic approaches in the use of this technique. In the first approach the problem may be posed in "paper and pencil" form, with suggested alternatives, or pupils may be asked to supply the alternatives. They are then asked to select the best or most appropriate alternative and to justify their choice. A question-and-answer and discussion session may be useful as a follow-up to help children rationalize why one answer is better than another. The immediate and long-range consequences of each alternative should be brought out in such a follow-up. In the other approach to problem solving, children actually identify a sociohygienic problem in the community as a field project and then proceed to solve it. The procedure in both approaches is the same, except that the latter is a long-lasting field experience, whereas the former is theoretical in nature and short in duration. Both approaches should be used.

Children may solve problems by working individually or in teams. If a health problem has social overtones, the peer-group process will be more effective in not only solving the problem, but also having the students become aware that the problem exists.

The steps of problem solving may be identified as follows:

1. Develop an awareness and admit that the problem exists.
2. Gather information about the problem.
3. Apply facts to the problem—analyze the problem.
4. List possible trial solutions or alternatives.
5. Apply personal and social values to the alternatives and indicate immediate and long-range consequences for each of the alternatives.
6. Select the best alternative as a solution to the problem.
7. Verify or try out the alternative. If it fails to work, select another alternative.

Almost all problems of living may be effectively solved by following the steps suggested above. The only way children will be able to solve problems is by actually applying the guidelines above.

Experiments

Experiments are procedures or operations undertaken to discover suggested truths or to prove or disprove a specific point, usually for the first time. Such an undertaking generally attempts to demonstrate how things are done, how they work, or what the truth is by employing exacting and precise controls so as to validate results. The purpose of an experiment is to illustrate and thus help a group or an individual understand the content or concept under consideration. Experiments have the potential of helping children to internalize, investigate health phenomena, and weigh and sift the evidence from the conclusions and the results. This process enables them to evolve their own concepts.

The following steps are helpful in conducting experiments:

1. Define the problem to be solved.
2. Select methods or procedure to be used.
3. Identify and assemble necessary materials and apparatus needed.
4. Conduct the experiment.
5. Collect and record data.
6. Select, organize, and interpret data.
7. Prepare conclusions.
8. Discuss the outcomes of the experiment and what was learned. Identify key concepts and relate to everyday living.

Experiments may be demonstrated by the teacher or pupil or conducted individually by each pupil. They are an excellent way of arousing class interest in a health topic and solving problems. Along with demonstrations, experiments provide an excellent opportunity to help the slow learner while also challenging the rapid learner. The elementary teacher should continually involve the children when doing the experiments. However, if the procedure involves a hazard or a risk of accident, the teacher should perform the experiment or avoid it altogether. The wise teacher keeps the experiment simple and stimulating enough to encourage children to think. He or she uses it as a way of helping children to answer a question or to understand an idea or a concept.

Demonstrations

A demonstration, similar in nature to an experiment, is usually considered a way of illustrating what is already known. On the other hand, an experiment is usually considered to be a way of learning about or discovering a scientific fact or a health concept for the first time. A demonstration may also be interpreted as a process of graphic explanation of a selected idea, fact, relationship, or phenomenon.

Demonstrations provide a visual explanation. Children like to be entertained; they like to see things done before their eyes, especially if there is an element of the mysterious which they do not understand. The teacher who describes some phase of the body function through skillful demonstration encourages the class to want to do it themselves. Demonstrations may be conducted by the teacher, the pupil, or the group. Any demonstration requires preplanning to be effective.

Sociodramas

Children like to play. They like to pretend, to imagine, and to imitate others. It is part of growing up socially. To the child, play is real. Through such natural expression, learning takes place, and life takes on social meaning. By use of sociodrama and simulation games, children gain knowledge about living. Children play, for example, house, school, doctor and nurse, cowboys and Indians, cops and robbers, and other life roles. Pretending at play is a natural part of being young. By pretending, the child is going through an interesting learning experience—trying out the various real-life or fantasy-life characters. By pretending to be a firefighter, the child sees or dreams about what it is actually like to be a firefighter. Dramatic play of this sort may be utilized by elementary teachers to gain insight about their pupils and to help the children to discover "the art of living" for themselves. Sociodramas having a natural appeal to children are simulation, let's pretend, role playing, puppet shows, plays and skits, and storytelling.

Most sociodramas may be utilized effectively by observing the following suggested procedures.

1. *Selecting the situation.* The situation should be a fairly simple one, involving one main idea or issue. It should also involve personalities. The issues should be those that arise because people have different desires, beliefs, hopes, and aspirations or ones that arise from the inability of people to understand the point of view of others.

2. *Choosing participants.* When first trying out role playing, the teacher should select students who are fairly well informed about the issue to be presented and who are imaginative, articulate, and self-assured. After the students have become familiar with the technique, the teacher should ask for volunteers.

3. *Preparing the audience.* Prior to initiating the sociodrama in class, the teacher should direct the class to observe for certain feelings, behaviors, and happenings.

4. *Acting out the situation.* The teacher should facilitate the learning experience by allowing children to become actively involved as much as possible. As a cross between director and audience, the teacher should, when necessary, remind the students of their role in the sociodrama and then withdraw into the audience. The sociodrama should be challenging, mentally stimulating, and fun for everyone.

5. *Following up.* A good sociodrama will generate interest and arouse comments and questions. Follow-up has to do with effective completion of the learning process. The valuable concepts conveyed through sociodramas need to be "nailed down" by means of reviews, discussions, and question-and-answer sessions. This kind of follow-up is essentially a part of all good learning experiences.

The teacher should express pleasure at how well the players performed. He or she should have thought out a series of questions to guide the ensuing discussion. An attempt should be made to identify main ideas and emotional reactions and to stimulate class involvement through questions, comments, and observations. At the end, the key points should be summarized. Ideally, the students will be able to internalize the main idea of the sociodrama and to evolve their own life-mediating concept. With slow learners and especially primary children, follow-up activities emanating from the sociodramas might include creative writing and individual drawing and construction work.

Role Playing

Role playing is the spontaneous, unrehearsed, ad lib, acting out of a situation or a problem. It is a form of improvisation in which the participants assume the fictitious identity of other persons and then react as they perceive their behavior in a particular set of circumstances. On the spot "acting out" can portray a concept or dramatize a problem-solving situation. Two or more people may participate, and ordinarily a short amount of time is allowed for planning. This learning experience has great potential to evolve an awareness of, to change, or to modify attitudes. It may also be used to introduce a health topic, to give students an opportunity to use what they have learned by applying some principle to the solution of a problem, or to illustrate the impact of tradition, values, or social pressure on individual behavior. Role playing differs from the usual type of dramatic experience in that no script, memorization, and rehearsal are needed. In fact, the value of role playing as a teaching device lies in the spontaneity of presentation. The action comes directly from the individual's creative use of his or her own experience.

The problem should be relevant to the health topic under study and should deal with a significant idea, concept, or issue involving personalities in a real-life situation. The problem selected should encourage the involvement of feelings and attitudes rather than straight factual information. A certain amount of teacher/pupil preplanning is necessary. The problem and the roles to be acted out need to be identified. The specific roles and a limited background regarding the personalities and attitudes to be projected should be briefly described on slips of paper. The time to be allotted should be short—one to three minutes. Two to five players are usually needed for a single episode. The roles assigned to students may be either congruent to or opposite from their real-life feelings. In either case the roles should be portrayed as the children perceive them and as the plot develops. The role playing should be stopped at the end of a specified time, when the idea or point has been reached, or when the dramatization begins to lag. The teacher should thank the participants for their performances and allow them to engage in the discussion which should follow. The teacher should follow up the role playing by attempting to identify the main ideas and emotional reactions presented.

Plays and Skits

A play is a carefully rehearsed dramatization that involves a predetermined script, costumed performers, and scenery. It can be extremely useful in portraying important concepts of a social nature. Play scripts may be obtained in professional form or developed as a class project. The latter has the advantage of student involvement and the discovery and application of knowledge to individual and group problems.

The skit or playlet is a relatively brief dramatic presentation. It too may be a planned satirical, comic, or humorous story, but requires little or no rehearsal. It has great appeal to primary children, for it is usually of short duration and may be used to help children explore problems in human relations. It may be presented in the classroom by simply providing scripts to students and asking them to "act out" as they read the script.

The emphasis in both examples should be on attaining and maintaining healthful living and not on dramatization. Humor and mild ridicule in the script may be used to influence student behavior. The play, probably more appropriate for the intermediate grades, should last from five to ten minutes, whereas the skit may last from three to five minutes and be used at both the primary and intermediate levels. Intermediate-grade pupils should be encouraged to write a skit or play and present it to primary-grade children or to their own class.

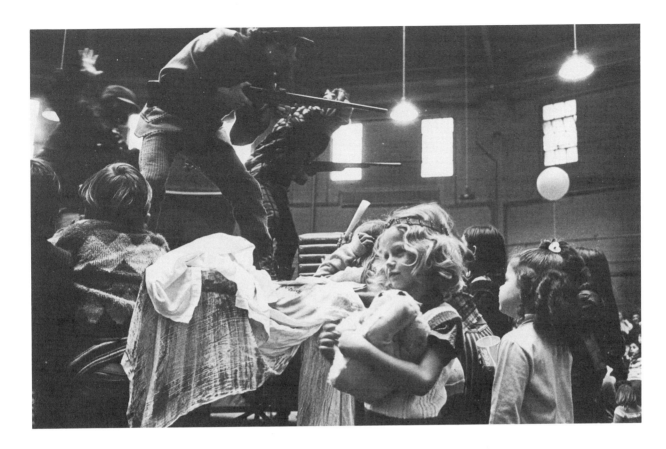

After the presentation, the class can analyze the meaning of the skit or play and its relationship to them, their needs, and their lives.

Fig. 12.3 Plays and skits help children to discover how others feel about well-being and life situations. (Daniel S. Brody/Editorial Photocolor Archives)

Puppets

Puppets are small figures or dolls. Marionettes are constructed with jointed limbs that can be manipulated from above by attached strings or wire. Hand puppets are made from cloth or paper and are pulled down over the hand. Movement of the hand gives the puppet movement and expression.

Puppets are fascinating to the average child. Puppets can make statements that will be remembered longer than those made by the teacher. Interest may be maintained at an even higher level when the puppets are made by members of the class and spontaneous dialogue added. Puppets have great attitudinal effect on primary children, as well as allowing for creativity.

A puppet show may be presented very effectively by the pupils' putting on the whole show. The teacher merely facilitates the learning process. A health theme or situation should be selected by the class and teacher for dramatization. A variety of methods may be used in the actual construction; consider, for example, hand puppets, stick puppets, paper-bag puppets, sock puppets, *papier-mâché* figures, and one- and two-string puppets. The characters assumed by the puppets may be taken from *Sesame Street* or other familiar television shows as well as favorite storybook situations. The stage should be inexpensive and may be of two types—a sheet or blanket stretched out as a curtain with the puppet manipulators hidden behind the curtain and the audience on the other side, or a large cardboard box with a curtain as a stage. The extended sheet as a curtain has appeal because it is quick and easy to rig up and adds to a relaxed and informal setting. An added advantage is that it provides space for mass participation of the pupils. One group can manipulate the puppets, another can hold the curtain, and the third group can spontaneously verbalize the roles of the puppets. The use of puppets in this way provides an ideal opportunity for creativity and subject correlation with art, English, drama, and health science. As with all sociodramatic techniques, a follow-up is necessary.

Storytelling

Storytelling as a pedagogical technique has been used by the world's greatest teachers. Jesus used it, as did Plato, Confucius, and other great philosophers and teachers. It has great appeal to primary school children in that it provides an opportunity for them to experience living language—language that communicates at a level above and beyond that of everyday usage. Storytelling is defined by Means (1968, p. 35) as the narration to a class of incidents or events, true as well as fictitious, which is read, told, or presented through various forms of expression. Its general aim is to present a message, interpret the literature, or inspire reading and expression. Anderson (1970), Chambers (1970, pp. 14-43), and Means (1968, p. 35) point out that one tells stories to children to:

1. Entertain and charm them. Life is made rich by sharing the adventures of others, finding new solutions to old problems, and seeing the familiar in a new way.

2. Explain about human nature. As the child identifies with characters, he learns to recognize his own feelings about health topics.

3. Give reassurance that life is good. With news of today stressing violence and the exceptional, children especially need reassurance that most people are kind and thoughtful, that most persons have only good intentions, or that most people feel the same about work, play, and well-being.

4. Give meaning to the big ideas of life. The good, the true, and the beautiful are learned concepts. Storytelling creates a concrete situation in which ideas and judgments can be tested and applied to personal experiences.

5. Give children a sense of competence to face each day, an appreciation of our environment, or an understanding of self.

6. Encourage the development of good listening skills and provide for aesthetic enjoyment.

7. Stimulate the imagination and provide opportunities for creative expression.

The storyteller needs to be honest, relaxed, and tell the story in a sincere manner. The story should possess substance and involve content related to the topic under study. The beginning storyteller

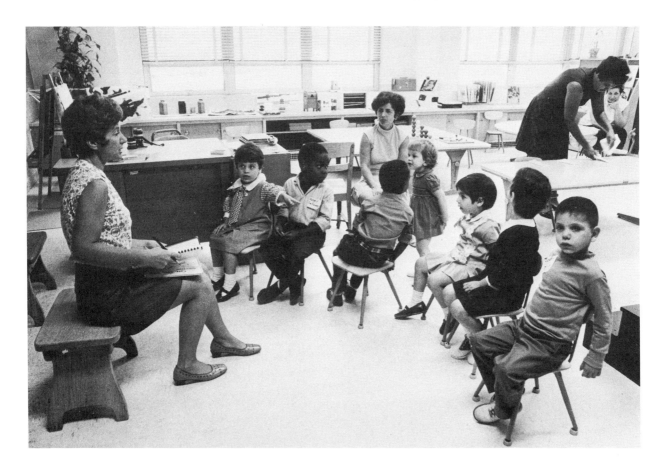

Fig. 12.4 Instead of teacher reading, have teacher telling and use of feltboard illustrations. Children should be encouraged to tell health stories. What is the teacher doing wrong in this picture? (Editorial Photocolor Archives)

should explore the children's collection in the library for suitable stories and should review the story in detail so as to know it well, but should avoid rote memorization. The storyteller utilizes his or her own personality as a teller—that is, his or her own choice of words, voice, pace, gestures, facial expressions, and so on—sending it to the ears and imagination of the listeners. When desirable, visual aids should be used to stimulate imagination, but not so that they distract from or interfere with the story. There is a need to create a visual picture of the story, to project into its character, and to consider

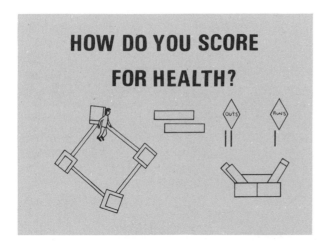

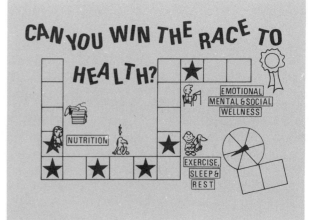

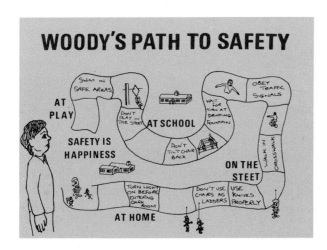

Fig. 12.5   Teacher/pupil–made health games allow for pupil participation. They may be used as bulletin boards or adapted for groups of four to five students.

ways in which effectiveness might be enhanced. The teller selects and arranges supplementary materials which will be used. Pictures are an important aid in helping primary children to understand stories. The storyteller should also arrange the seating so that there is a closeness and relaxed atmosphere. Visual aids and materials should be set up so that they communicate at the children's eye level.

The class needs to be motivated to listen attentively to the story. One way of doing this is to use an "eye-catching" or "ear-catching" technique to ensure initial attention and a warm emotional climate. The teller then proceeds to unfold the story by dramatizing it enthusiastically. The teller avoids interrupting the story unnecessarily, but allows for some student reaction and response. As with other learning experiences, there is a need to provide for follow-up activities emanating from the story.

Health Games

These are board games, similar in nature to Monopoly®, Concentration®, checkers, ludo, fox and geese, and other commercial games for adults and children. The format and process of playing these board games may be adapted to the health area. Health games should be designed with the idea of helping children to: become more knowledgeable, clarify misconceptions, reinforce positive attitudes, and reinforce or evolve constructive health habits or practices. A good health game has a main theme, such as drug misuse, ecology, water or air pollution, disease control, or other health topics. Tokens, symbols, or colors may be used to represent the players on the board. The purpose of the game is to win while competing against other opponents. The players take turns by throwing dice, spinning an arrow, moving marked staves, or some chance technique. The game should provide for risk taking and acknowledge the consequences of good and bad decisions. Good decisions are rewarded with success; bad decisions need to be penalized by

loss of reward or disaster. The progress of the game should be based on emotional and psychological factors, cultural values, and the benefits of maintaining one's optimal well-being. The game should: be educational in nature, allowing for victory, success, or reward; attempt to solve problems; provide for varying degrees of skill and chance; and be bound by simple rules that allow the game to be completed in a short period of time. Children in the intermediate grades are mature enough to play with and to learn from such games. In playing out the games, children act out their feelings and wishes, and project their understandings of social and health situations.

Teachers and their pupils should create their own games. The quality of a game will depend on the psychological background of the teacher and his or her creativity, knowledge of the subject matter, acquaintance with gamesmanship, and interest in games. For more on this teaching technique, see Sleet and Stadsklev (1977).

Matching Bees

Matching bees may be used to motivate cognitive learning. There are two approaches in the use of matching bees—teacher and pupil. In the teacher matching bee the teacher uses the bee as a visual aid to supplement a lecture. For example, the teacher may use the bee to explain how the digestive system works. A life-size outline drawing of the body is made on a large piece of cardboard. Each part of the digestive system is of a different color, life size, and mobile. The name of each part may be printed on 3" x 12" mobile cards. The function of each part, described in one to three key words, is also printed on a separate mobile card. As the teacher comes to a part of the digestive system, she or he matches the colored part with the proper location on the body, places the name of the part adjacent to it, and finally places the function of the part alongside the name. This procedure, repeated for each of the parts, should not last more than three to four minutes. In

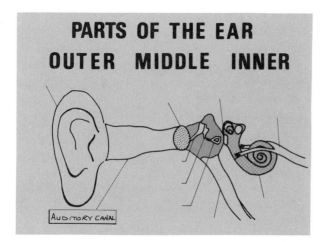

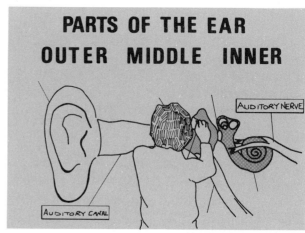

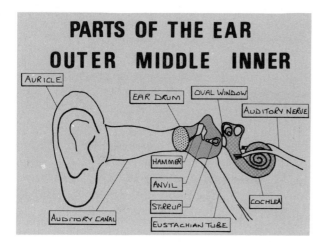

Fig. 12.6   A matching bee on parts of the ear. All of the parts, their names, and the functions are mobile. The three sequences illustrate the progression of the matching bee.

this way the audible explanation is visually reinforced.

The pupil matching bee is similar in technique to the teacher bee. One pupil matches a part, another the name, a third the function, a fourth spells the word, and so on until all of the parts have been matched and all the pupils have had a chance to participate. Pupil matching bees may be run off as competitions, with the class organized into two teams. Rules for playing the matching bee as an educational game may be structured by the class and teacher. It is important that competition not be allowed to destroy the matching bee as an educational game. Winning should be deemphasized.

Matching bees are educational in that children can be motivated to acquire cognitive health skills on their own initiative. They may be adapted to teach about body organs and systems, food groups

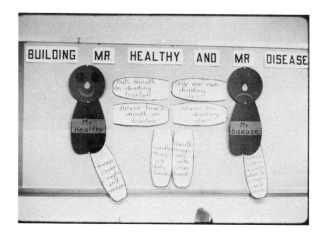

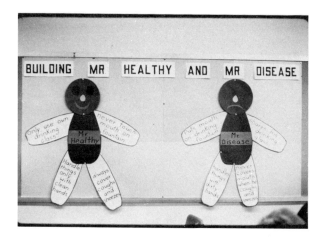

Fig. 12.7 Adapting the matching bee to teach about diseases.

and dieting, and most health topics. As a learning experience, the matching bee surpasses the lecture approach, for pupils are actively involved in this learning process.

INTRODUCTION OF LESSON PLAN

Success in presenting learning experiences effectively is often influenced by how the teacher starts the lesson. An introduction of one to three minutes should create a classroom-topic atmosphere for the main body of the lesson. It should capture the minds, interest, and attention of the children. A few ways of introducing health topics prior to teaching the main body of the lesson are:

1. a simple show-of-hands survey about a behavior or habit;
2. a short quiz and analysis;
3. reading a newspaper clipping or picture reaction;
4. referral to a TV story or film;
5. referral to an accident or happening;
6. referral to readings in a book;
7. carry-over of topic from previous class period;
8. creation of curiosity about the topic through audiovisual materials;
9. demonstration (e.g., disclosing tablet staining unbrushed teeth);
10. follow-up of a homework assignment;
11. asking key questions.

RELATIONSHIP BETWEEN METHODS AND MATERIALS

Materials and teaching aids are part of the process of methodology. It is often difficult to distinguish between the two. A film by itself is a teaching aid. It becomes a part of methodology when children discuss what they saw and heard. Likewise, colored cutout pictures of foods may be used with a flannel board or bulletin board as teaching aids. When these items are used to demonstrate a balanced daily diet, they structure an organized teaching approach, or method. Obviously, materials may be used to facilitate a method. They should make the method more meaningful. Good teachers use a variety of materials and methods. Perhaps, in conclusion, it is wise to think of methods and materials as both contributing to more effective pupil learning experiences. Use of both helps children to make well-being a dynamic and valued force in their lives.

Teaching Aids and Materials

Teaching aids and materials should be used to enrich and to supplement learning experiences. They do not replace the teacher. They are sensory aids to methodology and constitute a medium of communication.

Various terms have been used in reference to teaching materials: supplementary materials, audiovisual aids, multisensory materials, perceptual aids to learning, and instructional materials. Perhaps the safest way of categorizing materials is to say that these are: (1) *printed materials,* such as textbooks and pamphlets, overhead transparencies, workbooks, songs and poems, graphs, flip-charts, flash-cards, and cartoons; and (2) *audiovisual aids,* including motion pictures, filmstrips, various projectors, records, tapes and recorders, photographs, slides, mobiles, models, posters, specimens, bulletin boards, flannel boards, and so on. Printed materials are like a "second" teacher, for they may temporarily remove the burden from the teacher. The latter aids are used by the teacher while actively engaged in teaching.

Materials and aids enrich learning experiences by facilitating communication. They should give the spoken word and printed symbols meaning and life and help children to discover and to extend understandings. They should further help to crystallize sociohygienic concepts, thereby motivating the children toward positive attitudes and habits.

Materials should be varied from time to time. Such change avoids boredom, adds spice to the learning process, and brings forth new freshness and interest. The elementary teacher should also remember that some aids are better than others in doing the job at various grade levels. To children who cannot read, a flat or plain photograph may be more effective than a cluttered-up poster.

The teacher should use materials that help pupils attain desirable outcomes. Materials should be selected with the following criteria in mind. They should:

1. be relevant to the topic and to the grade or maturity level of the students;
2. be clear and focused in presenting the message or idea and not splattered and confusing, with each single message having a central theme or focus.
3. be free from bias;
4. be free from commercial advertising;
5. be attractive and in color, to emphasize highlights and to add interest;
6. present accurate information;
7. use vocabulary and type appropriate for the maturity of the children;
8. be free from sensationalism;
9. help children to conceptualize for well-being;
10. serve a specific purpose, such as to clarify an abstract idea, show a sequence, explain a relationship, or magnify a small part;
11. not have a lot of distracting written information or small pictures (splattered);
12. have balance and proper proportion;
13. be based on identifiable behavioral objectives (pupil outcomes);

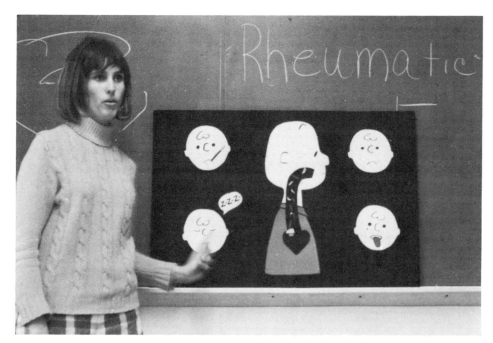

Fig. 12.8 Teaching about the symptoms of rheumatic fever, using Charlie Brown and his facial expressions as the communicatory technique between teacher and class.

14. be short and concise (most films being too long, with most of it cluttered with nonessential and irrelevant information);

15. be prepared with the time limit of the teacher in mind;

16. extend the range of stimuli to several senses.

The elementary teacher should keep in mind that all materials are aids to learning. How valuable and effective an aid is depends on how it is used with children. Many films, filmstrips, and charts have been abused by showing them too often. Likewise, good posters and pictures may have been employed to put a point across, but were not clearly explained to the viewers and hence were not used effectively. Obviously, beginning teachers and others need to be aware of how to use teaching aids properly. Guides for using materials and aids are similar to those suggested for use of sociodramas: (1) selection, (2) preparation, (3) presentation, and (4) follow-up.

Up to now, we have assumed that children will be coming into contact with materials and learning aids inside the classroom. With the advent of television and mass media being consumerized, the classroom has moved outside the school. Commercial television has become a major medium for propagandizing health products. Children can often be expected to learn more about health topics from watching television than from a classroom teacher. Teachers should be aware that this competitive force has the potential of evolving destructive as well as constructive attitudes and habits.

It is virtually impossible to cover adequately all of the health materials and teaching aids and their utilization. There are just too many of them. Instead, prospective teachers are referred to standard books on audiovisual education and other publications for detailed discussion of the various materials and where to obtain them. A list is included at the end of this chapter.

REVIEW QUESTIONS

1. Define teaching, method, and learning experience.
2. How should teachers use teaching strategies?
3. All methods have a basic commonality. What is it?
4. What variables affect the teacher's choice of a method?
5. Is one method of teaching better than another?
6. Which method would you select to teach "coping with problems of living"? Why?
7. How would you teach "effect of vitamins on humans"?
8. Which method is most appropriate to teach "how children feel about cigarette smoking"?
9. What is the difference between a role play and a skit?
10. At what grade level is storytelling most effective?
11. How would you teach parts of an ear? Why?
12. How can you introduce or begin a health lesson?
13. What should you do before showing a film to your students?

REFERENCES AND BIBLIOGRAPHY

Anderson, Paul S. *Story Telling with the Flannel Board*, Book Two (Minneapolis, Minn.: T. S. Denison, 1970).

Berelson, Bernard, and Gary A. Steiner. *Human Behavior: An Inventory of Scientific Findings* (New York: Harcourt, Brace and World, 1964).

Blough, Glenn O., and Julius Schwartz. *Elementary School Science and How to Teach It* (New York: Holt, Rinehart and Winston, 1969).

Broudy, Harry S., and John R. Palmer. *Exemplars of Teaching Method* (Chicago: Rand McNally, 1965).

Chambers, Dewey W. *Storytelling and Creative Drama* (Dubuque, Iowa: W. C. Brown, 1970).

Davis, Morton D. *Game Theory* (New York: Basic Books, 1970).

Gage, N. L. *Handbook of Research on Teaching* (Chicago: Rand McNally, 1965).

Goodwin, Arthur B. *Handbook of Audio-Visual Aids and Techniques for Teaching Elementary School Subjects* (West Nyack, N.Y.: Parker, 1969).

Hilgard, Ernest R., and Gordon H. Bower. *Theories of Learning* (New York: Appleton-Century-Crofts, 1966).

Hoyman, Howard S. *Teacher's Manual: Your Health and Safety* (New York: Harcourt, Brace and World, 1963).

Huey, J. Frances. *Teaching Primary Children.* (New York: Holt, Rinehart and Winston, 1965).

Humphrey, James H., Warren R. Johnson, and Virginia D. Moore. *Elementary School Health Education* (New York: Harper and Brothers, 1962).

Hyman, Ronald T. *Ways of Teaching* (Philadelphia: Lippincott, 1970).

Irwin, Leslie W., Harold J. Cornacchia, and Wesley M. Staton. *Health in Elementary Schools* (St. Louis: C. V. Mosby, 1966).

Klausmeier, H. J., and K. Dresden. *Teaching in the Elementary School* (New York: Harper and Brothers, 1962).

Means, Richard K. *Methodology in Education* (Columbus, Ohio: Charles E. Merrill, 1968).

Oberteuffer, Delbert, Orvis A. Harrelson, and Marion B. Pollock. *School Health Education* (New York: Harper & Row, 1972).

Phenix, Philip H. *Realms of Meaning* (New York: McGraw-Hill, 1964).

Platt, Ellen S., Ellen Krassen, and Bernard Mausner. "Individual Variation in Behavioral Change Following Role Playing," *Psychological Reports* 24 (1969): 155-170.

Rash, Keogh J. *The Health Education Curriculum* (Bloomington: Indiana University Press, 1965).

Selberg, Edith M., Louise A. Neal, and Mathew F. Vessel. *Discovering Science in the Elementary School* (Reading, Mass.: Addison-Wesley, 1970).

Sleet, David A. and Ron Stadsklev. "Annotated Bibliography of Simulations and Games in Health Education," *Health Education Monographs* **5** (1977): 75-90.

Veneker, Harold, ed. *Synthesis of Research in Health Education* (Washington, D.C.: School Health Education Association, and National Education Association, 1964).

Victor, Edward. *Science for the Elementary School* (Toronto: Macmillan, 1970).

Weaver, Gilbert G., and Louis Cenci. *Applied Teaching Techniques* (New York: Pitman, 1960).

Willgoose, Carl E. *Health Education in the Elementary School* (Philadelphia: Saunders, 1969).

Audiovisual Resources for Health Instruction

Beyrer, Mary K., Ann E. Nolte, and Marian K. Solleder. *A Directory of Selected References and Resources for Health Instruction* (Minneapolis, Minn.: Burgess, 1966).

Brown, J. W. *et al. Instruction, Materials and Methods* (New York: McGraw-Hill, 1964).

Children's Record Reviews, Box 192, Woodmere, New York.

Dale, E. *Audio-Visual Methods in Teaching* (New York: Holt, Rinehart and Winston, 1964).

Educational Film Guide, ed. Joseph S. Antonini (New York: H. W. Wilson).

Educator's Guide to Free Filmstrips, ed. Mary Foley Horkheimer and John W. Diffor (Randolph, Wis.: Educators Progress Service, 1971).

Hulfick, James W., Jr. *The Audio-Visual Equipment Directory* (Fairfax, Va: National Audio-Visual Association).

Hunter, Donald C., and Henry C. Wohlers. *Air Pollution Experiments for Junior and Senior High School Science Classes* (Pittsburgh: Air Pollution Control Association, 1969).

Perry, Margaret. *Rainy Day Magic* (New York: Evans, 1970).

Schultz, Morton J. *The Teacher and Overhead Projection* (Englewood Cliffs, N.J.: Prentice-Hall, 1965).

The Educational Media Index (New York: McGraw-Hill).

UNESCO. *UNESCO Source Book for Science Teaching* (Paris: Place de Fontenay, 1962).

Weaver, Elbert C., ed. *Scientific Experiments in Environmental Pollution* (New York: Holt, Rinehart and Winston, 1968).

Textbooks

Elementary Health

Bauer, W. W., *et al. Curriculum Foundation Series* (Grades 1-8) (Chicago: Scott, Foresman).

Byrd, Oliver E., *et al. The New Road to Health Series* (Grades 1-8) (River Forest, Ill.: Laidlaw Brothers).

Cornwell, Oliver K., and Leslie W. Irwin. *My Health Book Series* (Grades 3-8) (Chicago: Lyons and Carnahan).

Hallock, Grace T., *et al. Health for Better Living Series* (Grades 1-8) (Boston: Ginn).

Irwin, Leslie W., *et al. Dimensions in Health Series* (Grades 1-8) (Chicago: Lyons and Carnahan).

Schneider, Herman, and Nina Schneider. *Health Science Series* (Grades K-8) (Boston: D. C. Heath).

Wilcox, Charlotte E., *et al. The Health Action Series* (Grades 1-8) (Chicago: Benefic Press).

Wilson, Charles C., and Elizabeth A. Wilson. *Health for Young America Series* (Grades 1-8) (Indianapolis: Bobbs-Merrill).

References Supplying Enrichment Ideas in Health Science

Children's Journals and Magazines

Child Life

Jack and Jill

Ranger Rick's Nature Magazine

Sesame Street

Wee Wisdom

Textbooks

Barrows, Marjorie, ed. *The Children's Hour: First Story Book* (New York: Grolier, 1966). (Series of 17.)

Childcraft. *Poems and Rhymes*, Vol. 1 (Chicago: Field Enterprises Educational Corporation, 1972).

———. *Stories and Fables.* Vol. 2 (Chicago: Field Enterprises Educational Corporation, 1972).

Rees, Ennis. *Fables From Aesop* (New York: Oxford University Press, 1966).

Plays

The Drama Magazine for Young People

Films

Proper Use of Films

Before showing a film to a class, the teacher should prepare as follows:

1. Order the film at least a month before scheduled date of showing so that the film will arrive a few days early and allow the teacher to:

   a) Preview the film the first time, in order to:

      (1) Become acquainted with it.

      (2) Decide whether it is appropriate for the class level.

   b) Preview a film a second time to:

      (1) Pin-point just what the students should look for.

      (2) Discover the main points of the film.

      (3) Be able to draw up a questionnaire, test, or work sheet based on this film.

2. Before showing film to the class:

   a) Explain what to look for.

   b) Give a questionnaire or work sheet to the class and then collect these at the end of the period; the results will help the teacher to evaluate the film.

3. During the film:

   a) Stop the film to correct facts.

   b) Stop the film to clarify facts.

   c) Give a work sheet to the class to respond to during the film.

4. After the film has been shown:

   a) Plan to have a short discussion or question-and-answer period about the film (follow-up).

   b) Relate the film to the topic or unit taken up in class.

   c) Have the class complete the preplanned work sheet, test, or questionnaire.

    d) Be prepared to show the film a second time if there is an additional need and time permits.

5. DO NOT:

    a) Show the film without any previous preparation.

    b) Show the film only and avoid discussion after it.

    c) Show the film unless you have told the students what to look for in the film.

    d) Show the film as a substitute for teaching a subject.

    e) Show the film if there is a better way of presenting the same information.

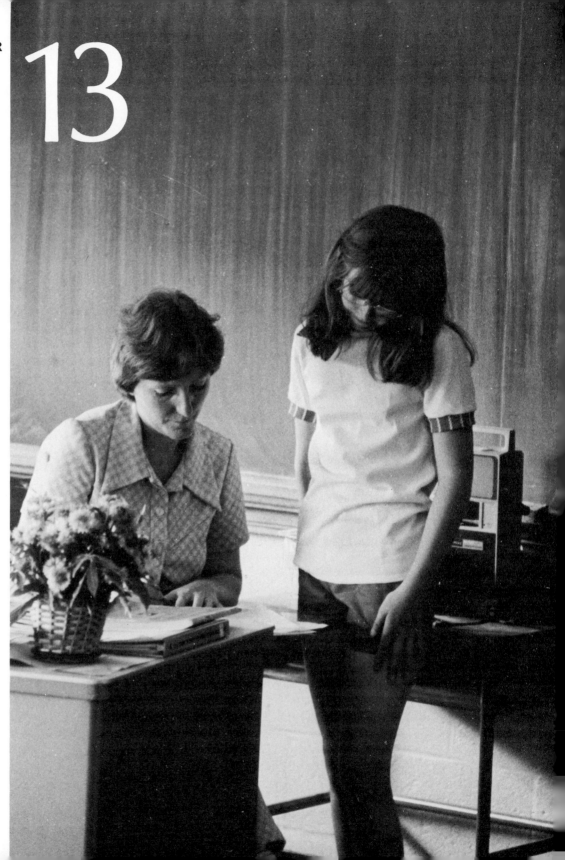

instructional accountability

INTRODUCTION

Assessment is one of the most controversial topics in American education. The already overburdened average tax-paying parent is more than ever concerned about the quality and quantity of the education his or her child receives. Administrators are continually under pressure to literally prove the effectiveness of their programs. Institutions of higher learning are presently taking a harder line than ever on admission requirements, much to the dismay of open-admission advocates. Younger and younger students are rebelling against the traditional grading system and avidly advocating such alternative approaches as a credit/no credit system of grading, which removes the pressure of grades and allows the student to explore those learning experiences most appropriate to his or her needs and interests. One thing is for sure: As a prospective teacher, you are undoubtedly destined to be confronted with your share of difficulties directly related to evaluation. It is our opinion that you will find your personal philosophy relative to evaluation changing numerous times as you progress through your neophyte years of teaching.

In an effort to explore this important issue, we must first come to grips with some of the more basic questions relative to the concept of evaluation. Thus we will attempt to determine just what evaluation is, why it is important, and how it is implemented.

EVALUATION DEFINED

Unfortunately, the term "evaluation" is more often than not misused by many educators. What is often referred to as evaluation is little more than testing or the score obtained by a student responding to a test instrument. For clarity, we need to differentiate among the terms testing, measurement, and evaluation (see Table 13.1).

Testing

Testing can and should be defined as the actual process of utilizing tests. Emphasis is placed on the instrument used in the process. Such techniques as observation, checklists, inventories, question-

209

Table 13.1   Interrelationship of testing, measurement, and education.

Term	Definition	Concept	Point of reference
Testing	Procedure of systematizing observations, e.g., a 25-question multiple-choice nutrition examination for fifth graders.	Instrument (tool)	Tests, check lists, rating scales, observation, etc.
Measurement	Assigning symbolic significance, e.g., a score of 95 percent.	Score (quantity)	Rank, status, classification comparison, etc.
Evaluation	Determining the worth of measurement, e.g., the number of scores above 95, the mean score for the test, etc.	Value (quality)	Goals, objectives, expected outcomes

naires, rating scales, interviews, tests, etc., are accented. The administration of a 25-question multiple-choice test about nutrition to a fifth-grade class would exemplify "testing."

Measurement

Measurement implies making a quantitative expression in answer to the question "How much?" Essentially, we are assigning numerals to a criterion according to a preconceived set of rules. Functions such as ranking, classification, comparison, description of status, or change and prediction are all implied by the definition above. A multitude of techniques or test instruments may be employed to fulfill these functions. One might consider the use of several kinds of tests such as rating scales and score cards as well as systematic observation to measure achievement. When all is said and done, measurement is probably best referred to as a condition of quantity. For example, if the highest score on the multiple-choice nutrition test discussed above is 95 percent, the score 95 can be termed a measurement.

Evaluation

Evaluation is far more complex than either testing or measurement. Compared to the quantity connotations of measurement, evaluation can be said to be more related to value and quality. The suggestion is that evaluation deals with questions and judgments of worth rather than amount. Evaluation should be thought of as a much more inclusive process, a process whereby quantitive statements are incorporated en route to ultimate value judgments.

When you actually think about it, the evaluation of public schools is an age-old process. Right or wrong, good or bad, evaluation finally is taking place around us. Anyone who has ever attended school—and all of us have—will in most cases find it quite easy to discuss the drawbacks and merits of American education. The average person on the corner can tell you exactly how he or she thinks schools ought to be run and will most likely add, "it ain't like it used to be in the good old days." There never has been, and surely never will be, a lack of both good and bad evaluation in education.

PURPOSES OF EVALUATION

Education is frequently conceptualized as a process comprised of three major elements: the determination of objectives, the planning and organization of learning experiences and materials for fullfilling these objectives, and the evaluation of the educational program. Figure 13.1 shows the interplay among these major elements and their relationship to the ongoing process of elementary health education.

The premise above raises many evaluative-type questions about elementary health education. For example, what is happening as a result of our instruction? Are we accomplishing what we set out to achieve? Is what we are doing helpful to students? Most authorities would agree that effective evaluation can answer these questions. However, there has been a great deal of controversy and mixed emotion as to just what is the best, most productive technique for answering assessment-type questions. More on approaches to evaluation later.

Being specific, let us now explore some of the more obvious reasons why we evaluate health instruction.

1. Perhaps one of the most important purposes of evaluation is to assist in the *diagnosis* and/or *classification* of pupils who are in need of special help. In addition to indicating a need for help, evaluation might also determine the specific kind of help needed by the youngster.

The health services aspect of the school health program provides an excellent reference point. The youngster failing to meet the minimum standards for the Snellan Eye Test (most often administered by the school nurse as a screening device) is referred for a more comprehensive eye examination. Let's say that the youngster is found to be nearsighted and is required to procure corrective glasses. The conscientious teacher would take advantage of this evaluatory information and seat the child in the front of the classroom so as to assist the youngster in dealing with his or her affliction.

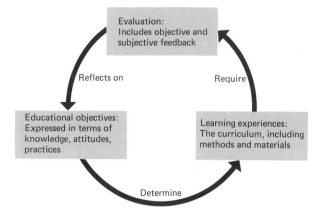

Fig. 13.1 Interplay of the three major elements of the educational process and their relationship to elementary health education.

The concept of diagnosis can also be viewed in another way. The teacher may very well want to use an examination to introduce a unit of study in an effort to determine just what the class already knows and does not know about the topic. Data of this nature can be helpful in determining where the greatest amount of instructional emphasis should be placed. Periodic evaluation of this nature can also be helpful with updating a course of study.

2. Evaluation can be thought of as *accountability*. Without some form of accountability, we can never really be sure whether or not our preconceived educational objectives have been attained. With reference to health education, we are concerned with whether our students are improving their health behavior, attitudes, and knowledge. The dedicated teacher wants to know if his or her teaching has been effective. Meaningful evaluation of instruction can be helpful in providing a valid indication of the effectiveness of the teacher's effort.

The task is one of assessing pupil progress. True appraisal of changes in health knowledge, attitudes, and practices resulting from organized classroom learning experiences is no easy task. Building on the concept of evaluation as diagnosis, the teacher could administer the same test instrument at both the beginning and end of the unit and then determine if there was any change in the domain being evaluated. There is no question but that such an approach lends itself in a more realistic fashion to the cognitive domain. Objective measurement of change in the affective and action domains is very difficult. In fact, it is next to impossible to objectively assess attitudes and behavior, a subject we will address later.

3. For those still operating within a traditional numerical-oriented grading system, sound knowledge tests provide *objective information on which to base grades*. This particular approach to evaluation has come under the greatest criticism of late at the elementary school level. Today, there appears to be a strong trend away from the categorical approach to grading at the elementary level. Instead, more and more emphasis is being placed on the descriptive analysis of each child's academic progress, thus eliminating the traditional grading approach. However, it is obvious that it is still necessary to effectively measure cognitive progress if any meaningful descriptive evaluation is to be employed. So although letter grades may be eliminated, testing may very well still play a large role in the evaluation process.

4. Some educators steadfastly assert that evaluative devices (tests) are excellent *motivational devices* for students. Certainly tests can be challenging and educationally rewarding for many students—perhaps all students under the right conditions. But by the same token, tests can be a most deadening influence on other students. Needless to say, then, this purpose of evaluation is highly controversial. All too often our opinion is influenced by our own past success with educational measurement. It is indeed sad to see the teacher who attempts to use testing as a prime motivating force for his or her students. If tests were taken away from this type of teacher, what control would she or he have over the class? Misguided rationale such as this on the part of the teacher is most unprofessional.

Summary

Evaluation should be thought of as a means to an end, not an end in itself. The greatest value of evaluation lies in the use to which it is put. Properly implemented evaluation in health education can be diagnostic in nature, provide for accountability, be used as a basis for letter-grade assignment if necessary, and perhaps even be motivational if realistically approached. Keep in mind that evaluation in health education is far more than *how much* the child knows.

Just as important is how the child feels and what she or he does about health matters. This is what makes meaningful evaluation of health education such a difficult task. Although most teachers easily develop the ability to measure students' health knowledge, much skill is required to develop effective techniques that can validly measure their health practices and attitudes.

Health knowledge has long been considered a basis for health behavior. Proponents of this theory have argued that what the child knows will have a strong bearing on how she or he feels and will act in health matters. No doubt a person adhering to such a philosophy would place a great deal of emphasis on how much the child knows about health. However, there is little evidence to support such a theory. Knowledge is just one of the many influential factors affecting health behavior, and given the multitude of avoidable health problems clearly evident in our enlightened American culture today, one wonders how important it really is. No doubt knowledge is important, but just as important are how the youngster feels and actually behaves. Ideally, we should strive to evaluate students' health practices and attitudes as conscientiously as we do their health knowledge.

PRINCIPLES OF EVALUATION

It is impossible to list a standard set of evaluation procedures that can be applied to health education. The variety of conditions and situations unique to each health teaching assignment precludes the establishment of a step-by-step format to evaluation. However, it is possible to discuss the generally accepted principles of evaluation. The neophyte teacher would do well to ponder the following considerations before endeavoring to assess any aspect of the school health program. Ask yourself:

1. Have I formalized myself with the instructional objectives or expected outcomes of the lesson, unit, or course I am attempting to evaluate?

2. In light of my response to question 1, have I precisely defined what it is I want to measure and eventually evaluate?

3. Do I have the insight and ability to select the most appropriate form of measurement?

4. Do I possess the skill to develop reliable and valid assessment tools?

5. Am I capable of analyzing, interpreting, and eventually evaluating the results of my measurement activities?

6. Am I dedicated enough to apply my findings and conclusions to future situations when applicable?

Failure to consider the principles above will more than likely yield faulty evaluation. This is unfortunate, given the importance of evaluation in terms of the time it consumes and the ultimate influence it has on the student. Indeed, poor and misguided evaluation is probably worse than no evaluation at all.

Although we cannot here present the fine points of sound tests and measurement, we are in no way minimizing the importance of educational assessment. To the contrary, we encourage every prospective teacher to develop competencies in the area of measurement along the lines of the principles listed above. Should your teacher-education program not require a measurement course as a prerequisite to your degree, we would encourage you to seek a measurement course that will assist you in procuring the necessary competencies in this important area.

METHODS OF APPRAISING HEALTH ATTITUDES AND PRACTICES

If you were asked to list the most popular form of evaluation utilized by teachers today, what would your answer be? If it is paper-and-pencil knowledge tests, you are right. In many instances this is the only form of evaluation utilized by the teacher. Such an inflexible approach is unacceptable in health education. Health is a way of life, and mere knowledge is only one aspect of the health-educated person. To rightfully do the topic justice, it is necessary to assess student health practices and attitudes as well as knowledge. Following are several suggested approaches to the evaluation of health education at the elementary level.

Observation

One of the easiest and most meaningful forms of evaluation is observation. Actions do speak louder than words, and the observant teacher can perceive a great deal about a youngster's health practices and attitudes. The creative teacher can even go so far as to foster environmental situations that will provide for the opportunity to observe students' health behavior. By critically observing typical everyday situations, we can determine if our instruction has had any significant impact on our students' health behavior.

The implications for such an approach are endless and far-reaching. Whenever beginning a health unit, the teacher simply decides what he or she would regard as a change in student health behavior after the unit has been completed. Since the expected outcomes listed for each lesson plan are for the most part behaviorally stated, they offer the type of direction needed to determine the observable behavior for which the teacher might watch.

From a more practical standpoint, let us consider the following example. You are undertaking a unit of study in nutrition with your fourth-grade class. One of the expected outcomes of the day's lesson is stated: "Is capable of selecting a balanced meal." Once the instruction is complete, the teacher merely observes the quality of the eating practices exhibited by the students in the lunchroom. Due to the fact that cafeteria lunches purchased by the child are already balanced, it would be advantageous to reserve evaluation for the days when the youngster brings his or her own lunch.

The possibilities for evaluation of this sort are unlimited. Every content area of elementary health education offers an opportunity for teacher observation and subsequent evaluation. Perhaps the only drawback of observation is that it is subjective in nature and more prone to error and bias. However, every effort can be made to clarify and define observation by knowing precisely what one is looking for. By adhering to the previously stated principles of evaluation and maintaining a critical and precise attitude about what is being observed, the elementary teacher can ascertain a great deal about the health practices of his or her students.

Conferences

A one-to-one conference can be a most effective technique for learning about a youngster's health attitudes and practices. In keeping with Glasser's comments relative to "involvement" (1969), the warm, empathic teacher is capable of establishing a rapport with students, becoming both friend and confidant. Such a relationship is conducive to learning about a student's health behavior. It also provides an excellent opportunity for the teacher to determine if there are any hidden problems. Oftentimes the student will refrain from discussing his or her health feelings or behavior in front of the class for fear of being embarrassed. By the same token, the teacher should be careful not to purposefully raise any question about a student's health behavior in front of the class if it might prove embarrassing for the youngster. Such inquiries are better left to individual conferences. The teacher's job is to assist young people in developing their maximum health potential. If individual conferences can contribute to this goal, they are worthy of implementation. Based on the results of such a conference, the teacher will, ideally, be able to evaluate any problems and proceed accordingly.

Self-Evaluation

Student input is becoming more of an issue with each passing day, and rightfully so. A student who is allowed to be a part of the evaluation process cannot help but be motivated to get involved. When the measurement activity is developed by the student or as a result of a group endeavor, it is likely to be much more meaningful to the student.

Primary-grade children are entirely capable of developing simple checklists or rating scales for evaluating individual or group health behavior. The teacher simply intervenes to act as the class facilitator for developing the instrument to be utilized in the self-evaluation process. Once the instrument is developed, the students simply introduce it and rate their own health behavior.

Intermediate and junior high school students find it more challenging to develop their own expected outcomes, learning experiences, and accountability techniques. Much to the amazement of many teachers, students will often be more difficult on themselves than the teacher would have been. Motivation can also be greatly enhanced. Care should be taken when such an approach is pursued to be sure that students build in feasible and attainable accountability factors. It is relatively easy for students to become overzealous and set their sights too high. The teacher's role is one of mediator and guide.

Even with all that has been said above, do not be surprised if your first attempt at introducing self-evaluation falls far short of your expectations. This will be especially true if the students have never attempted it before. Keep in mind that students are academically socialized to expect direction from the teacher. When the roles are reversed, most students are overwhelmed with the situation and respond rather erratically.

However, the more that students are subjected to such an approach, the more proficient they will become in dealing with self-evaluation. In the long run, the benefits in terms of motivation and personal satisfaction will far outweigh the detriments of any initial confusion and uncertainty. Modern psychology and democratic social values both hold that important educational strides can be achieved by eliciting student participation in evaluation. The present trend in education will continue to place more and more responsibility on students themselves for evaluating their own achievement. If such an endeavor is taken seriously by both the teacher and student and every effort is made to make it as valid as possible, there is no question but that self-evaluation can be a most desirable activity.

Checklists and Rating Scales

Checklists and rating scales are excellent questionnaire techniques of evaluation, especially when used to supplement self-evaluation. In essence, they serve as self-inventories and can be easily developed to assist in the evaluation of health practices. Use of a checklist or rating scale makes assessment more objective. Hence order and continuity are added to the evaluation process.

Health checklists and rating scales are similar in nature. Both are designed to ultimately seek an indication of the quality and quantity of the student's health behavior. The main difference lies in degrees of measurement. More precisely, the checklist requires only a simple yes or no answer. The respondent either is or is not performing a particular health practice.

We can turn our attention to the various charts and checklists presented in this text for examples of this type of evaluative tool. The Well-being Inventory in Chapter 16 requires the children to make a self-assessment of their physical, emotional, and social fitness. In Chapter 21 the chart entitled "Are My Meals Balanced?" asks the child to judge the degree to which his or her diet is well balanced. The picture quizzes on bicycle safety in Chapter 23 and the picture quiz on how to avoid a cold (Chapter 24) provide examples in which a variation on the theme has been developed. The inventory "Do You Help?" in Chapter 25 also reflects the pictorial approach to self-evaluation.

In addition, key questions of the type suggested following various lesson plans are direct-questioning techniques which can be aimed at making the students evaluate their own health practices.

Rating scales differ from checklists in that more response latitude is provided. The factor of degrees is introduced. Often a straight yes or no response does not completely or correctly answer the question being asked. Rating scales attempt to offset such a possibility by adding more response categories. The traffic safety education rating scale for the primary grades shown on the following page provides us with an example.

If all of the statements are expressed in a positive manner, numerical values can be easily assigned to the response alternatives. Such an approach adds a quantitative aspect which can be helpful to the evaluation process. The category "always" can be assigned three points; "usually," two points; "seldom," one point; and "never," a zero. A total score can be determined by simply adding the values for each response. With "always" being the most desirable response, the best possible score becomes 27 points. The teacher and students

	Always	Usually	Seldom	Never
1. I cross streets only at marked crosswalks and refrain from jaywalking.				
2. When I do cross at a marked intersection, I am sure that all traffic is stopped and that I can make the entire crossing safely.				
3. I obey "walk" and "don't walk" signals.				
4. I obey the safety patrol and traffic officers.				
5. I walk my bicycle across intersections.				
6. I do not play in the street.				
7. I enter and get out of cars on the curb side.				
8. If I must walk in the road, I do so facing traffic.				
9. If I am out at night and near traffic, I wear white or carry a light.				

could then establish ranges for evaluation purposes. It might look something like the following:

1. A perfect score of 27: Excellent traffic safety practices.
2. 22-26 points: Good traffic safety practices, but room for improvement.
3. 21 and below: You are an excellent candidate for an accident, and you will probably have one unless you quickly improve your traffic safety practices.

In conclusion, the use to which checklists and rating scales are put is most important. Only the most naive teacher would ask students to engage in such an activity and then use the results for grading purposes. Such an approach would only encourage students to be dishonest in their responses, and both the student's and the teacher's time would be wasted. To the contrary, students should be made well aware of the fact that such an undertaking will not be graded and that the entire experience is designed for them to assess their personal health practices and benefit from recognition of their particular levels of well-being. Obviously, the teacher can and should derive some input in terms of secondary evaluation by viewing the responses of the students. The results do reflect on the effect of the teaching that has preceded the checklist or rating scale.

Any evaluation that is derived should be twofold. On the one hand the teacher can ascertain the status of the student's health practices with regard to a particular aspect of health education. In light of these findings, future instruction can be altered if necessary. On the other hand, the child is afforded an opportunity to truthfully evaluate his or her own health practices and, ideally, make adjustments where necessary.

Summary

It is no secret that health attitudes and practices are exceedingly difficult to measure and evaluate accurately. Nevertheless, the overall importance of positive health attitudes and practices requires assessment, if only to assist in the evaluation of the health instruction taking place in terms of content, learning experiences, and teaching aids. Rationale such as this is based on the premise that health practices reflect health attitudes and understandings. As the child grows older, this statement takes on added meaning. The concept of developmental tasks (see Chapter 2) can be considered the ''key'' to successful teaching for health attitudes and practices. The most successful instruction is that which is timely. By introducing those activities (health practice learning experiences) that are most appropriate to the youngster's developmental level, there is an excellent chance of fostering positive health habits that very well may last a lifetime.

Evaluating all of this is another story. Unfortunately, all one can really do is attempt to evaluate the immediate behavioral results of health instruction. From a practical standpoint, the best the teacher can do is to evaluate the change in student health behavior over the span of the academic year. But this can be deceiving, because health behavior hardly begins or ends in the classroom, and worse yet, some health behavior cannot even be evaluated during the school years. The outcome of some health instruction may not be measurable for years to come and consequently never is evaluated. To add to the dilemma is the fact that health behavior is so greatly influenced by elements outside the classroom. Peer-group pressure, advertising, parental influence, the church, and all other environmental forces have an effect on health behavior. The direct health instruction that takes place in the classroom is only one of the many factors influencing students' health behavior. Ideally, the other factors influencing the child's health practices and attitudes will supplement and reinforce the school's activities.

In conclusion, it can be said that carefully planned, systematic, and ongoing evaluation of students' health practices and attitudes can be helpful in providing guidance and direction for classroom learning experiences. Use of the preceding methods of appraisal should prove helpful to the teacher in performing such a task.

METHODS OF APPRAISING HEALTH KNOWLEDGE

The assessment of health knowledge presents far less of a problem than does the challenge of evaluating health attitudes and practices. It is in the cognitive domain that the teacher can be most effective in evaluating. However, the basic philosophical question is: How useful and meaningful is evaluation in this area? We have already discussed the argument that knowledge alone does not necessarily mean that the student will practice wise health behavior. But then again, no one has yet conclusively proved that knowledge is not a prerequisite to an intelligent decision regarding health behavior. For example, it is logical to assume that if a person does not know that a vaccine exists for polio he or she may never become immunized or see that his or her children are inoculated. Such an outcome is as unfortunate as the one for the person who knows better, but still fails to act in a positive fashion. Keeping in mind the ultimate goal of health education (intelligent self-direction in health matters), it follows that students should acquire certain basic knowledge that will, ideally, influence their health behavior in a favorable way. This acquisition of knowledge is truly an objective of health education and rightfully should be subjected to evaluation as are the other areas.

In substance, the point of importance is that the evaluation of health knowledge is only one aspect of health education evaluation. Actually, it can be thought of as sharing equal billing with the evaluation of health practices and attitudes.

Constructing Teacher-Made Tests

Teacher-made paper-and-pencil tests are the most common approach to evaluating pupil health

Table 13.2 Summary of the advantages of essay and short-answer tests. A plus sign indicates the type judged to be superior as far as the factors listed are concerned.

Factor	Essay	Short-answer
Reliability of scoring		+
Adequacy of sampling student achievement		+
Labor required to prepare	+	
Labor required to score		+
Providing opportunity for student to select, organize, and integrate	+	
Providing opportunity to test effective writing	+	
Possibility for bluffing, "writing around the topic"		+
Opportunity for guessing	+	
Freedom from distortion of grading by skill in expression and quality of handwriting	+	

From p. 223 of *A Practical Introduction to Measurement and Evaluation,* 2nd Edition, by H. H. Remmers, N. L. Gage, and J. F. Rummel, Copyright, 1943, 1955 by H. H. Remmers and N. L. Gage. Copyright © 1960 by Harper and Row Publishers, Inc. Copyright © 1965 by H. H. Remmers, N. L. Gage, & J. Francis Rummel. Reprinted by permission.

knowledge. Examinations developed on the basis of recognized principles of test construction can be an effective means of evaluating both health knowledge and understanding. The teacher-made paper-and-pencil test can take one or two forms, or a combination of both if so desired. We refer specifically to the *short answer*–type test and the *essay* examination.

Both types of examinations have their merits, as pointed out by the summary comparison table (Table 13.2) found in Remmers, Gage, and Rummel (1965).

The following discussion is an attempt to examine precisely both essay and short-answer tests, with the express purpose of exploring the philosophy underlying each.

Essay Examinations

A good essay examination requires the student to organize his or her thoughts in a logical sequence and to support that position. It requires the student to reveal his or her general grasp of the subject matter being tested and to organize and express facts and documented opinion forthrightly.

In an effort to explore the type of essay questions that can be used for evaluation purposes, Monroe and Carter's (see Remmers, Gage, and Rummel, 1965, pp. 225–226) list of the types of essay questions was modified to apply to health education and is presented below:*

1. *Selective recall—basis given:* How can heart disease interfere with a normal lifestyle?

2. *Evaluative recall—basis given:* What do you consider are the five most important dental health practices in helping to prevent caries?

3. *Comparison of two things—on a single designated basis:* Compare the effects of stimulants and depressants on the central nervous system.

4. *Comparison of two things—in general:* Compare the definitions of chronic and communicable diseases.

* Excerpts from *A Practical Introduction to Measurement and Evaluation,* 2nd Edition, by H. H. Remmers, N. L. Gage, & J. Francis Rummel, Copyright 1943, 1955 by H. H. Remmers and N. L. Gage. Copyright © 1960 by Harper & Row, Publishers, Inc. Copyright © 1965 by H. H. Remmers, N. L. Gage, & J. Francis Rummel. Reprinted by permission.

5. *Decision—for or against:* Should marijuana be legalized? Support your opinion.

6. *Causes or effects:* How can cigarette smoking cause lung cancer?

7. *Explanation of the use or exact meaning of some phase in a passage:* Explain how digestion takes place.

8. *Summary of a unit of the text or of an article read:* Explain briefly the definition of mental health as stated by the National Association for Mental Health.

9. *Analysis:* Analyze the tobacco-smoking controversy. How did a health practice that is so harmful become so popular?

10. *Statement of relationship:* Why is health behavior important to lifestyle?

11. *Illustration or examples of principles:* Illustrate the correct procedure for mouth-to-mouth resuscitation.

12. *Classification (usually the converse of number 11):* Classify the following drugs according to category and cite their effects: heroin, amphetamine, barbiturate, LSD, etc.

13. *Application of rules or principles:* If one is attempting to lose weight, what principles of caloric intake must be applied?

14. *Discussion:* Discuss the functions of the skeletal system.

15. *Statement of aim:* Why is it important to understand how to select a proper diet?

16. *Criticism:* What is wrong with the following meal, and what would you add or delete to improve it?

17. *Outline:* Outline the four food groups and list two examples of each.

18. *Reorganization of facts:* After gleaning the following list of factual type statements about nutrition (some are not true), select the most appropriate and organize them into a paragraph.

19. *Formulation of new questions:* Based on your response to question 13, what other factors could theoretically influence weight control?

20. *New methods of procedure:* How would you approach the problem of drug abuse in the United States?

Note that several of these essay-type questions can also be easily converted to short-answer questions in the form of completion or simple-recall items.

Once the essay examination has been formulated and administered, the teacher is confronted with the issue of grading the essay examination. In an effort to make the process as objective as possible, the teacher should consider:

1. Grading the papers on an anonymous basis. That way the factor of teacher-student relationship is reduced, and the papers are graded on merit. The object is to eliminate as much prejudice as possible. By simply asking the students to sign their examinations on the back, the teacher does not know whose paper he or she is grading. (Unfortunately, as the year progresses, the teacher becomes more familiar with students' writing ability and style, and this approach may not be of as much value.)

2. By grading only one question at a time, the teacher can more precisely compare one student's answer to a given question with all other answers to that question.

3. It is important that prior provisions be made relative to sentence structure, paragraphing, spelling, and writing ability. If we are to consider such criteria in an evaluation, we must decide whether such an approach is consistent with our educational objectives or expected outcomes. If it is not, such variables should not be considered in the grading process. In any event, the teacher should consciously make a decision on this point prior to administration of the examination and tell the students of the decision.

4. Questions to be included on the essay examination should be given careful thought by the teacher during the construction process and be worded so as to call for definite and precise answers. Once this task is complete, the teacher should prepare model answers to the questions. The model answers are developed in an effort to establish pertinent points. Ideally, the student will provide each of the pertinent points in his or her answers. To score each question, the teacher simply compares the main points made by the student on each question with those formulated for the key (teacher's copy). A quantitative value is then awarded on the basis of the student's response.

Conclusion.   Even when the suggestions above are implemented, the essay examination is still notoriously difficult to score fairly and consistently. Most of the many inherent factors that will bias the grading process are not at all related to the quality of the student's answer to the question—e.g., spelling, handwriting, general appearance of the paper; when examination is graded; the scorer's fatigue, knowledge about the student's previous performances and overall ability; the student's ability to academically write around the question with eloquence rather than facts. All of these factors can drastically influence the subjective process of grading essay examinations. Keep in mind that it is also a laborious and time-consuming job to grade a number of essay examinations. Not to mention the fact that when compared to short-answer tests, much less of a sample of student achievement is obtained from essay examinations.

Obviously there are many drawbacks to essay examinations. But there are also advantages that should be considered. Essay examinations provide the student with a splendid opportunity to display his or her ability to analyze a situation and prepare a well-founded solution. It is this kind of thought process that students appear to be particularly weak in today. Apparently students are afforded less and less of an opportunity to react to the essay-type examination. The skill of organizing one's thoughts and expressing them in written form is like any other skill; it must be practiced if it is to be maintained and improved. As teachers, we are failing to contribute to the overall academic development of our students if we totally shun essay-type examinations in favor of short-answer tests. Perhaps the most sensible and helpful approach is a careful blending of the two types.

Short-Answer Examinations

Ebel (1965) discusses two major types of short-answer test items—the *supply* and *selection* types. The student is asked to provide the words, numbers, or symbols in the first case and to choose an answer from given alternatives in the latter.

Supply-Type Questions.   This type of question is best constructed as either a simple question or a completion-type statement.

> *Direct question:* What overt effect do alcoholic beverages have on the central nervous system?_____
> _____ .
>
> *Completion:* From a nutrient standpoint, bread is best classified as a _____.

The supply-type test item has both advantages and disadvantages. On the plus side, this type of item almost entirely eliminates the possibility of guessing. It is also relatively easy to construct because it is merely the extension of a natural question. The testee simply answers the question or completes the statement.

In terms of the disadvantages, the supply-type item slights the handling of complicated concepts. It is somewhat limited to identifying, naming, or associating facts. In other words, it tends to be shallow in achievement sampling. In addition, some objectivity can be easily lost when a student answers a question in a manner different from the suggested form (the answer on the test key), and his or her answer is every bit as correct as the teacher's answer.

Selection-Type Items. This type of examination can take several forms.

> *Constant alternatives (true-false):*   T   F   It is always best to cross the street where there is a marked crosswalk.

The true-false test item is well suited to test the pupils' ability to decipher the difference between facts and misconceptions. It can be especially helpful when applied in health education, where so many misconceptions abound. The true-false test allows the teacher to present a large number of items in a short period of time. Students can address themselves to more true-false items in a specified period of time than to questions of any of the other types of test items.

However, it is easy to misuse true-false tests. Some teachers lift sentences out of textbooks to provide true statements and every once in a while insert "not" to make a statement false. Another serious disadvantage of all constant-alternative test items is the influence of "response sets," whereby the testee develops an unconscious tendency to respond to all the test questions in a constant way unrelated to the purpose of the test. For example, many students tend to answer false (or vice versa) to a true-false question whose answer they are not sure of or do not know. Last, but not least, is the guessing factor. When only two alternatives are presented, one must seriously question exactly how many answers the student really knew and how many he or she was merely fortunate enough to guess correctly.

When constructing the true-false type test, the teacher should:

1. Have an approximately equal number of true and false statements.
2. Avoid trick-type questions.
3. Avoid involved and complex sentence structure.
4. Eliminate "specific determiners," e.g., always, never, no, all, only, etc.

Changing alternatives (multiple-choice): Of the following drugs, which one should be classified as a depressant?

a) Cocaine
b) Marijuana
c) Seconal
d) Dexedrine

By employing the changing-alternative type of test item, the teacher can test higher mental processes. In many instances the student is forced to employ inferential reasoning and fine discrimination. The possibility of the student's guessing the correct answer is substantially reduced, as is the interference of "response sets."

Obviously a good multiple-choice test item is much more difficult to develop than the constant-alternative test item. Often the teacher is hard pressed to devise plausible incorrect alternatives. The construction of a good multiple-choice test will easily involve four times the labor of preparing a true-false test of similar length.

Matching: Match the items by placing the letter of the *best* answer in the space provided:

1. _____ Largest bone of the body
2. _____ Bone of the upper arm
3. _____ Bones of the wrist
4. _____ Bone found on the thumb side of the forearm
5. _____ Largest bone of the lower leg
6. _____ Bones of the palm of the hand
7. _____ Bones of the ankle
8. _____ Bones of the ball of the foot
9. _____ Bones of the chest
10. _____ Bones of the fingers and toes

a) Tarsals
b) Metacarpals
c) Metatarsals
d) Radius
e) Humerus
f) Scapula
g) Femur
h) Fibula
i) Carpals
j) Phalanges
k) Ribs
l) Ulna

The matching approach to testing is efficient in terms of space utilized and amount of testing time required to respond to the item. It is also particularly useful for making a rapid survey of a specific aspect of a field of subject matter, as evidenced by the "bones of the body" example above. Perhaps the overall disadvantage of matching-type questions is the great care that must be taken to prepare them. Much forethought is necessary if the exercise is to be free of irrelevant clues, poor alternatives, and awkward arrangement.

Conclusion. When comparing and contrasting essay examinations with short-answer examinations, it is apparent that the short-answer approach does offer some advantages. More material can be covered, there is greater reliability and objectivity than with essay examinations, they are easier to score, and they tend to eliminate bluffing. However, the very nature of short-answer examinations limits them to the province of testing factual material and excludes their application to appraising important problem-solving skills.

To be truly effective, short-answer examinations must be carefully prepared, properly administered, and humanely interpreted. Just how accurately the answers can be evaluated depends largely on the skill and insight exercised by the teacher in preparing the test questions. It is one matter to reward rote recall and another to penalize creative student thinking when only *one* answer is considered correct because it is associated with a statement in the required text. Is it not possible that several responses could be correct, depending on the frame of reference assumed by the student?

Teachers should also strive to avoid falling into the trap of overemphasizing grossly trivial and meaningless information. Such facts are forgotten the minute (or sooner) the student leaves the classroom. Instead, the teacher should provide positive learning experiences (and tests can be just that) if only major concepts are tested.

APPROACHES TO GRADING

Based on the prior discussion of assessment and its many procedures, the next logical question is: "What do we do with our findings?" How do we ultimately evaluate what we have found to be the health attitudes, practices, and knowledge of our students? The answer is certainly not simple. There are as many opinions as there are educational authorities. Although the information that follows is intended to relate to health education, it can be applied just as well to every other content area found in the elementary education curriculum.

We do not pretend to have a "catch-all" answer; instead, we offer several alternative points of view regarding evaluation. We hope that this information will stimulate meaningful discussion among your class members as to the merits and drawbacks of each approach mentioned. From the elementary school to the graduate level, grading is surely one of the most controversial topics in American education today. Many school systems have already changed from what we refer to as the traditional A-B-C grading system to what they consider as more advantageous alternative approaches. The basic philosophical question at hand is simply: "Is the traditional system of grading the most educationally useful system of evaluation?"

Claims and counterclaims

More than 60 years ago, E. L. Thorndike (1918) asserted that "whatever exists at all, exists in some amount." Ever since that time (and surely before), educators have avidly been trying to measure that all-important "amount."

Since Thorndike's time, many other specialists in educational measurement have added strong support to the process of systematic evaluation in education. Their influence over the years is quite apparent today. Grades; grade-point averages; standardized tests of achievement, intelligence, and personality; proficiency tests; programed instruction; and measurement courses for prospective teachers all attest to the influence of their point of view.

To the testing enthusiast, the achieved score forms the basis for the definition of learning. The test score becomes the direct and complete evidence of learning. Validity is often considered in the narrowest context, and statistical reliability is substituted for evidence of relevance. The entire process at best must be considered within an extremely pragmatic and data-centered frame of reference. Keep in mind that we are discussing one of the most cherished and widely practiced aspects of American education. Without the fear of grades to hang over students' heads, many a teacher would be lost. How else would it be possible to coerce students into doing what the teacher wants them to do?

Several renowned educational authorities argue that the entire process of measurement and subsequent evaluation is literally useless and damaging to students. Hoffmann (1962), for example, charges that bright and creative students are actually penalized by contemporary test practices. Wernick (1956) suggests that the whole basis for employing tests is so shaky that tactics such as cheating and physical refusal to be tested are justifiable on the part of those subjected to the tests. Holt (1969) considers testing unnecessary, of no value, and inexcusable. He further states that testing does more harm than good and, at its worst, hinders, distorts, and corrupts the learning process. He believes that our chief concern should not be to improve testing, but to find ways to eliminate it. Glasser (1969) sees grading as being the most influential factor in producing failure among students. He points out the fact that grades do not truly motivate students at both ends of the scale. He feels that grades have become a substitute for real learning, a symbolic replacement for knowledge. One's transcript status becomes more important than his or her education.

So there you have it, a philosophical discussion of the merits of grading. Do you still think it is necessary to grade health education or, for that matter, any other subject in the elementary education curriculum? Is it possible to motivate students to learn without the fear of a grade hanging over their heads? Can we make health education as well as other content areas interesting and relevant enough to turn kids on to learning without the threat of grades? Is it possible to evaluate our teaching without testing?

Alternatives to Traditional Grading

Just in case you are not befuddled enough at this juncture, the following alternatives to the traditional grading system, which were compiled by Kirschenbaum, Simon, and Napier (1971), are offered as food for thought. No doubt many of you will enter a teaching situation in a school district that has adopted an alternative approach. That alternative approach will more than likely resemble one of the following.

*A. Written Evaluations**

1. Description
The teacher uses all the letters of the alphabet to evaluate to parents, kept on file in the school and eventually sent to colleges and employers.

Frequently, teachers are provided with a form to guide them in their written evaluations. Such a form might have spaces for the teacher to discuss "strengths," "weaknesses" and "recommendations for improvement." Or it might have a more detailed breakdown of various aspects of a subject, e.g., reading, writing, discussion skills, etc.

Teachers' written evaluations are sometimes combined with the student's written self-evaluation, and both become part of the student's record and are sent to colleges and employers. When a checklist form of grading is used,

---

* From *Wad-Ja-Get? The Grading Game in American Education* by Howard Kirschenbaum, Rodney W. Napier, and Sidney B. Simon, copyright © 1971 by Hart Publishing Company, Inc., New York. Reprinted by permission.

there is often room for the teacher's additional comments. This would be a form of written evaluation.

One school has teachers send out evaluations throughout the year, rather than at specific marking periods. They also provide equal space for the parents' written response.

2. *Advantages*

   a) *These evaluations are much more helpful to the students than letter or number grades. They have an educational value.*

   b) *Written evaluations are much more meaningful to parents and admissions officers.*

   c) *They encourage the teacher to think more about each student as an individual, rather than as a set of numbers in the grade book.*

   d) *The school with ongoing evaluation and parent response says their system encourages ongoing attention to student needs, better school-community relations, and parental responses which help the teachers write more meaningful evaluations.*

3. *Disadvantages*

   a) *Written evaluations allow teachers to be even more subjective than usual in evaluating students. Teachers might unconsciously minimize the strengths and focus on the weaknesses of students they dislike. Test scores averaged out into a letter grade, in some ways, prevent this kind of subjectivity.*

   b) *Not all teachers know how to write meaningful, helpful individualized evaluations. Some teachers will rely on vague terms like "excellent," "fair," "poor," "needs improvement," "good worker" and so on; their evaluations will be no more meaningful than letter grades.*

   c) *This is a much more time-consuming method of evaluation for teachers.*

   d) *Written evaluations create extra work for the school's records office.*

B. *Self-Evaluation*

  1. *Description*

There is a need to distinguish between self-evaluation and self-grading. In a formal system of self-evaluation, the student evaluates his own progress, either in writing or in a conference with the teacher. In a system of self-grading, the student determines his own grade. Presumably self-grading cannot take place without prior self-evaluation. On the other hand, some schools have self-evaluation, but no self-grading.

An English department in a Michigan high school has its students write out their own evaluations each quarter. These evaluations then go to the teacher who writes his own comments and reactions to the self-evaluation, if he desires. These evaluations are then sent to the parents and included in the student's permanent records. There are no grades.

The student's self-grade can be combined with the teacher's grade for him and the two averaged out to determine the recorded grade. Peer evaluations can be included. Sometimes forms for self-evaluations are devised to guide the student's self-appraisal.

In some settings, students are given freedom to determine many of their educational goals and the means to achieve them. In these cases, students evaluate their progress toward their own goals. Where educational goals and activities are determined by the teacher, self-evaluation implies that students evaluate their progress toward the teacher's goals. Even here, students can help establish the criteria for evaluation, so they can more meaningfully evaluate themselves according to agreed upon criteria.

2. *Advantages*

   a) *It is an important learning experience for students to evaluate their own strengths and weaknesses.*

   b) *Most teachers who use self-evaluation and self-grading report that students are very fair and objective and often harder on themselves than the teacher would be.*

   c) *Self-evaluation might tend to encourage students to want and teachers to allow students more responsibility for setting educational goals and means of achieving them.*

3. *Disadvantages*

a) Initially, students may take the "experiment" of self-evaluation and self-grading very seriously, but once the novelty wears off, they may give less thought to their self-evaluation and grade. There is some research to show that, over time, students' self-grades become less accurate.

b) When students respect their teachers they want to grade and evaluate themselves fairly, so the teachers will respect them. When students do not respect or when they dislike their teachers, they might tend to abuse the opportunity of grading themselves.

c) Because of the enormous pressure on students these days to get high grades, self-grading makes honest self-evaluation extremely difficult.

C. *Give Grades But Don't Tell The Students*

1. *Description*

Students receive grades as usual, but they are not told what their grades are. A strong, personalized advising system keeps students apprised of their progress, informs them when they are in danger of failing, and gives them a clear perspective of how they stand in relation to their peers when they are ready to apply to college. At some schools students can find out their grades a certain number of years after they have left the institution.

2. *Advantages*

a) Once the students get used to the idea, tension over grades decreases.

b) Without grades, students stop comparing themselves to one another and begin to shift their focus away from grades and toward learning. Reed College has had this system for over 50 years, and periodic polls show that its alumni are in favor of keeping this system.

3. *Disadvantages*

a) Initially, it might increase tension. For some students, the tension always remains.

b) Although it may reduce tension and help the focus shift away from grades somewhat, many of the prob-

lems of traditional grades remain. Even at Reed, there is a movement to introduce pass/fail courses.

D. *The Contract System*

1. *Description*

There is a need to distinguish between contract grading applied to a whole class and contract grading applied separately to the students.

When applied to a whole class, the contract system means that if the student does a certain type, quantity *and, ideally, quality of work, he will automatically receive a given grade. For example, one teacher made the following contract with his class:*

> *Anyone who neither comes to class (type) regularly (quantity) nor turns in all (quantity) the required work (type) will receive an F.*
>
> *Anyone who only comes to class regularly or only turns in all the required work will receive a D.*
>
> *Anyone who both comes to class regularly and turns in the required work will receive a C.*
>
> *Anyone who comes to class regularly, turns in the required work, and the work meets the following criteria (quality) will receive a B.*
>
> *Anyone who comes to class regularly, turns in the required work that meets the following criteria and does the following extra report will receive an A.*

Sometimes the teacher alone states the terms of the contract. Sometimes they are reached by a group decision. In either case, the same contract applies to the whole class.

Another practice is to have each student *design his own contract to which the teacher must agree. This use of the contract system implies that students are setting their own goals and ways of reaching those goals, and therefore, different grading procedures will be appropriate for different students. For example, in one social studies class,*

> *Student X might contract to read three books on the United States' political system and write a report on the three books.*
>
> *Student Y might contract to study the process of how a bill becomes a law and to lead the class in a simulated exercise that would help the class to understand this process better. Student Z might contract to*

work two afternoons a week in the campaign head-quarters of a local political candidate.

Since each contract calls for a very different type of activity than the others, each contract needs to include its own agreement as to how the student's grade will be determined. One of the grading variables in this situation will be who will do the evaluating. In the case of student X, the teacher might be the sole judge of the grade. For student Y, the class' feedback on the simulated exercise might play a part in the grade. And the local candidate might evaluate the work of student Z. But in all cases, the method of evaluation is decided upon jointly by student and teacher and stated clearly in the original, written contract.

In some classes, the type and quantity of work are the only components of the contract. Ideally, a contract should also include a statement of how the quality of the work will be judged, what criteria will be used and what levels of proficiency are necessary to earn a given grade. To do this adequately requires use of the "mastery approach" toward grading, which is discussed in the next section.

2. *Advantages*

a) Much of the anxiety is eliminated from the grading process because the student knows, from the beginning of the year, exactly what he has to do to get the grade he wants.

b) To the extent the teacher specifies the quantity and quality required for each grade, some of the subjectivity is eliminated from the grading process, and students have a clearer idea of what is expected of them.

c) The contract system, when applied to students individually, encourages diversity in the classroom, encourages students to set and follow their own learning goals, and decreases unhealthy competition.

3. *Disadvantages*

a) The quantity of work is easily overemphasized in contracts and tends to become the sole basis for a grade. To use an extreme example, one English teacher stipulated that five-page compositions would receive an A, four-page compositions would receive a B, and so on. When the quantity of work becomes the sole criterion for the grade, the grade loses its meaning.

b) It is difficult to find creative ways to measure the quality of the different types of work students may contract to do.

c) There is a danger that teachers will be too ambiguous in attempting to state the qualitative distinctions between grades. To say that work of "excellent" quality will receive an A, work of "good" quality will receive a B, and so on, is no different than the ambiguous and subjective criteria we presently employ.

E. *The Mastery Approach or Performance Curriculum (Five-Point System)*

1. *Description*

The mastery approach is not only a different method of grading, but an entirely different approach toward teaching and learning. It may be practiced by one class or by an entire department or subject area. In a sense, it is not an alternative to traditional grading; rather, it is the traditional grading system, done effectively.

The mastery approach begins with the teacher deciding what his operational or behavioral objectives are for his students, that is, what exactly he wants them to be able to do as a result of their learnings. He then organizes these learnings into units of study and arranges the units in a logical sequence, each unit serving as a necessary or logical building block to the unit succeeding it. Then the teacher determines how he will measure the extent to which his students have mastered the body of knowledge and skills in each of the units.

For each unit, the teacher designates levels of mastery or proficiency. Thus, if a math teacher wants his students to be able to solve a quadratic equation, he stipulates what the student must do to demonstrate a C level of proficiency, what he must do to demonstrate a B level of proficiency, and so on.

At the very beginning of the course, the teacher provides the students with all this information—what they are expected to learn, how their learnings will be tested, what the criteria are for the different levels of *proficiency and what level of proficiency is required before they can move on to the next part of the course. In addition, he explains to the students what resources are available to help them achieve the levels of mastery they desire.*

Students are then free to master the course content in their own fashion. Some students will attend class lectures and discussions. Others will work independently. Many students will utilize the various resources the teacher has provided—learning packages, programmed tests, films, tapes, speakers, field trips, etc.

Each student proceeds at his own pace. One student may take a semester to accomplish what is normally done in a year. Another student may take a year to do a semester's work in a particular subject. Under this system the course is oriented much more to the individual student, and the professor spends most of his time in review seminars and in individual tutoring, rather than in large group lectures.

Students ask to be examined when they think they are ready to move on. Usually, when a student has achieved a C level of mastery in one unit of a course, he can choose to go on to the next unit. However, students who want to earn B and A grades will stay with each unit until they have achieved that level of proficiency. A student may take an exam (a different form each time, of course) over again until he is satisfied with his grade.

Using the mastery approach, several teachers or an entire department can get together and plan their courses sequentially—one course building upon the next. This is sometimes called a performance curriculum, since course credits are no longer determined by the length of time a student spends with a given subject ("I had three years of French.") but by the level of performance he has achieved in a given area.

Bucknell's Continuous Progress Program is one example of the mastery approach and performance curriculum. Courses as different as biology, philosophy, psychology, physics, religion and education are all involved.

2. *Advantages*

   a) *A student's grade becomes more meaningful to him because it is tied to a performance level. In the*
performance curriculum, grades become more meaningful because, in several different classes, the same grade now means the same thing.

   b) *Much of the teacher's subjectivity in grading is eliminated.*

   c) *When students know where they are heading, they are likely to get there faster.*

   d) *The focus of this system is on success, not failure.*

   e) *The student has freedom to pursue his own path in mastering the course content.*

   f) *The teacher is held accountable for stating his objectives, providing many resources, and helping his students achieve mastery. Sloppy organization and ill-prepared teachers are readily noticeable.*

   g) *In the performance curriculum, the cooperation among teachers can generate better morale and the sharing of resources.*

3. *Disadvantages*

   a) *To utilize the mastery approach properly requires considerable skill on the part of teachers and administrators. Most educators were not trained in this method and a great deal of retraining will be necessary. The funds are not easily made available.*

   b) *The performance curriculum somewhat limits a teacher's freedom to run his classes in just his own way. In some cases this might be desirable; in other cases some creative teachers might be hampered.*

   c) *It is possible for teachers to use the mastery approach without allowing students to pursue their own ways of achieving the levels of proficiency. When this happens students might feel, more than many do now, that all their education means is jumping over a series of prescribed hurdles.*

   d) *Even when students have freedom to choose how they will achieve the teacher's goals, the mastery approach discourages them from setting and working toward their own goals.*

   e) *The total faculty must be involved in setting up a performance curriculum. The teachers in each subject* area would have to carefully study goals and methods and explore new approaches to the subject matter. This could take a very long time and might normally be impossible, since most teachers teach 5 classes, have supervisory duties, and are involved in one or more student activities. A long-term grant might be needed to hire additional personnel to free teachers to do the necessary research and curriculum development.

F.   Pass/Fail Grading (P/F)

1.   Description

At the beginning of the course, the teacher states his criteria for a passing grade, or else the teacher and students together decide on the criteria for a passing grade. Any student who meets these criteria passes; any student who does not meet these criteria fails. Students have the opportunity to redo failing work to bring it up to passing quality.

Pass/fail is a form of blanket grading, with the blanket grade being a P. P/F is also a form of the contract system, since the students know that if they meet the teacher's stated criteria for passing, they will automatically receive a P. Finally, it is also a form of the mastery approach, since the teacher designates the level of mastery needed to pass the course.

2.   Advantages

a) Students are more relaxed, less anxious, and less competitive.

b) There is a better learning atmosphere. Students feel freer to take risks, disagree with the teacher, and explore the subject in their own way.

c) There is no point to cheating or apple-polishing (except for students in danger of failing).

d) Students still have to meet the teacher's requirements to get the blanket grade, so plenty of work gets done. Freed from the pressures of traditional grading, some students do even more work than usual.

3.   Disadvantages

a) Some teachers will use blanket grading as an excuse to avoid all evaluation. This deprives the student of potentially helpful feedback.

b) The blanket grade does not distinguish between students of different abilities. Therefore, the grade is meaningless except to connote passing work.

c) Freed from the pressures of traditional grading, some students do less work than usual.

d) Just as it is difficult for teachers to distinguish between the different levels of mastery in the performance curriculum, it will be difficult to clearly state and measure the level of mastery needed to earn the blanket grade.

e) The student in danger of failing still labors under all the pressures normally associated with traditional grading. P/F is no help to our poorer students.

4.   Note

The system of pass/fail grading has two kinds of variations:

a) Modified Pass/Fail which adds one category to denote outstanding work. This is called Honors/Pass/Fail (H/P/F).

b) Limited Pass/Fail in which the student may take only some of his courses on a pass/fail basis.

G.   Credit/No Credit Grading (CR/NC)

1.   Description

This system works precisely the same way as pass/fail grading, except the two categories are "credit" and "no credit" instead of pass and fail. CR/NC also can be practiced on a modified or limited basis. It is important for systems using CR/NC to note right in their transcripts that NC does not connote failing work.

2.   Advantages

Same as those for pass/fail but with one additional advantage: "No Credit" does not connote failure; students simply do not get credit for the course. With this fear of an E removed from those students on the borderline, they, too, can feel freer from the need to cheat and con their way to a passing grade. It is a small difference, but significant for those on the borderline.

3.   Disadvantages

Same as those for pass/fail, except for "e."

H. Blanket Grading

1. Description

The teacher announces at the beginning of the year that anyone in the class who does the required amount of work will receive the blanket grade. Usually, the grade is B. Sometimes classes use the blanket A to make a protest statement to the school. Sometimes a blanket C is used, as a way of saying to the school, "See, this is how little we care about grades. The focus in this class will be on learning."

If a student's work is of such poor quality that the teacher does not feel justified in giving him the blanket grade, he allows the student to keep trying until the quality improves.

This is a form of contract grading. It is also a form of the mastery approach, since the teacher is saying, "Anyone who achieves this minimum level of mastery will receive the blanket grade."

Blanket grading is used in individual classrooms only; it is never used by a whole school.

2. Advantages

Same as those for Pass/Fail Grading.

3. Disadvantages

a) Same as those for Pass/Fail Grading.

b) Although teachers frequently use blanket grading without any repercussions, this system would violate most school's written or unwritten grading policies and, therefore, be a risk for the teacher.

Same of those for blanket grading.

REVIEW QUESTIONS

1. Differentiate among the terms testing, measurement, and evaluation.

2. Why evaluate students? Support your answer with facts.

3. Discuss some principles that should be basic to any form of evaluation.

4. The appraisal of health attitudes and practices is no easy task. Cite and discuss some techniques that might be implemented by the classroom teacher to evaluate students' health attitudes and practices.

5. Discuss the relative merits of both the essay examination and the short-answer examination.

6. Select three alternatives to the traditional system of grading and explain the merits and drawbacks of each.

REFERENCES AND BIBLIOGRAPHY

Dizney, Henry. *Classroom Evaluation for Teachers* (Dubuque, Iowa: Wm. C. Brown, 1971).

Dobbin, J. E., and Henry Chauncey. *Testing: Its Place in Education Today* (New York: Harper & Row, 1963).

Ebel, R. L. *Measuring Educational Achievement* (Englewood Cliffs, N.J.: Prentice-Hall, 1965).

Glasser, William. *Schools Without Failure* (New York: Harper & Row, 1969).

Green, J. A. *Teacher-Made Tests* (New York: Harper & Row, 1963).

Hoffmann, Banesh. *The Tyranny of Testing* (New York: Crowell, Collier & Macmillan, 1962).

Holt, John. *The Under-Achieving School* (New York: Pitman, 1969).

Kirschenbaum, Howard, S. B. Simon, and R. W. Napier. *Wad-Ja-Get? The Grading Game in American Education* (New York: Hart, 1971).

Marshall, Max. *Teaching without Grades* (Portland: Oregon State University Press, 1969).

Remmers, H. H., N. L. Gage, and J. F. Rummer. *A Practical Introduction To Measurement and Evaluation* (New York: Harper & Row, 1965).

Thorndike, E. L. "The Nature, Purposes and General Methods of Measurements of Educational Products," *The Measurement of Educational Products*—17th Yearbook of the National Society For the Study of Education, 1918, Part II.

Wernick, Robert. *They've Got Your Number* (New York: Norton, 1956).

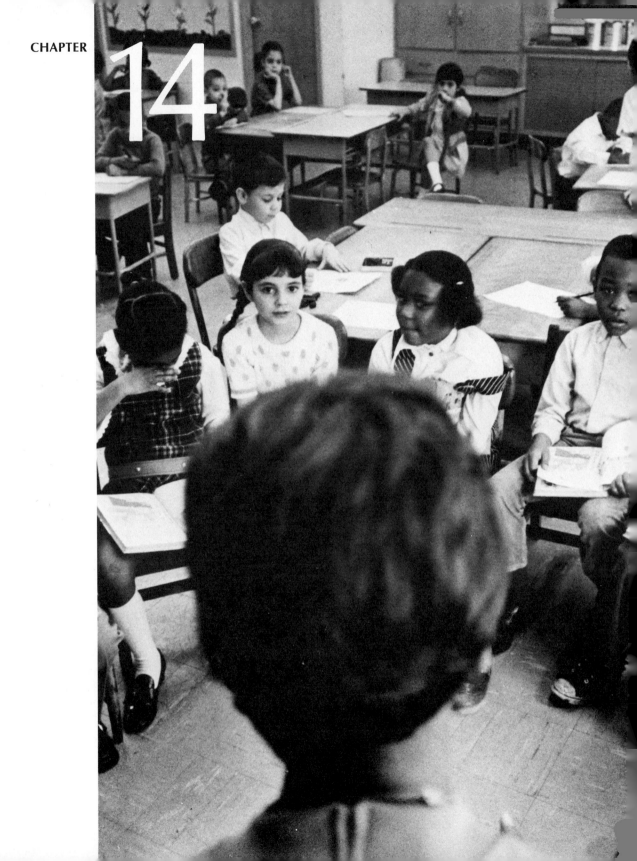

14

organizing for health instruction

Among the essential basic elements of health instruction are concept formation, objectives instruction, content cognition, method and technique selection, evaluation skills, and unit and lesson plan organization. Failure to master these skills leaves the instructor without the essential process skills so vital to effective health instruction.

This chapter is concerned with organizing the previously presented material dealing with concepts, objectives, methods, and techniques into a blueprint for learning—the unit and daily lesson plan. This approach is a theoretical model to be used as a guide. Under no circumstances does the effort required to develop such a plan ensure that learning will take place. On the contrary, unit and lesson plans serve only to assist in the organizational process that normally accompanies effective health instruction.

The material in this chapter is adapted from Walter D. Sorochan and Stephen J. Bender, *Teaching Secondary Health Science,* New York: Wiley, 1978. By permission.

CONCEPT UNIT PLANNING

Modern education has fostered the change from memory-centered education to problem-solving learning. Elementary health education is no exception to this rule. Effective elementary health education is so designed to provide a systematic organization of activities, experiences, and situations that all contribute to the optimal health development of the youngster.

In an effort to accomplish this task, it is necessary to have a well-perceived plan of educational experiences. Such a plan initially takes the form of a unit plan. The health education unit plan consists of a number of interrelated concepts, objectives, learning experiences, content, evaluation procedures, and references. Although the literature yields various forms for presenting the unit plan, we have found that the parallel-column form possesses considerable merit. See Fig. 14.1.

Unit Title

The title of the given unit should be short, clear, and concise. Every effort should be made to convey clearly to the reader the nature of the topic to be

Unit title _____

Grade level _____

Instructor _____

Date _____

Concepts	Behavioral objectives	Learning experiences	Content	Evaluation procedures	Resources

Fig. 14.1   Suggested format for a unit plan.

discussed. The title should also be so stated that it stimulates the interest of the reader. It is not necessary to spend an inordinate amount of time developing a catchy unit title; however, an effort should be made to assemble a title that both clearly informs and motivates the reader about the topic selected for a given unit.

Concepts

The concepts serve as the framework for the unit plan. Concepts are the big ideas that will be emphasized in the unit. They serve as focal points for the development of the remainder of the unit and the entire instructional process. The concepts act as guides to the competencies that are to be demonstrated eventually by the learner.

Concept formation is invaluable with reference to the service such an action provides. Careful concept formation forms the very basis for formalized health education.

Behavioral Objectives

The unit plan should be comprised of statements that clearly describe what students will be able to do after completing the prescribed unit of instruction. Theoretically, the objectives add further direction to the instructional process once the concepts for a given unit have been developed. The objectives suggest what should be taught and how the material should be taught.

Behavioral objectives can be stated in various ways: as objectives, expected outcomes, goals, aims, and/or competencies. Behavioral objectives are referred to in this text as *expected pupil outcomes*. They are what children are expected to attain as skills or to acquire as a level of competence in a skill. Expected outcomes may be of three types:

1. *Cognitive:* pertaining to knowledge and intellectual or thinking skills, such as recall and recognition;
2. *Affective:* pertaining to feelings, emotions, interests, values, and the development of appreciation and adequate adjustment or attitudes;
3. *Action:* relevant to acting, manipulating, or motor skills or acts of overt behavior.

The elementary teacher should possess the ability to develop appropriate outcomes in all three domains (see Chapter 11).

Content

The content section of the unit plan outlines the subject matter to be taught in satisfying the desired objectives of the instructional process. More often than not, several content items will be required to ensure the proper development of each objective. The content items should be carefully selected to enhance the development of the desired objectives.

Without content, there is literally no concept development. Specific details of a topic make up content. Content is a collection of facts and information. Such facts need to be relevant to a concept and expected outcomes. Obviously, numerous facts may be difficult for the child to assimilate and to categorize. Indeed, the child may forget the specific details making up the content in a few minutes. When this happens, the details are overwhelming, and the child will not be able to analyze and categorize the information. The content cannot be internalized.

Teachers may help to make the content meaningful to children by providing the proper learning experiences. The learning experiences should help the child to internalize the content and to evolve his or her own concept. Although most of the minute details of information (content) will be forgotten in 24 hours, the big idea, or concept, structured by the details will be retained. There are no concepts without content. Concept provides the fuel for the discovery of concepts. The spark for igniting such a discovery comes from the learning experience.

In selecting content, the teacher should start out at the pupil's level, then select and present the content in a progressive manner. This approach sustains pupil interest and provides intrinsic motivation to learning.

Methods and Techniques

Once the concepts have been developed, the behavioral objectives established, and the content for each objective determined, suitable instructional methods and techniques must be selected. The methods and techniques selected for each content item should be carefully selected to ensure that individual factors such as class differences, strengths, weaknesses, time allotment, and so on, are all considered. Due to such factors, it may be necessary to develop more than one learning experience to choose from.

Teachers are the facilitators of these learning experiences. Teachers help children to make information meaningful and to evolve concepts. Concepts, in turn, can be mediators of behaviors. Whether such an internalized process in the child occurs depends to a large degree on the kind of learning experiences that teachers provide. Learning experiences should help children to "discover for themselves" the big ideas, or concepts.

Teachers should keep in mind that concepts are classified information and gradually arise from per-

Table 14.1   Relationships among behavioral domains, health instructional aims, expected outcomes, behavior, and learning experiences.

Domain (behavioral)	Aims (health instruction)	Outcomes (expected)	Behavior (overt/covert)	Learning experiences
Cognitive	Impart facts	Knows, writes, recites, recalls, lists	Think	Lecture, discussion question-answer (Q-A), group reports
	Develop understandings	Understands, reasons, perceives, realizes, recognizes, analyzes, identifies		Discussion, Q-A, demonstration, field trip, experiment
Affective	Evolve attitudes	Is aware of, is sensitive to, accepts, likes to, believes, values, appreciates, feels	Feel	Role play, debate, sociodramas, panel-group reports, discussion
Action	Develop habits	Does, brushes, eats	Act (does)	Teacher demonstration
	Develop practices	Visits, relaxes, exercises, sleeps, plays		Pupils practice habit or skill

cepts, experiences, and images of observations. The child perceives by acquiring an awareness of self, the environment, and that which he or she is trying to relate to sensually. Through experience, the child synthesizes information and gives meaning to the information. For example, a kindergarten child watching guppies swimming in an aquarium eventually sees small dark spots in the mother guppies' transparent stomachs and later locates baby guppies; the child synthesizes impressions of color, shape, content and structure, and growth characteristics derived through the light receptors of his eyes. The child perceives an answer to the question, "Where do babies come from?" Learners see, touch, and hear about fish, babies, and other objects to formulate an image of an understanding of their nature. Crucial to learning for elementary school children, then, is the selection of basic experiences appropriate to the concept to be developed.

Some learning experiences are more appropriate than others in evolving specific concepts. Although good research is still lacking in this area, the basis for this is suggested in Table 14.2. The four basic aims of health science instruction are to: (1) impart facts and knowledge; (2) develop understandings; (3) evolve attitudes; and (4) develop habits and practices. Table 14.1 also summarizes the behavioral objectives, or expected outcomes, and suggests learning experiences that may help to attain the outcomes.

Learning experiences are very much like the "how" of where you want to go. How do you want to travel to your destination (expected outcome)? Do you travel by car, train, ship, or airplane? Each is a different mode of transportation and places a different priority on time and experience. And so it is with learning experiences. Learning experiences are vehicles for not only attaining expected outcomes, but also helping children to evolve desirable concepts in the interim.

Teaching Aids

It is important to list many materials, essential supplies, and aids necessary to carrying out instructional process. Films, projectors, screens, models, specimens, transparencies, overhead projectors, opaque projectors, slides, and slide projectors are all typical teaching aids. The aids listed provide the instructor with a quick inventory of the items necessary to carry out the instructional process.

Evaluation Procedures

It is important to implement some form of measurement and evaluation to determine whether or not the established objectives have been attained.

Accountability can take on many different forms. Several of the more common techniques are knowledge tests, attitude scales, practice inventories, checklists, rating scales, observations, oral and written reports, and so on. It is important that each objective be measured with an appropriate measurement technique. (See Chapter 13.)

References

It is helpful to have one list of references for the instructor and, depending on the grade level, another list of references for the student. The student list can be explicit to the point of providing exact page numbers if necessary. In some instances it might be a more valuable experience to provide students with general references and leave the task of isolating the most relevant material to them. In any event, it is important that reference lists be kept current.

CONCEPT LESSON PLANNING

Once the unit plan has been established, the *daily lesson* plans must be made. In other words, the daily lesson plans become the day-by-day progression toward the ultimate goal of realizing the established objectives of the unit. Effective lesson planning requires that the instructor have a clear understanding of the total learning package presented in the unit. With that understanding in mind, the instructor carefully separates the unit into the separate daily lesson plans.

It is entirely possible that a lesson plan, by design, might extend into more than one class period. As might be imagined, it is also likely that a daily lesson plan designed for completion in one class period may well have to be extended into another class period due to the instructor's miscalculation of the time allotment. A most important consideration surrounding the daily lesson plan concept is that a sense of continuation be observable from one class period to the next and that ultimately the objectives of the unit are met and the concepts realized. Table 14.2 shows the suggested format for the daily concept lesson plan.

The theoretical daily concept lesson plan should be structured so that each component reinforces the other components. For example, the content should reinforce the concept, which in turn should reinforce the outcome. The learning experience(s) should specify how each part of the content may be "internalized" into a concept. Indirectly, the learning experience contributes to the outcome by helping children to discover the concept.

Sequentially, the theme topic and expected outcome for the lesson plan should be initially identified by a developmental task. The specific information relevant to the outcome should be selected next. Third, a concept should be evolved from the content by the teacher in such a way that it helps to mediate for the outcome. Finally, the learning experience should be "plugged" into the lesson plan.

In addition to the suggested four major components of a lesson plan, the following may be added:

1. Key questions (for review to help children to internalize the content and structure the concept);

Table 14.2   Suggested format for a daily concept lesson plan.

Topic: ———————————————————

Outcome (Behavioral objective):

Concept: ———————————————————

Content:	Learning experiences:
1.	A.
2.	1.
3.	2.
4.	3.
5.	4.
6.	5.
7.	6.
	7.
	B. Key words:
	C. Evaluation:
	1. Key questions:
	a)
	b)
	c)
	2. Observe behaviors
	3. Pre-/postquiz
	4. Skills?

2. Key words;
3. References for pupils and the teacher;
4. Visual aids and materials;
5. Evaluations, such as pre-/postquiz, observations of behavior.

Inclusion of these elements in the lesson plan is left to the discretion of the critic teacher and prospective teachers. Examples of concept lesson plans for various topics on well-being are given in Chapters 15 through 25.

Health instruction, like the practice of medicine, is both an art and a science. It is a science in that it has content that is interdisciplinary and relies on the principles of educational and developmental psychology. As a science in terms of the knowledge, techniques and methods employed, it is similar to medicine. But which techniques to use and how to use them becomes an art in medicine as much as it does in teaching. Medicine becomes an art of diagnosing, prescribing, and treating. Selecting appropriate learning experiences to attain expected outcomes becomes a process of decision making as well as manipulating human behavior. Teaching is an art because the teacher becomes a social engineer of having his or her pupils evolve new health habits and behaviors and accept new public health practices. Dealing successfully with children to attain these outcomes is an art. Thus the conceptual lesson plan is a scientific approach, and its execution becomes an art.

REVIEW QUESTIONS

1. Differentiate between the concept unit plan and the concept daily lesson plan.
2. Explain the components of the concept unit plan.
3. Explain the key components of the concept daily lesson plan.
4. Develop an acceptable concept unit plan and one acceptable concept daily lesson plan relevant to the unit.

REFERENCES AND BIBLIOGRAPHY

Bloom, Benjamin S., ed. *Taxonomy of Educational Objectives*, Handbook 1, Cognitive Domain (New York: McKay, 1968).

Bourne, Lyle E. *Human Conceptual Behavior* (Boston: Allyn and Bacon, 1966).

Broadbeck, May. "Logic and Scientific Method on Teaching," in N. L. Gage, ed. *Handbook of Research on Teaching* (Chicago: Rand McNally, 1965), pp. 44-93.

Gage, N. L., ed. *Handbook of Research on Teaching* (Chicago: Rand McNally, 1965), pp. 48-72, 884-887.

Hurlock, Elizabeth B. *Child Development* (New York: McGraw-Hill, 1964).

Kibler, Robert J., Larry L. Barker, and David T. Miles. *Behavioral Objectives and Instruction* (Boston: Allyn and Bacon, 1970).

Klausmeier, Herbert J., and Chester W. Harris. *Analyses of Concept Learning* (New York: Academic Press, 1966).

Mager, Robert F. *Preparing Instructional Objectives* (Palo Alto, Calif.: Fearon, 1963).

Phenix, Philip H. *Realms of Meaning* (New York: McGraw-Hill, 1964).

Rash, J. K. *The Health Education Curriculum* (Bloomington: Indiana University Press, 1970).

Sorochan, Walter D., and Stephen J. Bender. *Teaching Secondary Health Science* (New York: Wiley, 1978).

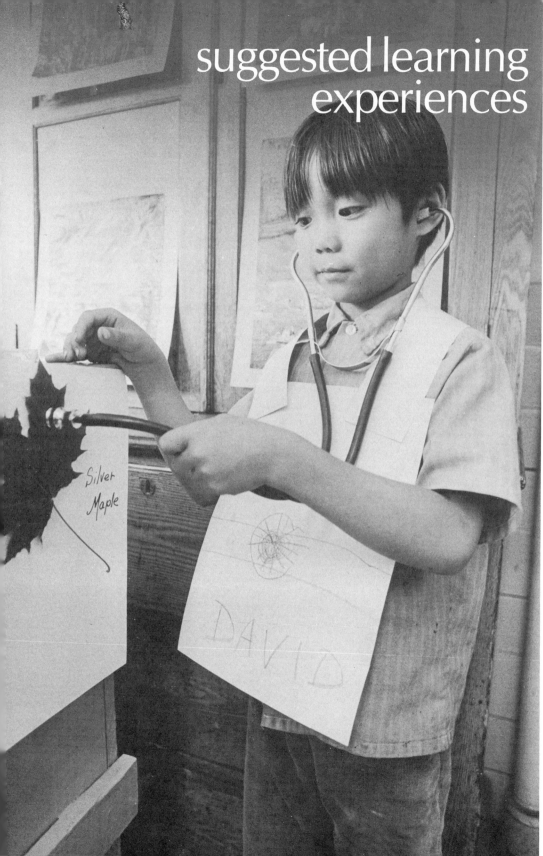

suggested learning
experiences

PART V

CHAPTER 15

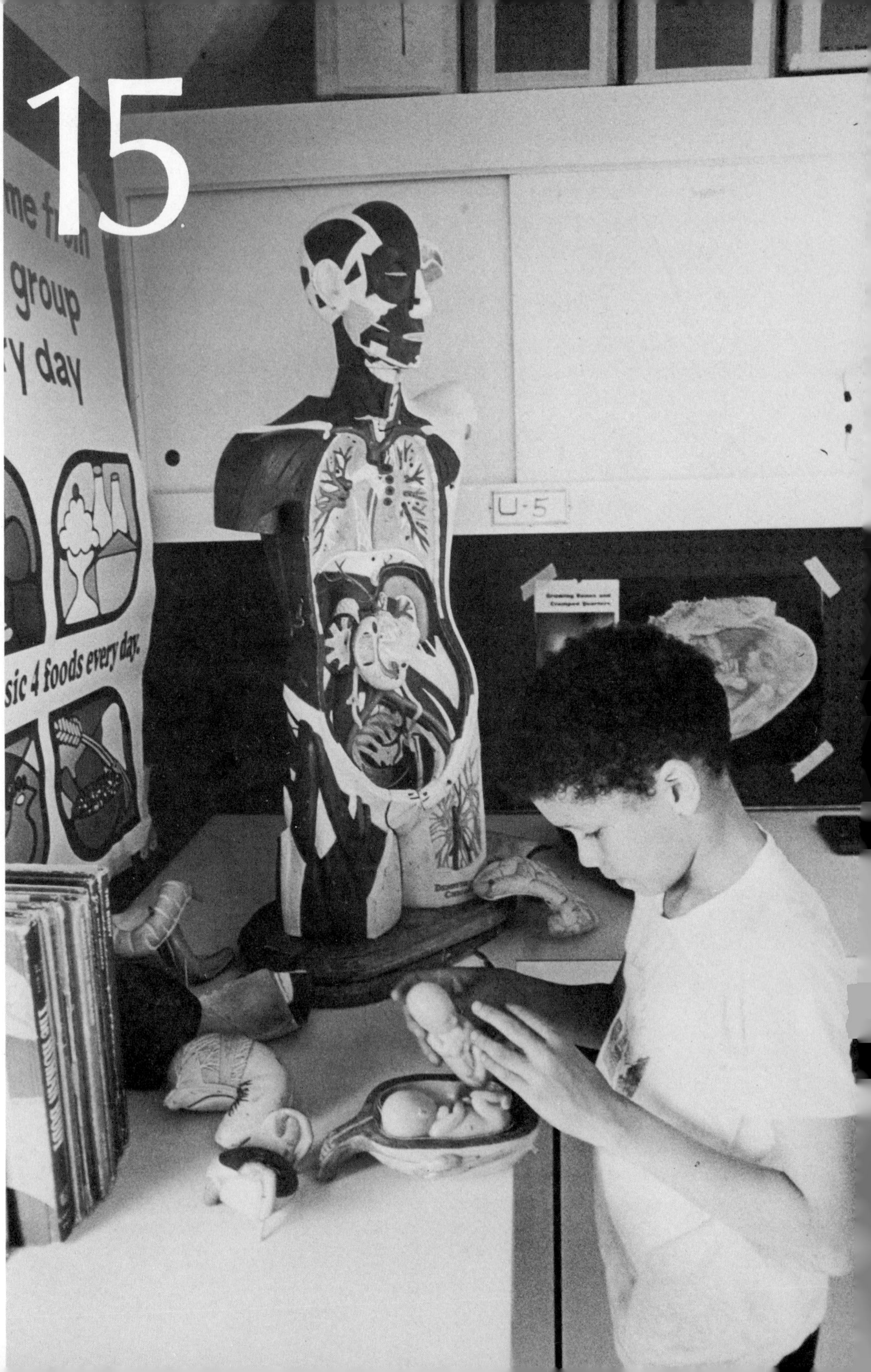

teaching about the human body

INTRODUCTION

The human body is literally a marvel of nature. The human physiological machine consists of ten body systems and their numerous organs. The nervous system facilitates communication; the glandular system regulates body function and provides a stress-defense mechanism; the skeletal system gives us appearance and protection; the muscular system allows for locomotion; the cardiovascular system transports blood and other substances; the respiratory system allows for gaseous exchange; the digestive system provides fuel; the excretory system removes wastes; the reproductive system procreates the species; and the lymphatic system protects the body. Collectively, these systems make the human body a complex living organism. Its different parts act and react on one another in a mutual operation quite impossible of any other machine.

The heart is one of the most fascinating organs of the body. One of the strongest muscles of the body, it pumps blood through the arteries to all parts of the body. Exercise and stress make the heart beat faster, increasing blood-volume per minute by as much as ten times in trained athletes. During a night's sleep, the heart does work equivalent to carrying a 30-pound pack almost to the top of the Empire State Building—not bad for an organ the size of a clenched fist.

The five quarts of blood in an average adult are replaced once a month. It takes about 23 seconds for the blood to complete a circuit of the systematic circulation. During this time, the blood holds enough oxygen for about five minutes or so during rest; the same amount is used in a fraction of a minute during strenuous exercise. Yet when 10 percent of the blood is lost over a short period of time, the body goes into a state of shock and death results when 40 percent is lost.

In the average male the blood vessels will, when stretched out side by side, reach a length of 100,000 miles or more. It is in the smallest vessels, the capillaries, that the exchange of substances takes place between the blood and the rest of the body. Although the vessels are elastic, the arteries readily lose their elasticity if the body is not exer-

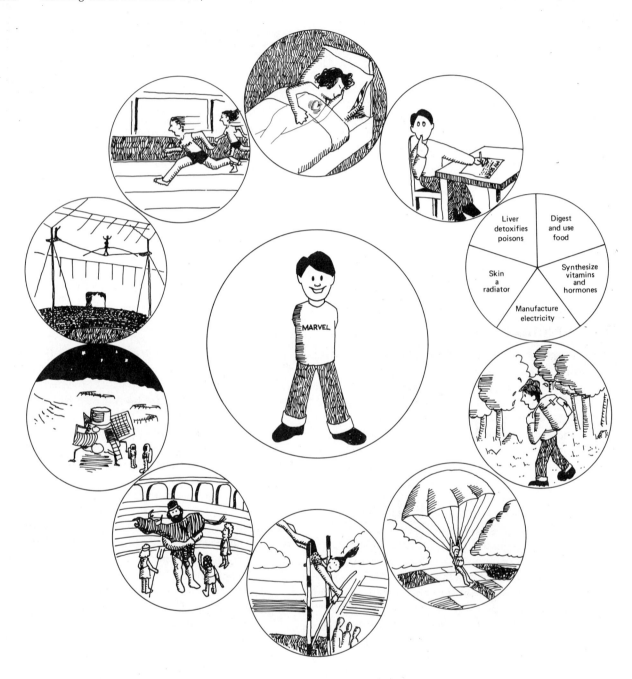

Fig. 15.1 The marvel of the human body.

cised regularly and when the diet is rich in fats. No wonder physiologists say that you are as old as your blood vessels.

Nature designed the body so that the cardiovascular system is complemented by the respiratory system. Oxygen is necessary every minute that the human body lives. The lungs, where exchange of gases takes place, contain 700 to 800 million air sacs, or alveoli. The inner surface of the lungs in an adult is equivalent to the size of a tennis court. Lungs help us to breathe about 12,000 liters of air each day.

One of the first organs to receive the oxygenated blood is the kidney. The kidneys work in much the same way as a screen does in separating rocks from sand. The waste products of cell and liver metabolism are screened out by the kidneys, stored in the bladder, and excreted as urine. Through filtration, the kidneys control body fluids and maintain a stable fluid environment. Of the 180 quarts of blood filtered by the kidneys each day, only one to two quarts are excreted as urine. Every 20 minutes the entire volume of the blood passes by a set of molecular filters in the two million glomeruli of the kidney. Many vital substances, such as salts, minerals, and vitamins, are retained and recycled by the kidneys.

The liver can be thought of as a chemical factory in the body. Besides storing fat-soluble vitamins and maintaining about a 12-hour energy supply of body sugar, the liver synthesizes bile for the small intestine. Perhaps the liver's most important function is to detoxify poisons and complex body chemicals. When these chemicals are broken down into simpler substances, they can then be excreted by the kidneys. Many poisons and/or drugs, such as alcohol, caffeine, and nicotine, are detoxified by the liver. The liver is also capable of making antibiotics, as when it converts the chemical prontosil into sulfanilamide as needed in the fight against bacteria and viruses.

In addition to synthesizing hormones, enzymes, and drugs of various kinds, the body also synthesizes vitamins. The skin harnesses the sun's rays to manufacture vitamin D, and the bacteria in the large intestine make vitamin K.

The blood supply to the muscles varies in proportion to the amount of muscle work. Active muscle on one side of the body will have from 40 to 100 times more capillaries than the inactive muscle on the opposite side of the body. About 750 major muscles are attached to more than 205 bones. After stretching, twisting, and squeezing, muscles return to their original length and shape. In so doing, they oxidize glycogen (body sugar), help with body balance, and generate heat, energy, and minute electrical currents. Muscles have enormous strength. Some, like the biceps in the arm, are capable of lifting a weight 1500 times their own weight. In addition to doing work, muscles support the skeleton and refine body posture and personal appearance. They allow for locomotion. The human being's greatest speed is about 22.2 mph, the equivalent of running 220 yards in 20.3 seconds. In spite of these potentialities, people over 70 years of age have diminished work capacities; these are estimated to be only 50 percent of the values of a 17-year-old youth.

It is little wonder, then, that many doctors and physiologists believe that exercise helps to control body weight. Exercise burns food, which in turn is measured as calories. To lose one pound of body fat, one must burn off 3500 calories. In so doing, the heat produced, if not checked, would rise and coagulate the protein in muscles. A heat-regulating apparatus keeps body temperature almost constant. This radiator is the skin, which dissipates about 80 percent of the excess heat. This cooling/heating system in the human body is completely self-regulating.

In order to survive, the human body has made numerous physical adaptions through the years of evolution. A general defense mechanism automatically immobilizes the body against damage, infection, and injury. The lymphatic system is supplemented by the endocrine system in this work. The adrenal glands, about 1/7000th of the total body weight, synthesize numerous stress-regulating hormones from cholesterol and vitamin C. These are called into play whenever needed.

A highly developed nervous system and brain, more efficient than the best communication systems yet devised, including radio and television, coordinate all of the body systems and organs just described. The nervous system has powerful transmitting equipment, sensitive receivers, and durable trunk lines to control and coordinate messages from one part of the body to another in a fraction of a second. The brain alone has over 17 billion cells; the eye has 1,000,000 private telephone lines in the optic nerve. Although the average person has the capacity to think, create, and remember, he or she uses only about 10 percent of that brain power. Use of the brain for reasoning is complicated by the activity of the endocrine system; emotionality is the product of the interplay between these two systems. Hence one's intellectuality is often textured with shades of mood—sadness and happiness, love and hate. When compared to a simple machine, human behavior becomes very complex, difficult to interpret, and many times unpredictable.

In spite of these limitations, a person is still the world's most miraculous mechanism, capable of taking a lot of punishment and still functioning. A person can get along without a gall bladder, the spleen, the appendix, the bladder; can give up one kidney, one lung, two quarts of blood, a piece of brain, both eyes and ears, and all of the teeth and still live. A human can survive 30 days without food, three days without water, but only about three minutes without air. This living wonder is also sensitive to lack of rest and sleep, administration of drugs, physical and emotional stress, and malnutrition. Like a worn-out battery, it needs to be psychologically and physically recharged from time to time. It needs a balanced blending of nutrition, exercise, rest, and social interaction to keep going. Exercise especially tunes up and regulates all the body processes. Without it, the body slowly withers.

Good body functioning is a basis for medical diagnosis. It is a doctor's yardstick for assessing one's health. With physiological growth, changes occur almost every day in children. It is no surprise to observe children taking a keen interest in their bodies at this time. "How big is the heart?" and "How does it work?" reflect the natural curiosity of children. It is in the second and third grades that children become fascinated by sense organs and how they work. When children get to the awkward and clumsy stages of development—at about grades five, six, and seven—they once again develop a natural curiosity about body systems. It is at these crucial times in the child's life that information about the body becomes relevant, important, and meaningful. Many teachers defer teaching about the body until high school. Children need to become conscious of their physiological needs early. Such consciousness includes how to maintain and conserve the body through sound sociohygienic habits. It is through healthy physical education activities (see Fig. 15.2) that such awareness may best be developed. Muscular strength and endurance may be improved through strenuous activities. Participation in such endeavors also hones the sense of balance, and improves general body coordination. Elementary school children need opportunities to appraise themselves through self-testing activities and a chance to relate success in motor activities to personal health habits. Thus the emphasis in elementary school physical education should be on helping children to develop neuromuscular coordination, general motor skills, and how to attain and maintain physical fitness. These raw ingredients are the foundations for lifetime sports and activities.

As the child participates in regular physical activities, she or he should be evolving a future lifestyle. By performing continuous, progressive, and

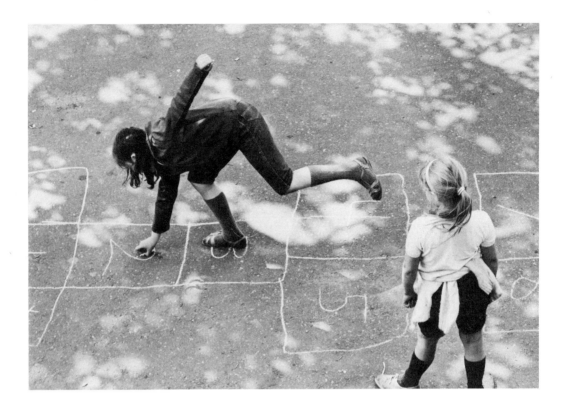

Fig. 15.2 What skills do children develop through an activity such as hopscotch? (Marion Bernstein/Editorial Photocolor Archives)

rhythmical exercises and activities for half an hour or more each day, the child learns how to acquire and maintain a high level of physical fitness. Such awareness is a preparation for adult living. Participation in vigorous physical activities during adulthood becomes an essential process for conserving well-being, thereby extending longevity and creating a more abundant life.

Physical education of the body needs to be reinforced by direct health instruction. The following sample lesson plans provide suggestions for helping the child to discover the wonder and beauty of his or her body. Because of the natural concern all children have in trying to manage their bodies, teaching about the human body should be one of the most exciting and rewarding experiences for both children and the teacher. The subject is all the more important since other topics of health are facilitated by an understanding of our physiological makeup.

TOPIC: THE GLANDULAR (ENDOCRINE) SYSTEM

(See Chapter 21, on nutrition, for a lesson plan on the digestive system.)

Grade Level: Intermediate

Note: This lesson topic may be taught as an introduction to the reproductive system, as emotional well-being, and as a part of a series of studies of the body systems.

Outcome I: The student will be able to name the parts, locations, functions, and products of the endocrine system.

Concept: Seven endocrine glands regulate the body.

Content: The seven regulatory glands are:

1. Pituitary: located at base of brain; function—produces master hormones, regulates growth and size. Produces various hormones.
2. Adrenals: location—top of kidneys; function—produce stress hormones, or adrenaline.
3. Islets of Langerhans: location—behind stomach; function—regulate sugar use. Produce insulin.
4. Thyroid: location—neck region; function—regulates body use of food (metabolic rate). Produces thyroxin.
5. Parathyroid: location—on thyroid gland; function—regulates calcium-phosphorus balance, regulates muscle tone.
6. Thymus: location—lower neck; function—protects body from early childhood diseases-immunity.
7. Gonads: location—groin and lower pelvic area; function—produce reproductive hormones, regulate sexual development.

Learning Experiences

1. *Matching bee:* (teacher and pupil playing a matching game)
2. *Overhead projections*
3. *Work sheet* as review
4. *Film: The Endocrine Glands,* AMA, No. 141.

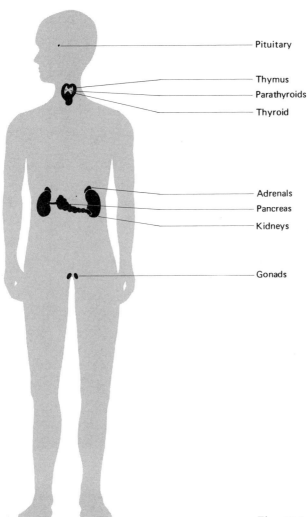

- Pituitary
- Thymus
- Parathyroids
- Thyroid
- Adrenals
- Pancreas
- Kidneys
- Gonads

Fig. 15.3 Glands of the endocrine system.

Outcome II: The student will be able to describe how to take proper care of the glandular system.

Concept: Good health habits help our glands to function properly.

Content: Good health habits aiding the glandular system are:

Learning Experiences

1. Frequent rest periods.
2. Flush the body out with water.
3. Don't lose your cool (keep emotional stability).
4. Exercise to relieve tensions.
5. Eat balanced diet regularly.
6. Have regular medical checkups.

1. *Question* and have students suggest proper health habits.
2. Pupil lists these on the blackboard.

Key Questions

1. What is the function of the _____ gland?
2. Where is it located in the body?
3. How many major glands are there?
4. Which is the gland that produces the master hormone?
5. Which gland helps you adapt to the stresses of life (when you get frightened or mad)?
6. What habits of life help you to keep the glandular system in good health?

TOPIC: THE LIVER—A CHEMICAL FACTORY

(Similar lesson plans may be evolved for other body organs.)

Grade Level: Intermediate, junior high

Outcome I: The student will be able to describe how the liver works like a chemical factory.

Concept: The liver works like a chemical factory.

Content: Ways the liver is a factory are:

1. a) Detoxifies drugs and poisons.
   b) Enzymes in the liver convert poisons (e.g., drugs, alcohol) into harmless substances that the kidneys can excrete from the body.
   c) If drugs (poisons) are continually imbibed, the liver is forced to overwork unnecessarily.
2. Stores vitamins A, D, E, K, B_{12}. Vitamins regulate body processes.
3. Stores sugar (provides quick energy for body).
4. Produces and stores bile. Bile used to break down fats in small intestine.

Learning Experiences

1. *Demonstration:* an experiment to conceptualize chemical changes taking place in body. To a test tube of dilute sulphuric acid (colorless), add phenolphthalein (red). Observe the white, sodium, settling as a precipitate. Phenolphthalein may be conceptualized as the poison and the white precipitate as the detoxified poison. The visible color change should simulate a chemical factory.
2. *Simulate* vitamins (in capsule form) and adhere to picture of liver. Or, identify each vitamin with food source and adhere these to picture of liver.
3. Adhere sugar cubes to picture of liver.
4. *Demonstration:* Show the action of soap and water in dissolving butter in a plastic bag. Demonstrate first without soap. Soap could be conceptualized as the bile.

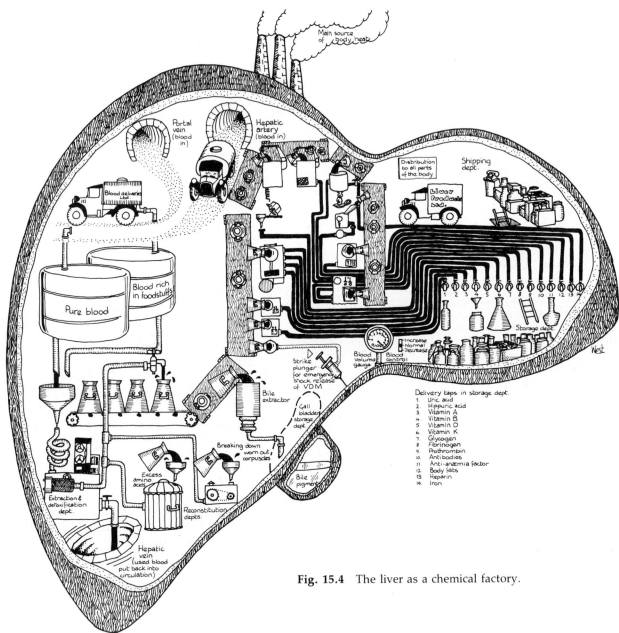

Fig. 15.4 The liver as a chemical factory.

Outcome II: The student will be able to state how to keep the liver healthy.

Concept: Healthful living keeps the liver functioning properly.

Content: Ways of keeping the liver healthy are:

1. Avoid alcohol.
2. Avoid drugs.
3. Avoid cigarette smoking.
4. Avoid excess of soft drinks.
5. Avoid coffee.
6. Eat balanced diet regularly.
7. Get plenty of exercise.
8. Get plenty of rest.

Learning Experience

1. Teacher brings sample bottles and packages of substances hazardous to the liver.

Key Questions

1. What is one function of the liver?
2. Why is drinking beer harmful?
3. How does the liver provide energy?
4. What are four main functions of the liver?
5. Why must we protect the liver and not abuse it?
6. How can we keep the liver healthy?
7. In what way is the liver a chemical factory?

. . . .

TOPIC: HOW WE SEE—VISION

(A similar lesson plan can be developed for hearing, touch, smell, and taste.)

Grade Level: Intermediate

Outcome I: The student will be able to describe how we see!

Concept I: Light transmits image (picture) through eye to nerve.

Content: Parts of the eye and their functions are:

1. *Iris* muscles (e.g., blue, brown) control amount of light entering lens.
2. *Pupil* is black center of iris through which light passes.
3. *Lens* focuses light rays on retina.
4. *Vitreous humor* helps focus light on retina.
5. *Retina* receives image upside down.

Learning Experiences

1. *Matching bee* using chart and model of eye.
2. *Demonstration:* Obtain beef eye from slaughter house and dissect an eye for the pupils. Let each pupil dissect an eye.

How to dissect an eye.* A bull's or a sheep's eye can be used. Remove the clear front skin, or cornea. This will reveal the iris and behind it the crystalline lens. This lens divides the eye into two parts, the front containing a thin liquid called aqueous humor *and the back a jellylike liquid, the* vitreous humor.

Removing the lens and vitreous humor, the retina or sensitive surface can be seen. It is more richly served with sensitive cells at a spot opposite the lens called the yellow spot. The nerves carrying the sensations pass out through a hole in the outer sclerotic membrane; this spot is therefore not sensitive to light and is called the blind spot.

Other body organs, like the lung, heart, and kidney, may be obtained from the local slaughter house and dissected for the class.

*Excerpted from *700 Science Experiments for Everyone* by UNESCO. Copyright © 1956, 1962 by UNESCO.

Concept II: The nerve sends message to brain, where image becomes picture.

Content: Transmission of light occurs as follows:

1. Optic nerve changes light image into message.
2. Optic nerve transmits message to brain.
3. Brain makes message meaningful as picture.

Learning Experience

1. *Demonstration:* Use electric cord and light or TV set to simulate function of nerve (see Fig. 15.5b).

(a)   Concept I: Light transmits image of object through eye

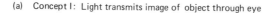
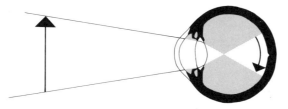

(b)   Concept II: Nerve (conceptualized by electric cord) sends message to brain

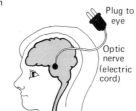

(c)   Concept III: Parts of the eye work like the parts of a camera

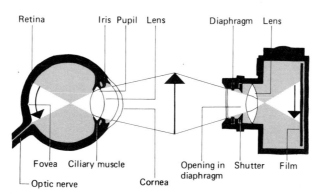

Fig. 15.5 How we see.

Concept III: Parts of eye work like a camera. (The brain interprets the light impulses visually.)

Content: Ways the camera is similar to the eye are:

1. Shutter acts like iris.
2. Lens of camera focuses light on film as in eye.
3. Film as retina records image upside down.

Learning Experiences

1. *Matching bee* comparing diagrams of camera and eye (see Fig. 15.5c).
2. Comparing models of eye and camera.
3. Essay: How eye works.

Outcome II: The child will be able to protect his or her eyes in daily life.

Concept: Eyes are precious and need to be protected.

Content: Ways of protecting eyes are:

1. Avoid bright light.
2. Avoid looking directly at the sun.
3. Do not allow glare in room.
4. Keep sharp objects away from eyes.
5. Protect eyes when participating in an activity that could be hazardous to the eyes.
6. Visit eye doctor once a year.

Learning Experiences

1. *Problem solving:* How to make room a safer place for eyes.
2. Make appointment with ophthalmologist.
3. Check vision of pupils by using Snellen Eye Test.

Key Questions

1. What does the *(pupil)* do?
2. What part focuses the light?
3. What does the optic nerve do?
4. Do you often frown when reading?
5. Do your eyes get sore often?
6. How do you see things?
7. How can you protect your eyes?

TOPIC: MAJOR ORGANS OF THE BODY (GENERAL INTRODUCTION)

Note: Body systems may be taught in similar fashion.

Grade Level: Primary, intermediate

Outcome I: The student will be able to state the names, locations, and functions of the major body organs.

Concept: Body organs are essential to optimal well-being.

Content: Major body organs are:

1. Brain: location—skull; functions—switchboard of the body, coordinates everything, communication center.
2. Heart: location—middle chest cavity; function—pump blood throughout body.
3. Lungs: location—in upper chest cavity; function—exchange gases CO_2 and O_2.
4. Kidney: location—one on each lower side of vertebral column; function—filters wastes from blood and maintains fluid balance.
5. Liver: location—right side of abdominal cavity below lung; function—detoxifies poisons and body wastes, stores body sugar, produces bile.
6. Spleen: location—behind liver and to left of stomach; function—although not well understood, it appears that the spleen has much to do with the formation and destruction of blood cells.

Learning Experiences

1. *Matching bee* and/or *human torso* (see Fig 15.6). Conceptualize function of brain with electrical telephone switchboard.
2. Heart can be compared in size to a clenched fist; function—conceptualized by a bicycle tire pump.
3. Lungs: function and appearance conceptualized by balloon.
4. Kidney: physical comparison of kidney shape to bean shape. Conceptualize function by putting chopped carrots through strainer (action of strainer simulates kidney function).
5. Refer to previous topic: "The Liver—a Chemical Factory."
6. Conceptualize function of spleen to water sponge.

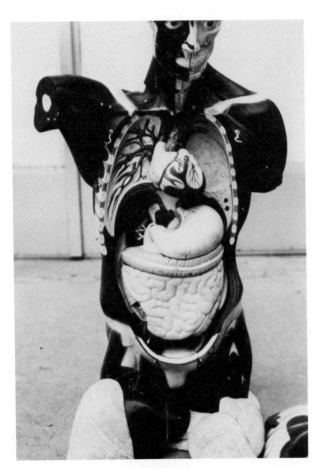

Fig. 15.6 A life-size human torso. Parts may be dismantled.

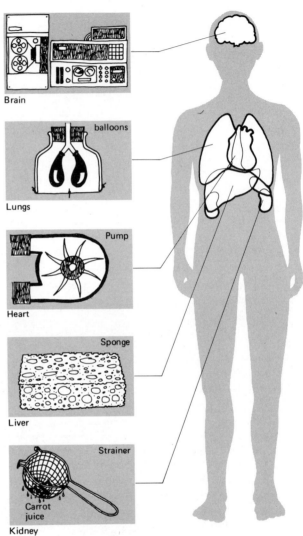

Fig. 15.7 Organs of the body, the locations, and their functions conceptualized.

Outcome II: The student will be able to take regular care of his or her body organs.

Concept: Regular care keeps body organs healthy. (Good style of living conserves body organs.)

Content: Ways to keep body organs healthy:

1. Avoid habit-forming substances.
2. Exercise regularly.
3. Eat a balanced diet regularly.
4. Have regular habits of elimination.
5. Avoid emotional stresses of living.
6. Find time to rest and sleep.
7. Relax often and regularly.
8. Drink plenty of fluids.
9. Have regular dental and medical checkups.

Learning Experiences

1. *Pictures* of good and bad health habits. Have student identify habit and match each to condition of good or poor health.
2. *Crossword puzzle* (Fig. 15.8), followed by *discussion.*

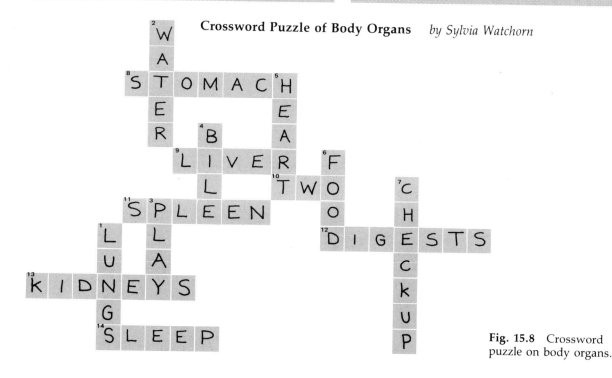

Crossword Puzzle of Body Organs *by Sylvia Watchorn*

Fig. 15.8 Crossword puzzle on body organs.

Directions: Each sentence below contains a missing word. Fill in the blank space with the words provided. Then place the word in the crossword puzzle space with the same number, either down or across.

Down:

1. L __ __ __ __ are shaped like balloons.
2. Your body needs 4-5 glasses of W __ __ __ __ daily.
3. You should P __ __ __ outdoors.
4. The liver secretes B __ __ __ .
5. The H __ __ __ __ is the size of your fist.
6. The right F __ __ __ is good for your body.
7. You need a health C __ __ __ __ __ __ once a year.

Across:

8. The S __ __ __ __ __ __ can hold one quart of food.
9. The largest glandular organ is the L __ __ __ __ .
10. The heart has T __ __ pumps.
11. You can live without your S __ __ __ __ __ .
12. The stomach D __ __ __ __ __ __ food.
13. The K __ __ __ __ __ __ are shaped like beans.
14. You need plenty of S __ __ __ __ and rest.

Use these words:

Water	Checkup	Sleep	Liver	Kidneys	Heart	Digests
Food	Play	Bile	Spleen	Two	Stomach	Lungs

Key Questions

1. What is the function of each of the organs?
   a) lungs
   b) heart
   c) liver
   d) spleen
   e) kidneys
   f) brain
2. Which are the essential organs? Why?
3. Where are the kidneys located?

4. How big is your heart?

5. Three ways to take care of your organs are . . . ?

3. *Alternative learning experiences**

a) *How the lungs work.* Cut the bottom off a large bottle. Fit a cork to the neck with a Y tube in it. On each of the lower limbs of the Y tie a rubber balloon or some small bladder. (See Fig. 15.9.)

Tie a sheet of brown paper or sheet rubber around the bottom of the jar, with a piece of string knotted through a hole and sealed with wax. Pulling this string lowers the diaphragm and air enters the neck of the Y piece causing the balloons to dilate. Pressing the diaphragm upwards has the opposite effect.

The rubber balloons represent the lungs, the tube represents the windpipe and the open bottom jar represents the bony thoracic girdle. Lowering the diaphragm reduces the pressure inside the chest cavity and air flows into the lungs. Raising the diaphragm reverses the flow of air. Try moving the diaphragm with the clamp closed.

b) *What is your lung capacity?* Pupils may be interested in finding the volume of air that the lungs can displace. This can be determined quite easily. (See Fig. 15.10.)

Fill a jar with water and fit a two-hole stopper. Insert a rubber tube through one hole; the other hole serves as an outlet. Invert the jar in a larger vessel and have a pupil make one exhalation through the tube. Place the fingers over the outlet and remove it from the large vessel. Use the graduated jar to measure the amount of water needed to refill the jug. The amount of water needed

---

* Parts (a) through (c) are excerpted from *700 Science Experiments for Everyone* by UNESCO. Copyright © 1956, 1962 by UNESCO.

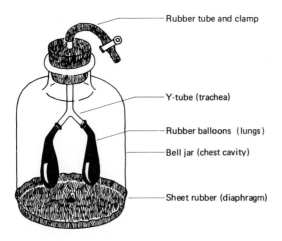

Fig. 15.9 Equipment set up to simulate how lungs work.

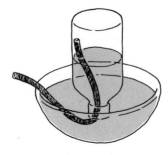

Fig. 15.10 Simple classroom spirometer set up to help children to discover their lung capacity.

will equal the volume of air that was exhaled.

Adjust the level of the water in the bowl so that the pressure of the air in the bottle is the same as that of the atmosphere, and stick a piece of gummed paper on the side of the bottle. Remove the bottle and measure the volume of water required to fill it to this mark.

c) *To show that expired air contains carbon dioxide.* The two flasks are connected so that when you breathe through the T piece, all the air bubbles through the lime water in the flasks. One tube is closed with the finger while the air is drawn in; the other tube is closed when it is expelled. (See Fig. 15.11.)

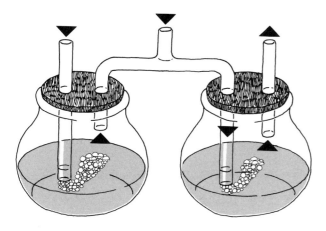

Fig. 15.11   Equipment set up to demonstrate that expired air contains carbon dioxide.

d) *Demonstration:* Beef lung inflation. Obtain a beef lung intact with the trachea (see Fig. 15.12a). Seal the upper end of the trachea to the end of a tire pump hose. Pump air into the trachea.

   Dissect a small section of the lung, and using a drinking straw, work it into a small bronchiole and inflate. The alveoli should become small bellows. Have each pupil try this demonstration. (See Fig. 15.12b.)

e) *Films: The Digestive System,* 13½ min.; *The Circulatory System,* 13½ min.; *The Excretory System,* 13½ min.; *The Respiratory System,* 13½ min.; *The Nervous System,* 13½ min. These films are available from Coronet Films, 65 East South Water St., Chicago, Illinois 60601.

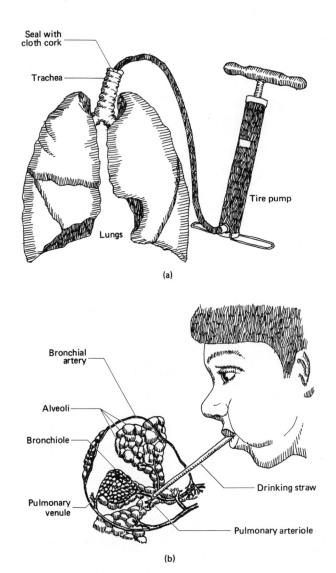

Seal with
cloth cork

Trachea

Lungs

Tire pump

(a)

Bronchial
artery

Alveoli

Bronchiole

Pulmonary
venule

Drinking straw

Pulmonary arteriole

(b)

Fig. 15.12   Experiments to demonstrate beef lung inflation.

REFERENCES AND BIBLIOGRAPHY

Best, C. H., and N. B. Taylor. *The Living Body* (New York: Holt, 1963).

Guyton, Arthur C. *Textbook of Medical Physiology* (Philadelphia: Saunders, 1966).

Kirchner, Glenn. *Physical Education for Elementary School Children* (Dubuque, Iowa: Wm. C. Brown, 1970).

Rush, F. L. *Psychology and Life* (Chicago: Scott, Foresman, 1948).

Scientific American, Reprints of Body Organs (San Francisco: Freeman, August 1958).

The Wonderful Human Machine (Chicago: American Medical Association, 1961).

"The Working of the Human Body," *Life,* October 26, 1962, p. 76.

Your Body and How It Works (Chicago: American Medical Association, 1961).

CHAPTER

16

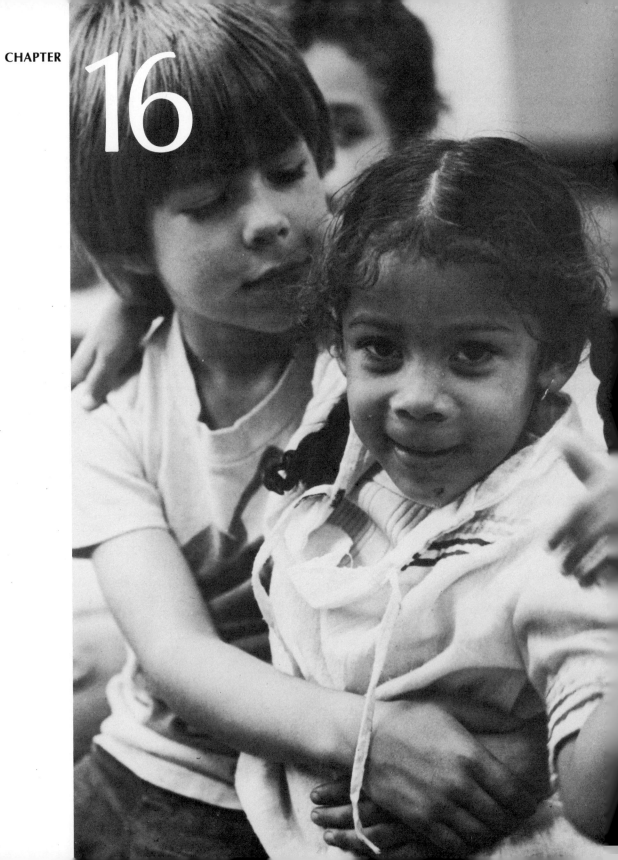

teaching about emotional and social well-being

INTRODUCTION

Emotional well-being is a fascinating topic; in essence, it is life itself. Our whole approach to life is literally dependent on the state of our emotional well-being. Some of us excel in this vein and lead happy, wholesome, and well-adjusted lives. Others approach each day as sheer drudgery and find life a chore. All too often these unhappy individuals spend a lifetime in misery. Their coping behavior becomes negative in nature, and they enter a downward spiral that may eventually lead to a form of mental disturbance or end in suicide.

All of us know that meeting life's demands is no easy task. One does not inherit good mental health, but rather has to work at it. Life is a series of minor and major developmental tasks (see Chapter 2) requiring mastery. When we are successful in fulfilling these tasks, our self-esteem receives a boost, and we move closer toward becoming fully functioning persons. When we fail, our course—for better or worse—becomes altered.

The nature of emotional well-being was explored in Chapter 5. It is a complex, multifaceted concept of total well-being. Emotional well-being may be interpreted as how one feels, thinks, acts, and behaves. In real life, these four are intermeshed and so integrated into the personality makeup that we find it most difficult to recognize them separately. Perhaps for purposes of simplicity, we should think of emotional well-being in terms of the three concepts evolved by the National Association for Mental Health: (1) feeling comfortable about self, (2) feeling right about others, and (3) being able to meet the demands of life. The interpretation of such concepts is culturally determined.

All people have the same fundamental emotional needs. Understanding ourselves and adjusting to others is primarily an emotional task. Stated in another way, if you understand the emotional needs of others, you will not only get along better with them, but come to a greater realization of your own self. Everyone wants to: be loved, feel secure, be independent and successful, and be recognized and accepted for what he or she is. To understand that all human beings have precisely these same emotional needs is probably the most fundamental step toward both maintenance of good mental health in yourself and fostering sound emotional development in others. In addition to understanding the basic emotional needs, elementary teachers should also make an effort to contribute to the satisfactory fulfillment of these needs in children. Good emotional well-being is truly based on giving as well as receiving.

Two approaches to emotional well-being education have already been implied. The indirect approach is concerned with evolving and maintaining a socioemotional climate, or environment, that is favorable to both learning and the development of emotional well-being. The well-adjusted teacher is part of this environment and becomes involved with his or her students. The direct approach provides for planned and relevant instruction that assists the children in: finding their self-identities, managing their emotions, having positive attitudes or thoughts about life in general, coping with the problems of living, and behaving in socially acceptable ways.

Obviously, this kind of instruction becomes meaningful only in a social setting, where behavior arises from coping with others. Direct teaching can help children develop responsibility for self and others. The child should learn to value a "synergic" social approach, which is predicated on the notion that one becomes a better person by helping others to be better persons—thereby attaining good feelings about self and others. The synergic concept is socioemotional in nature. It helps us to demonstrate that emotional well-being permeates all avenues of life. That is, emotional well-being is interrelated with a child's attitudes toward school and work, feelings toward sex and family living, behaviors in sports and play, and so on. It is for this reason that many educators justify inserting sex education into the mental health unit.

The teacher should structure the learning process as part of the emotional climate of the school.

The environment—social, physical, and academic—should ensure more successes than failures for all children. Indeed, every child should succeed in the elementary school, for it is at this level that attitudes toward life are structured and grafted. From this time on, the child's behavior becomes either social or antisocial, he or she either copes or does not cope with life, either withdrawing or mixing with society, either has or does not have identity, either feels comfortable about self and others or does not, and so on. As the child progresses through the secondary school system, the die that was cast in the formative years merely hardens and then comes to direct the child's destiny into adulthood.

The emotional climate in the elementary school is important as a place where the child can try out what he or she learned in the direct teaching situation. It becomes a "proving ground" for the child, providing opportunities for finding self and for learning to control emotions, deal with problems and people, and generally acquire ways of becoming adequate and worthwhile as a person. Here we are reflecting on the concept of social competence that was explored in Chapter 5. Social skills arise from physical skills. Both allow the child to be academically successful. The emotional climate in the classroom is essential to reinforcing direct teaching. It is for these reasons that this unit deals not just with emotional well-being, but with social well-being as well. Teaching for emotional well-being should be so structured that it becomes a humanizing social process.

The prospective elementary teacher is asked to view this unit as an approach to initiating both direct and indirect teaching for well-being. With these thoughts in mind, scrutinize the following lesson plans. Their purpose is to stimulate your thinking, insight, and creativity in lesson-plan development.

TOPIC: COPING WITH CRISES (PROBLEMS)

Grade Level: Intermediate

Outcome: The student will be able to cope with situations and problems effectively (solve problems as they arise).

Concept: Most problems can be solved.

Content: Typical problems children face are:

1. Getting along with others (fighting)
2. Homework
3. Lying
4. Smoking cigarettes
5. Cheating

Learning Experiences

1. *Problem solving:* Teacher prepares a worksheet on problem situations.

Problem Solving
by Jaynee Lee

Problem 1: Getting along with others (fighting)

Bill and Gary are team captains. Both teams are playing softball. Bill says "out." Bill hits Gary. What should Gary do?

Alternatives

1. Hit Bill.
2. Tell the teacher Bill hit him.
3. Ask Bill if that made him feel better and suggest taking the play over.
4. Call Bill a name.
5. Run away from Bill.

Key Questions

The following questions are suggested as a follow-up for stimulating and guiding the discussion of each problem. The direction such questioning takes should be based on (1) the teacher's endeavoring to use each situation as a way of making pupils aware of the steps for solving problems, and (2) the reactions and needs of the pupils.

1. Is there a problem?
2. Who has it?
3. Is it a recurring problem?
4. How would you solve it? Why?
5. Is there a good immediate solution?
6. Is this the best solution for later on?
7. Do you agree with _____ and his solution?
8. How would you solve it differently?
9. Does anyone have a different solution?

Problem 2: Homework

Sue has just started working on her homework assignment. Lynn calls Sue to the telephone and asks her if she can play after supper. What should Sue do?

Alternatives

1. Close her book, forget about her homework, and go play with Lynn.
2. Copy Sally's homework and then go over to Lynn's house to play.
3. Tell Lynn she has to finish her homework, but if it's not too late, she can play afterwards.
4. Tell Lynn she's busy and will play with her tomorrow after school.
5. Go to Lynn's house to play, and then stay up late to do her homework.

Key Questions

Problem 3: Lying

Jim and some of the other boys are on the playground throwing rocks. Jim's rock hits a classroom window and breaks it. The classroom is empty. No one saw Jim throw the rock. What should Jim do when the teacher asks the class: "Who threw the rock?"

Alternatives

1. Admit he broke the window.
2. Say nothing.

3. Blame it on someone else.
4. Say nothing at school, but that evening tell his mother he broke a window at school.

2. Additional problem situations are suggested.

Additional Problem-Solving Situations

Problem 1: You see a classmate take money out of a girl's purse. What should you do?

Possible Alternatives

1. Tell the teacher on duty.
2. Confront the child and say that you saw the theft and that the child should give the money back.
3. Don't do anything.
4. Tell your friends that you saw the child take the money out of the purse.

Key Questions

Problem 2: The boys do not want Jane on their baseball team because Jane cannot play well. What should Jane do?

Possible Alternatives

1. She could try to form a team of her own.
2. She could pretend she did not care and is not bothered by the whole thing.
3. She could not speak to any of the boys.
4. She might ask her father to help her practice her batting and catching.
5. (You suggest an alternative.) _____.

Key Questions

Problem 3: You arrive at school upset because you just had an argument with your parents. No one in your family gets along. You try to help your parents with their problems because you are the oldest. They only become angry at you. What should you do?

Possible Alternatives (helpful hints)

1. You decide to forget the whole incident.
2. You decide not to tell anyone because of embarrassment.
3. You decide to tell your teacher to see what he or she can do.

4. You try to talk to your parents again.

5. You tell your friends and see what they say.

6. (You suggest an alternative.) _____.

3. Small *group buzz sessions.*

Additional problems:

1. Stealing

2. Rejection

3. Mishandling money

4. Quarreling with parents

5. Playing hookey from school (truancy)

. . . .

TOPIC: RULES CONTRIBUTING TO GOOD EMOTIONAL WELL-BEING

Grade Level: Intermediate

Outcome: The student will be able to practice the rules contributing to good emotional well-being.

Concept: A good lifestyle contributes to good emotional well-being.

Content: Fifteen rules of good living helping us to have good emotional well-being are:

Learning Experiences

1. Be cheerful.

2. Be calm about things you do.

3. Think before you do things.

4. Be dependable.

5. Be patient.

6. Practice self-control.

7. Respect rights of others.

8. Plan what you do.

1. Role playing.

2. Pictures depicting bad and good lifestyles. Pupils identify both.

9. Be fair.
10. Do your share.
11. Do unto others as you would have them do unto you.
12. Do something for others without any apron-strings attached.
13. Believe in yourself.
14. Develop skills in the 3 R's.
15. Develop social skills.

TOPIC: QUALITIES OF A GOOD FRIEND

Grade level: Primary

Outcome: The student will be able to recognize qualities of a good friend.

Concept: Good friends help us to be happy, better people (good friends help each other).

Content: Good friends are:

1. Honest
2. Kind and considerate
3. Thoughtful and polite
4. Helpful—do things for us
5. Cooperative and share things
6. Clean and neat
7. Cheerful
8. Interested in you
9. Responsible and dependable
10. Fun to be with
11. Good companions and listeners

Learning Experiences

1. *Role play and dialogue* of poor and good qualities of a friend. Teacher reads off statement, and two to four children act out roles; rest of pupils identify kind of quality projected.
   a) Poor qualities
      (1) You've got bad breath and unruly hair!! (mental cruelty, insulting, thoughtless)
      (2) If you don't give me a nickel, I'm going to hit you right in the mouth!! (mental cruelty, implies physical harm, bullying)

12. Able to bring out the best in you
13. Able to share secrets

    (3) Isn't that the same shirt you've been wearing all week? (mental cruelty, possible sarcasm, thoughtless, insulting)

    (4) When was the last time you brushed your teeth? (mental cruelty, possible sarcasm, thoughtless, insulting)

b) Good qualities

    (1) Let's eat lunch together today! (amiability, sharing)

    (2) I really like your new shoes! (thoughtful, complimentary)

    (3) I just got a new bike, would you like to ride it sometime? (thoughtful, sharing, amiability)

    (4) I'm sorry that you got a low grade in spelling, but maybe we could study together for next week's test! (tactful, sharing, sympathetic, amiability)

    (5) I enjoyed playing with you. You are a lot of fun. Let's do it again! (considerate, cheerful, fun to be with)

    (6) Gee, I didn't know I could ride a bicycle! Thank you for showing me how! (able to bring out the best in you)

    (7) How can _____ keep friends?

c) *Role playing: Sample situations*

Sample Situations

I. Two boys walking home from school behind a plump girl:

    Dale: Fatty fatty two by four, couldn't get through the kitchen door.

    Ronni: Don't say that.

    Virgil: Okay, Fatso.

    Dale: Yea Piggy!!!

    Ronni: My Mommy says I'm not fat and I don't have to listen to you. (and goes running off)

Key Questions

1. Why wasn't it nice for Virgil and Dale to tease Ronni?
2. Were Dale and Virgil being friendly toward Ronni?

II. Boy and girl on same kickball team and another girl is kicking:

Debby: Come on, Sandra, we need a homer!

Dan: Oh, Sandra is so bad, she'll make us lose for sure.

Debby: She's not either—come on, Sandra, you can do it!

Dan: She'll miss, she'll miss, you watch ol' clumsy, she's the worst . . .

Debby: Yea, Sandy, you can do it . . . you can . . . you can . . . WE WON!!!

Key Questions

1. Was Debby being a good friend? Why?
2. Was Dan being a good friend? Why?
3. Is it good to encourage your friends?

III. Two girls playing with one toy and another girl comes to play:

Susan: Come on, Kath, let's play dolls.

Kathy: Okay. (turns to Diane) Gimme that doll.

Diane: No, I had it first.

Kathy: I don't care, Susan and I want to play dolls, so give it!

Diane: No. (and tugs away)

Susan: Let's all three of us play together and share the dolls.

Key Questions

1. Was Kathy being a good friend?
2. Was Susan being a good friend? Why?

2. Story: *The Easter Rabbit*

The Easter Rabbit
by Elizabeth Brown

Once upon a time, many years ago, the winter had been long and cold.

"What makes Spring so late?" said all the little children. "Let us go to the woods and see if she has come yet."

But when they got there they found the woods bare and cold. There were no birds or flowers, anywhere, and only Jack Frost and North Wind were playing among the trees.

Poor children! They went back to their homes with sad hearts and faces.

At last Spring came. When Jack Frost and North Wind saw her, they waved good-bye and ran away.

Soon the birds were building their nests, the flowers were peeping up out of the ground, and the tree buds were bursting.

But the children—where were they?

"Why didn't the children come to the woods?" said Spring. "Last year and every other year they came to play with the birds and the flowers and the animals."

"It is lonely without them," said the birds. "They will not hear our beautiful songs."

"If they do not come soon," said the flowers, "our blossoms will all be gone."

All the baby rabbits and squirrels and foxes said, "We want to see the children. We want to hide in our holes and peep out at them as they pass."

"Perhaps they do not know we are here," said Spring. "Robin, will you tell them?"

"I am too busy building a nest for my little ones," said the robin. "Send the fox. His little ones are already here."

"Will you go, Red Fox?" said Spring.

"I dare not go," said the fox. "The people will think I have come to steal the chickens."

"That is true," said Spring, "We cannot send you. Black Bear, will you go?"

"I am so big and I look so fierce," said the bear, "that I would frighten the children. Besides, I am so thin and hungry after sleeping all winter that I must eat and eat all day long. Ask the rabbit to go. Children all love rabbits."

Now, the rabbit is very timid, but he felt so proud to hear that all the children loved him that he said he would go. Then he thought of the dogs. "Oh! But the dogs!" he said. "The dogs will catch me."

"You can go at night, when all their dogs are asleep," said Spring. "So I can," said the rabbit. "I will go tonight."

So they made a big basket of twigs and leaves, and lined it with soft green grass. Then each bird brought an egg from her nest, until the basket was nearly full.

There were blue eggs, and speckled eggs, and brown eggs. How pretty they looked! Then they covered and tied the basket on bunny's back.

When evening came, the rabbit set off for the town, hippity-hop, hippity-hop. How strange and quiet it was in the town when everyone was alseep.

Bunny went to the first house where a child lived. He made a little nest of the soft green grass, and put into it one pretty egg and one spring flower.

He put the nest on the doorstep, and hopped on to the next house, and the next. When the sun came up, he hopped back to the woods, a happy bunny.

"Why, Spring is here! Spring is here!" said the children when they saw the pretty nests on their doorsteps next morning. "We were afraid that she was not coming this year. But, see, here are the tracks of a rabbit's feet. He must have brought us the message."

So off they ran for the woods, crying with happy voices, "Hurrah for bunny! Hurrah for bunny! For Spring is here at last, and bunny has come to tell us!"

Key Questions:

1. What did the children long for?
2. Was Jack Frost a good friend?
3. Was the robin a good friend? Why?
4. Was the fox a good friend? Why?
5. Who was a good friend? Why?

....

TOPIC: DECISION MAKING (STEPS TO SOLVING PROBLEMS)

Grade Level: Primary

Outcome: The student will be able to demonstrate ability to solve problems.

Concept: There are seven steps to solving problems.

Content: Steps to solving problems are:

1. Recognize and accept the problem.
2. Get all the facts about the problem—study it.
3. Analyze the problem.
4. Interpret the facts in light of your values and those of society.
5. List alternative solutions.
6. Select best alternative.
7. Take action on chosen alternative.

Learning Experiences

1. *Group solves* a sociohygienic problem in the community.
2. Individual problem solving.

Problem sample: Cigarette smoking

George and Marty just started smoking cigarettes. They try to talk Lance into smoking a cigarette with them. What should Lance do?

Work sheet to accompany problem on cigarette smoking:

A. What is the problem?

B. Below is a list of the *consequences of cigarette smoking.*

   Rate the following consequences with numerical values according to this code:

   1 = good consequence of cigarette smoking

   2 = bad consequence of cigarette smoking

   3 = This consequence of cigarette smoking doesn't seem important.

   1. Acceptance and social status among one's friends.   _____

   2. Cigarette smoking is a cause of lung cancer.   _____

   3. Cigarette smoking will give you bad breath.   _____

   4. Cigarette smoking is a cause of heart attacks.   _____

   5. Smoking a cigarette gives a person something to do when he or she is nervous.   _____

   6. Cigarette smoking may make you feel like an adult.   _____

   7. Cigarette smoking is linked to the cause of respiratory diseases such as emphysema and bronchitis.   _____

List the alternatives (ways) of solving the problem:

1. _____

   _____

2. _____

   _____

3. _____

   _____

4. _____

   _____

5. _____

_____

Choose an alternative that is best for you and the other people involved.

_____

Key Questions

1. What is the first thing you should do when you have a problem?
2. Does worrying solve a problem?
3. How do you go about solving a problem?

. . . .

TOPIC: WELL-BEING (ORTHOBIOSIS)

Grade Level: Intermediate

Outcome: The student will be able to describe the concept of well-being.

Concept: Well-being evolves from a balance of many fitnesses.

Content: Fitness components of well-being are:

1. Physical fitness:
   a) exercise
   b) good posture
   c) rest/relaxation
   d) resistance to disease/disorder
   e) sleep
   f) eating balanced diet regularly
   g) having physical skills
   h) cleansing body regularly
   i) weight and height normal

Learning Experiences

1. *Mobile well-being ladder*—"How well am I?"—to conceptualize fitness components.
   Each of the fitness components is vertically mobile and of a different color. All are interrelated and raise or lower the fitness levels of the others (see Chapter 1).

2. Emotional—spiritual (emotionally stable):
   a) exercise self-discipline
   b) relieve tensions properly
   c) give and receive affection
   d) feel good about others
   e) feel good about self
   f) assume responsibilities
   g) cope with problems
   h) feel happy
   i) feel worthwhile and adequate
   j) enthusiastic about living
   k) have future goals
   l) flexible in social situations
   m) realistic about life
   n) confident
3. Sociocultural:
   a) participate in activities
   b) relate to others
   c) do things with others
   d) interested in others
   e) go to parties often
   f) have an active hobby (paint, play musical instrument, etc.)
   g) set up moral standards of conduct
   h) cultivate close friends

How Well Am I?
(Well-Being Inventory)

	Mobile ladder		
Fitness components of well-being:			
Physical	Emotional (and spiritual)	Social (and cultural)	Level of well-being
1. Exercise/play daily 2. Seldom sick (never see doctor) 3. Have all immunizations 4. Seldom have colds 5. Have good strength, endurance, coordination 6. Eat balanced meals regularly 7. No dental caries 8. Have lots of fresh energy 9. Have ideal weight and height for age 10. Take no medicines or drugs 11. Drink no soft drinks 12. Always eat breakfast	1. Do chores regularly 2. Do homework regularly 3. Always on time 4. Always keep promises 5. Always play by the rules 6. Give and receive affection 7. Always do things on time 8. Always exercise self-discipline 9. Always confident 10. Feel good about self most of the time 11. Have goals in life	1. Have many friends 2. Like everyone 3. Do things for others often 4. Do things with others 5. Go to sports events, plays, movies, parties regularly 6. Have active hobbies (play musical instrument, paint, etc.) 7. Never cheat 8. Always play by the rules 9. Never steal 10. Always considerate (waits for turn) 11. A good loser	Optimal (High)
1. Tired often 2. Sometimes sick (see doctor sometimes) 3. Have some immunizations 4. Get colds sometimes 5. Have average strength, endurance, coordination	1. Do chores sometimes 2. Do homework sometimes 3. On time sometimes 4. Usually keep promises 5. Usually play by rules	1. Have a few friends 2. Like a few people only 3. Do things *for* others sometimes 4. Sometimes do things *with* others	

6. Eat balanced meals regularly
7. Miss breakfast sometimes
8. Height and weight fair
9. Take medicines sometimes
10. Drink 2–3 soft drinks a day
11. Stay up late often
12. Exercise/play several times a week

6. Receive affection more than give it
7. Usually do things on time
8. Lose temper and get mad sometimes
9. Usually confident
10. Usually feel good about self
11. Not sure of future life goals

5. Go to sports events, plays, movies, parties once in a while
6. Play or do hobby sometimes
7. Cheat sometimes
8. Usually play by the rules
9. Steal once in awhile
10. Usually wait for turn
11. A poor loser sometimes

Average

---

1. Always tired
2. Usually feel sick (see doctor often
3. Have few/no immunizations
4. Get colds all the time
5. Have weak strength, endurance, poor balance, poor coordination
6. Eat same things all the time
7. Do not eat breakfast
8. Overweight
9. Take medicines regularly
10. Drink more than 3 soft drinks a day
11. Stay up late all the time
12. Seldom exercise or play

1. Never do chores
2. Never do homework
3. Always late
4. Break promises often
5. Sometimes play by rules
6. Have no affection and give none
7. Postpone doing things
8. Get angry often
9. Lack confidence
10. Don't feel good about self
11. Have no life goals

1. Have no close friends (a loner)
2. Hate people
3. Do things for others only if there is a reward
4. Withdraw from others
5. Do not go to sports events, plays, etc.
6. Have no hobbies
7. Cheat often
8. Never play by the rules (have own rules)
9. Steal often
10. Never wait for turn
11. Always a poor loser

Low

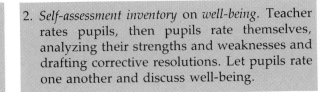

2. *Self-assessment inventory* on *well-being*. Teacher rates pupils, then pupils rate themselves, analyzing their strengths and weaknesses and drafting corrective resolutions. Let pupils rate one another and discuss well-being.

How Well Am I?
Well-Being Inventory for Elementary Children
by Walter D. Sorochan, H.S.D.

Introduction

This exercise will help you discover how well you are. You will find out your own level of well-being. If you are not clear about the directions, ask your teacher for help.

Well-being, or health, consists of many things. We can think about most of these things as either physical fitness, emotional (mental) fitness, or social fitness. Each of these fitnesses is measured by what happens to you, by how you feel, and by how you behave.

This is not a test. There are no right and wrong answers. Be honest in reacting to each statement.

Directions

1. Turn to the first page that describes the things that make up an optimal level of well-being. Eleven things make up each of the three fitness components.
2. *Rate yourself* for physical fitness first. Give yourself the number of points indicated in parentheses next to the item you chose.
3. Add your score and write it in the blank at the bottom.
4. Do the same for the emotional and social fitnesses.
5. *Analysis:* Add your scores for three fitnesses of well-being.

+ Total physical fitness score   = _____

+ Total emotional fitness score   = _____

+ Total social fitness score   = _____

Your well-being score   = _____

6. *Interpretation:* Interpret your well-being score by observing where this score falls on the scale:

Well-being scale	*Your level of well-being*
99-75	High (optimal)
74-49	Average
48-33	Low

A. *Physical fitness*

1. You exercise
___ (1) seldom
___ (2) twice a week
___ (3) each day

2. You are sick
___ (1) often
___ (2) sometimes
___ (3) seldom

3. You feel tired
___ (1) always/often
___ (2) sometimes
___ (3) never/seldom

4. You see a doctor
___ (1) very often
___ (2) sometimes
___ (3) never/seldom

5. You have colds
___ (1) 6 or more times a year
___ (2) 2-3 times a year
___ (3) once a year or seldom

6. Your muscle strength
   and body coordination are
___ (1) very weak
___ (2) average
___ (3) strong

7. You eat nutritional meals each day
___ (1) seldom miss breakfast
___ (2) usually
___ (3) always

8. Your weight for your age is
___ (1) too much
___ (2) fair
___ (3) ideal

9. You take medicines or drugs
___ (1) often (always)
___ (2) sometimes
___ (3) seldom

10. You drink soft drinks each day
___ (1) 3 or more glasses
___ (2) 1-2 glasses
___ (3) none

11. You have accidents
___ (1) often
___ (2) sometimes
___ (3) never/seldom

Total physical fitness score = ___

B. *Emotional fitness*

1. You do chores
___ (1) never/seldom
___ (2) sometimes
___ (3) often

2. You do homework
___ (1) never/seldom
___ (2) sometimes
___ (3) often

3. You are on time
___ (1) sometimes
___ (2) often
___ (3) always

4. You keep promises
___ (1) sometimes
___ (2) often
___ (3) always

5. You play by the rules
___ (1) sometimes
___ (2) often
___ (3) always

6. You give and receive affection
___ (1) sometimes
___ (2) often
___ (3) always

7. You do things on time
___ (1) sometimes
___ (2) often
___ (3) always

8. You get angry
___ (1) sometimes
___ (2) often
___ (3) always

9. You feel confident
___ (1) sometimes
___ (2) often
___ (3) always

10. You feel good about yourself
___ (1) sometimes
___ (2) often
___ (3) always

11. You plan ahead
___ (1) sometimes
___ (2) often
___ (3) always

Total emotional fitness score = ___

C. *Social fitness*

1. You have friends
   _____ (1) none
   _____ (2) few
   _____ (3) many

2. You like people
   _____ (1) hate people
   _____ (2) like few people
   _____ (3) like most people

3. You do things *for* others
   _____ (1) sometimes
   _____ (2) often
   _____ (3) always

4. You do things with friends
   _____ (1) sometimes
   _____ (2) often
   _____ (3) always

5. You see sports, movies,
   and go to parties
   _____ (1) sometimes
   _____ (2) often
   _____ (3) always

6. You play at a hobby
   (paint, play musical instrument, etc.)
   _____ (1) don't have one
   _____ (2) once a week
   _____ (3) three or more times a week

7. You cheat in games, at school,
   or on friends
   _____ (1) always
   _____ (2) sometimes
   _____ (3) never

8. You play by the rules
   _____ (1) sometimes
   _____ (2) often
   _____ (3) always

9. You steal things
   _____ (1) often
   _____ (2) sometimes
   _____ (3) never/seldom

10. You wait for your
    turn to do things
    _____ (1) sometimes
    _____ (2) often
    _____ (3) always

11. You are a poor loser
    _____ (1) often
    _____ (2) sometimes
    _____ (3) seldom

Total social fitness score = _____

3. *Alternative learning experiences*

   a) *Orthobiosis:* This lesson could be adopted to teach about orthobiosis, or right style of living. Components of orthobiosis could be interpreted as daily and weekly habits of living. Pupils could rate themselves on a simple rating scale and analyze and interpret their lifestyle, e.g.,

   (1) *Good citizenship quiz*

   (2) Administer a *physical fitness* test, analyze weaknesses, and recommend corrective exercise for each pupil.

   (3) *Picture quiz* on rules of good living.

Rules of Good Living

Name _____

Directions

One of each pair of the following pictures does not represent a good living habit. Which one is it?

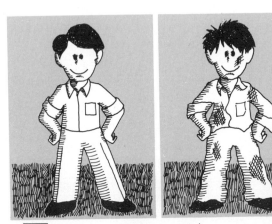 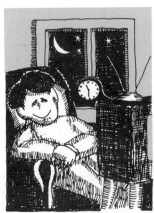

1. ☐   (Personal appearance)   ☐

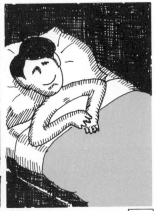

2. ☐   (Rest, sleep)   ☐

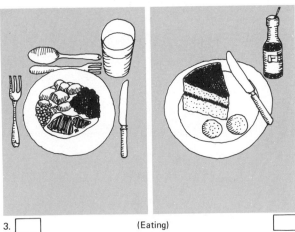 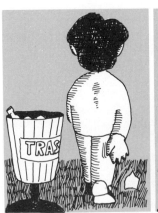

3. ☐   (Eating)   ☐

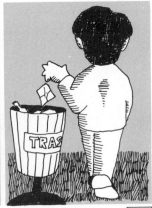

4. ☐   (Waste disposal and sanitation)   ☐

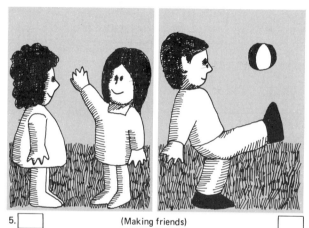

5. ☐   (Making friends)   ☐

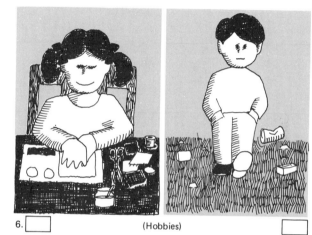

6. ☐   (Hobbies)   ☐

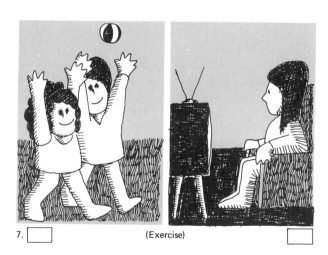

7. ☐   (Exercise)   ☐

(4) *Health heroes story:* value of good health.

Key Questions: (Emphasis at elementary school level should be placed on physical, emotional, and social fitness components of well-being.)

1. What does "body physical fitness" mean?
2. What is emotional fitness?
3. What do we mean by social fitness?
4. How do you know if you have_____ fitness?
5. What is well-being?
6. How do we get optimal well-being?
7. How can we maintain optimal well-being?
8. How can we conserve our well-being?
9. Why do we need optimal well-being?

REFERENCES AND BIBLIOGRAPHY

Arnspiger, Varney C., *et al. Personality in Social Process* (Dubuque, Iowa: W. C. Brown, 1969), pp. 174-176.

Erikson, Erik. *Growth and Crisis of the Health Personality.* pp. 5-100.

Gruenberg, Sidonie M. *Your Child's Friend* (New York: Public Affairs Committee, 1959).

Kaplan, Louis. *Mental Health and Human Relations in Education* (New York: Harper & Row, 1959), pp. 315-379.

Meninger, William C. *Making and Keeping Friends* (Chicago: Science Research Associates, 1952).

Remmers, Herman. *Your Problems: How to Handle Them* (Chicago: Science Research Associates, 1953).

Wilde, George, *et al.* "You and Your Friends," "Learning to Make Friends; Being a Likeable Person," in *About Your Health* (New York: American Book, 1959).

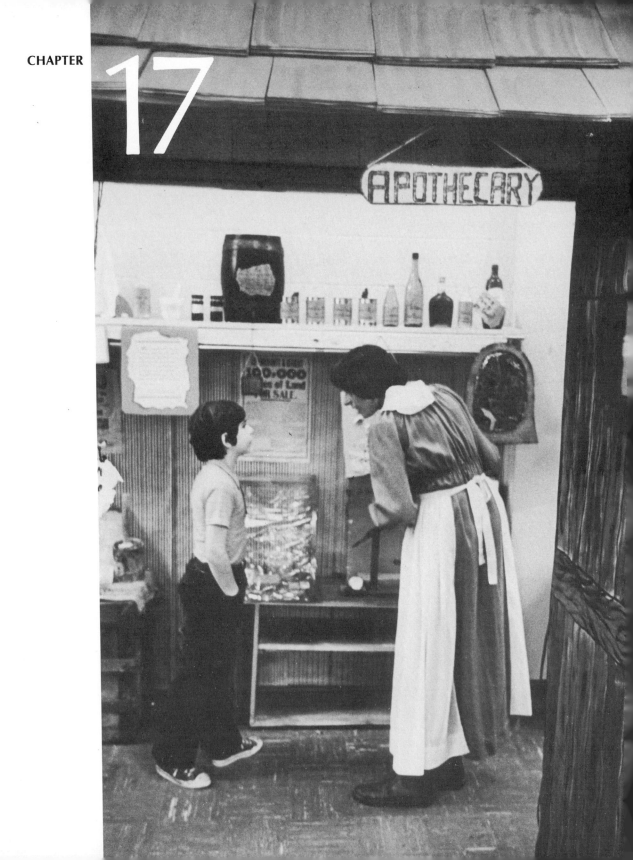

teaching about drugs

Perhaps no other health content area today commands more public attention than drug use and abuse. Nearly every school system has some form of a formal drug education program. However, effectiveness of many of these programs is debatable.

The classic assembly program at which a local narcotics officer lectures on the ill effects of marijuana while dragging on a cigarette may satisfy many an administrator's ego, but does little to impress students. The classroom teacher who adamantly denounces the popular hallucinogenic drugs but fails to discuss the shortcomings of alcohol and tobacco is not only naive, but hypocritical as well. Inviting a rehabilitated narcotic addict to "tell it like it is" can be impressive, but should hardly be considered as either all-encompassing or constituting the appropriate focal point of a drug education unit. The utilization of inaccurate or out-dated teaching aids is also a serious error. Youngsters are far more sophisticated in the area of drug use and abuse than one might believe. In many instances they may be far more experienced than you.

So what do we do? Is there one best way to approach drug education? Probably not. Surely many classroom teachers are doing an effective job of drug education, and chances are that each uses a different technique. However, there are underlying principles that can and should be considered basic to effective drug education. For example:

1. Only sound, scientific, and up-to-date information has a place in drug education.
2. Scare tactics have little long-lasting value.
3. Drug education includes instruction about *all* mood-modifying substances; alcohol and tobacco are no exception.
4. When expression of biases and/or moralizing become overly apparent, the objectivity of drug education suffers and instruction loses its impact.
5. Instruction about drug use and abuse should be handled only by a well-informed, empathic, competent teacher.

Identify drugs suggested by TV slogans:

Slogan	Drug
Come to ? County	(Cigarettes)
Mountain grown for better flavor ?	(Coffee)
? Works wonders	(Aspirin)
Take ? tonight and sleep — Safe and restful sleep, sleep, sleep	(Sleeping pills)
Tastes like a mint works like a miracle ?	(Antacids)
Made from spring water ?	(Beer)

Fig. 17.1 Matching drugs with TV slogans. The answers to the slogans are given in the "Drug" column.

6. Drug education is ongoing and comprehensive in nature. "One shot" endeavors are of little value.

7. Drug education encompasses far more than mere cognitive information. By its very nature, drug education deals with behavior, and this implies that the affective and action domains are explored.

By now it should be obvious that drug use and abuse is not just a passing adolescent fad. The complexities of our culture provide the basis for what in many instances is irresponsible, self-destructive, and/or escape behavior in the form of drug abuse. Actually such behavior is really not new. People have abused drugs for centuries and in some cases have been successful in legalizing the means for such abuse, as evidenced by the sale of alcoholic beverages. The only new thing many young people have done is to expand the horizon of the world of illusion and experiment with a wider variety of mind-altering drugs.

Surely our most important task at hand is to deal with the "whys" of drug abuse. We have already discussed the behavioral nature of drug education, and it follows that one of the greatest emphases in instruction should be on exploring the reasons why people chemically escape from reality. It is also important that we devote attention to meaningful alternatives to drug abuse. Last, but certainly not least, we should provide children with the most up-to-date, objective, and factual information relative to the physiological effects of drugs on the body.

As with previous chapters in this section, the lesson plans that follow are presented as exemplary models of what can be developed as a part of a drug education unit.

TOPIC: EFFECT OF DRUGS ON THE BODY

Grade Level: Intermediate

Outcome: The student will be able to describe how drugs affect the body in different ways.

Concept: Drugs can depress or stimulate the body.

Content

1. Ways in which some drugs slow down or depress the body are:
   a) destroy vitamins A, B₆, C, and E; make you feel depressed and tired
   b) make nerves sluggish
   c) make you lose your balance
   d) difficult to hear and see
   e) slow down heart rate
   f) slow down breathing
   g) lower blood pressure
   h) make you feel like sleeping

Learning Experiences

1. Students *simulate* depressed effects:
   a) relax muscles;
   b) close eyes and drift to sleep;
   c) count breathing and pulse rates (at rest).

Key Questions

1. How do you feel?
2. Are you relaxed?
3. How fast are you breathing?

2. Ways some drugs speed up or stimulate the body are:
   a) get nerves excited
   b) speed up heart beat
   c) speed up body use of energy
   d) increase blood pressure
   e) speed up breathing
   f) make you tired after a while
   g) stimulate adrenal glands

2. Students *simulate* stimulant effects:
   a) run in place for two minutes;
   b) recount breathing and pulse rates for one minute immediately after work;
   c) compare rest and work rates.

Key Questions

1. How do you feel?
2. How fast were you breathing?
3. How fast was your heart beating?
4. How can drugs stimulate your body?
5. How can drugs depress your body?

3. Have students complete crossword puzzle in order to learn the symptoms of drug use.

Crossword Puzzle

I. Symptoms

   A. Depressants—*ACROSS*

      1. Mixed up
      2. When one slides one's words together, one talks with slurred _____.
      3. Sleepiness
      4. Walks crookedly
      5. Unable to concentrate (two words; first word is a contraction)
      6. Too much alcohol will cause one to become _____.
      7. Unable to stand without swaying (two words; first word is a contraction)

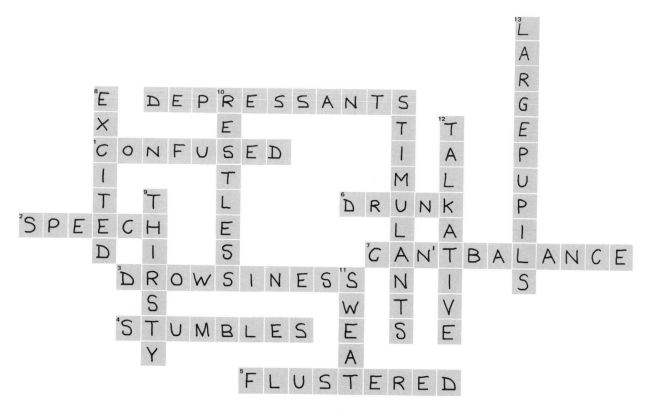

Fig. 17.2 A crossword puzzle to help children learn about the symptoms of drug use.

B. Stimulants—*DOWN*

8. Usually when one gets "butterflies" in one's stomach, it is because one is _____.

9. Craving a drink of water

10. Uneasy

11. To perspire

12. Talky

13. When one's dots in the middle of the eyes get big, one has _____. (two words)

. . . .

TOPIC: HOW TO USE MEDICINES SAFELY

Grade Level: Primary

Outcome: The student will be able to summarize the safe ways to use medicines.

Concept: Medicine helps keep us healthy only when we use it safely and properly.

Content: Safe ways to use medicines are:

1. Take under doctor's care.
2. Identify medicine in lighted room.
3. Have Mom or Dad read directions on label.
4. Follow directions.
5. Take exact amount.
6. Let Mom or Dad give it to you.
7. Keep in safe place.
8. Never share your medicine with others.
9. Don't borrow someone else's medicine.

Learning Experiences

1. *Storytelling:* "How Snoopy Got Better"

"How Snoopy Got Better" (Outline)

Introduction

It is Saturday morning and Charlie Brown wants to play baseball. He goes out to wake up Snoopy so that they can practice. Snoopy is the shortstop for the team. He finds Snoopy sick and does not know what to do. Then the other children come.

1. Sally offers aspirin.
2. Lucy says that only grown-up people should give medicine and only if the doctor says to do so.
3. Linus offers cherry-flavored medicine.
4. Lucy says that medicine should not be shared with others. Medicines are not toys even if they sometimes taste good.

Climax

Lucy suggests taking Snoopy to the doctor. Perhaps the doctor can help him. So Charlie, Charlie's mother, and the other children take Snoopy to the doctor.

1. The doctor helps Snoopy. He gives Snoopy a special medicine and gives special directions to Charlie and Charlie's mother.

2. The doctor says the medicine will make Snoopy's sickness go away because it will kill the bad germs.

3. The doctor says that the medicine will help Snoopy to feel much better.

4. The doctor gives Snoopy a shot so that the sickness will not come back.

Conclusion

Charlie's mother helps him give Snoopy the medicine by following the doctor's directions carefully. Soon Snoopy is all better and is playing baseball with the team once more.

Key Questions (follow-up)

1. Did you like the story?

2. Why didn't Lucy want to give Snoopy an aspirin?

3. Why didn't Lucy want to give Snoopy the medicine that tastes like cherries?

4. Why did the doctor say that the special medicine would make Snoopy's sickness go away?

5. Why did the doctor give Snoopy a shot?

6. Did Snoopy get better?

7. Would you like to be Snoopy?

· ·

TOPIC: VOLATILE SUBSTANCES ARE HAZARDOUS TO OUR HEALTH

Grade Level: Intermediate

Outcome: The student will be able to describe the harmful effects of volatile substances.

Concept: Volatile substances are physically harmful.

Content: Volatile substances cause the following symptoms:

1. Kill brain and liver cells.
2. Depress the brain and body.
3. Irritate the nasal passages.
4. Cause conditions similar to alcohol intoxication.

Learning Experience

1. *Demonstration:* Use hair spray to intoxicate rat—observe symptoms.

. . . .

TOPIC: TRIPPING WITHOUT DRUGS (ALTERNATIVES)

Grade Level: Intermediate

Outcome: The student will be able to discuss the many ways to trip without drugs.

Concept: One can get good and exciting feelings about the things one does without drugs.

Content: Nondrug ways of getting high are:

1. Imagination
2. Painting
3. Reading a book
4. Singing
5. Playing musical instrument
6. Playing sports
7. Going for a bike hike
8. Sewing
9. Surfing
10. Writing
11. Joining a club

Learning Experience

1. *Simulate* a trip through imagination and, if desired, by use of senses. Students may need to learn to relax and to concentrate on a single thought before being successful in this adventure of "tripping."

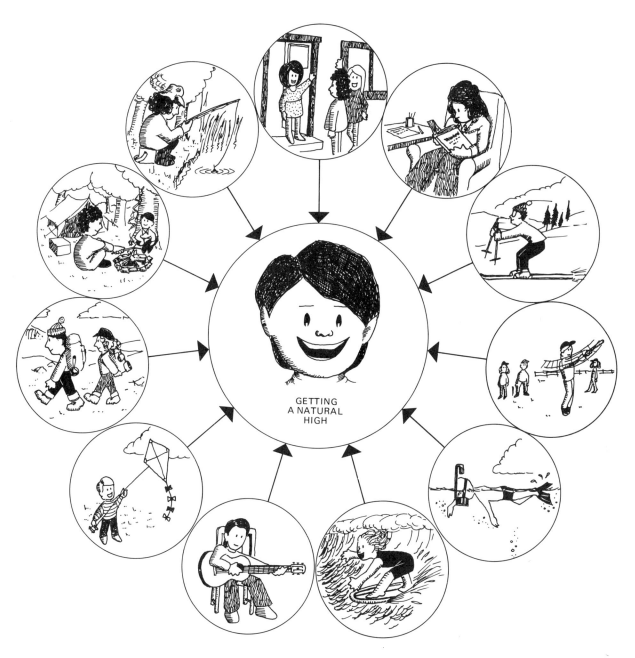

Fig. 17.3   A few "natural" ways of tripping without drugs.

A Trip Using the Imagination

Since it is early spring and the sun is out this morning, let's take a walk through a big, huge garden of flowers. Look at all the colors! There must be every kind of flower in the world in this garden. If you look real hard, back in the far left-hand corner, past the tulips and past the yellow daisies, go way back past the pink and white carnations, and you will find the roses. Do you see all the different colors of roses? Yellows, whites, pinks, reds? Let's take a closer look at that big rose bush in the middle—the one with the big, beautiful red roses on it. Now, look at just one of the roses. How about the big one on the right side? If you get real close to it, you can see it better. It is a deep wine-red and very beautiful. The petals are opening just a little because it is just now early spring. The stem and the leaves are a beautiful green, but don't touch the stem, because you might get hurt on the sharp thorns. Since it is early morning, we can still see drops of dew on the petals. Isn't it pretty? If you get close enough and use a whole lot of imagination, you might be able to smell the beautiful rose fragrance.

Can you think of other ways of tripping without the use of drugs?

Key Questions

1. Did you let your imagination carry you away?
2. How did you feel? Muscles? Body?
3. Were you able to imagine the color of the rose?
4. Did you smell the rose?
5. Could you paint a picture of the rose?
6. Did you enjoy the imagination trip?

REFERENCES AND BIBLIOGRAPHY

Bennett, James C., and George D. Demos. *Drug Abuse Among Youth—Implications for A New Approach to Education* (Riverside, Calif.: Riverside County Department of Education, 1969).

Carney, Richard E. *Risk-Taking and Drug Abuse* (Coronado, Calif.: Coronado Unified School District, 1970).

Girdano, Daniel A., and Dorothy Dusek Girdano. *Drug Education: Content and Methods,* 2d ed. (Reading, Mass.: Addison-Wesley, 1976).

Jones, Kenneth L., Louis W. Shainberg, and Curtis O. Byer. *Drugs and Alcohol* (New York: Harper & Row, 1971).

Lockheed Education Systems. *Drug Decisions* (Burbank, Calif.: Lockheed Aircraft Corporation, 1969).

McGrath, Richard F. *Narcotics Dangerous Drug Abuse: Instructor's Guide* (San Diego, Calif.: Winston Products for Education, 1968).

Teaching About Drugs: A Curriculum Guide Kindergarten Through Twelfth Year (Kent, Ohio: American School Health Association and the Pharmaceutical Manufacturers Association, 1970).

Weinswig, Melvin H., and Dale W. Doerr. *Drug Abuse: A Course for Educators* (Indianapolis: Butler University Press, 1968).

18

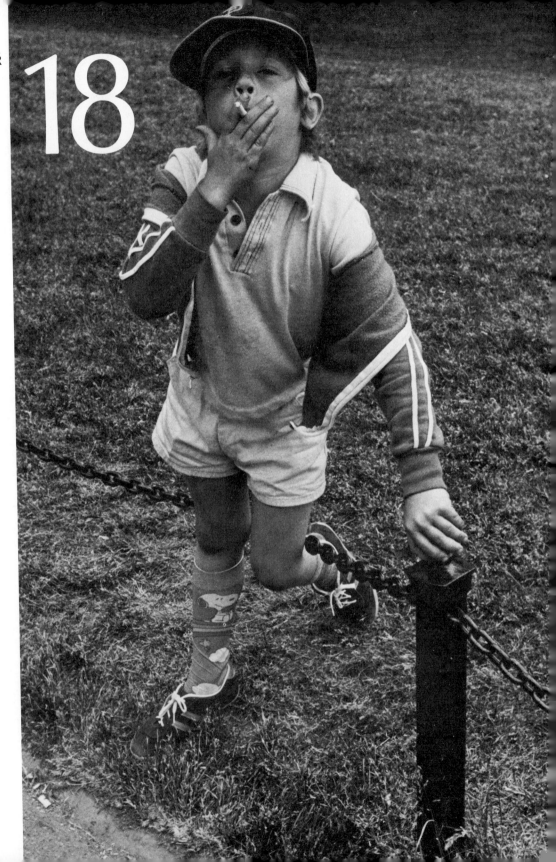

teaching about tobacco

INTRODUCTION

There is a cause-and-effect relationship between smoking and lung cancer. That's right, smoking *causes* lung cancer. In fact, if you're a chronic smoker, your chances of dying before your life expectancy are enhanced sevenfold. You have a seven in ten chance of never reaching your life expectancy, because you will most likely die as a result of a cigarette-related chronic disease. This is indeed tragic when you realize that cigarette smoking is surely one of the greatest preventable causes of illness, disability, and premature death in the United States today.

The logical question is *why*; why do so many people smoke in light of all the evidence linking the smoking habit with ill health? What entices the smoker to risk longevity and good health for the seemingly meager benefits derived from smoking? Certainly some smokers are ignorant of the facts. Some choose to ignore the evidence or rationalize their behavior; others assume a "devil may care" attitude and throw all caution to the wind. Whatever the case may be, it is obvious that smoking gives many Americans an indispensable pleasure.

Further analysis discloses that most smokers acquire their habit early in life. Initial smoking experiences are likely to take place during the late intermediate or early junior high years. This is unfortunate because in most cases youngsters have received very little, if any, formalized instruction about the health ramifications of smoking. All too often we are content to wait until the high school years before providing students with health information regarding smoking. In most instances we are four or five years too late.

Smoking is most often described as a form of coping behavior that can easily become habitual. Everyone has his or her own personal habitual-type coping behaviors. More than likely some are positive in nature, whereas others may be negative or harmful, like smoking. After a period of time these habits become a part of our nature and in many instances are next to impossible to change. How many times have you heard a person say, "I want to quit (smoking), but somehow I just don't have the perseverance to do it once and for all"? This type of person is most difficult to help. Unless she or he

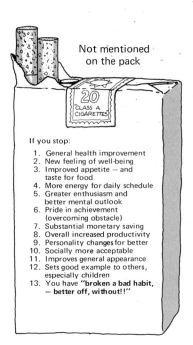

Not mentioned on the pack

If you stop:

1. General health improvement
2. New feeling of well-being
3. Improved appetite — and taste for food
4. More energy for daily schedule
5. Greater enthusiasm and better mental outlook
6. Pride in achievement (overcoming obstacle)
7. Substantial monetary saving
8. Overall increased productivity
9. Personality changes for better
10. Socially more acceptable
11. Improves general appearance
12. Sets good example to others, especially children
13. You have **"broken a bad habit, — better off, without!!"**

Fig. 18.1 Summary of the benefits of not smoking cigarettes.

truly wants to quit and is willing to pay the emotional price, there is little chance that the habitual smoker will ever achieve even token success in terms of completely giving up smoking.

Perhaps our effort would be better directed at attempting to discourage youngsters from ever starting to smoke. This is a difficult task, to say the least, but it is possible to have a positive influence on children's initial smoking behavior. Unbiased, sound, and scientific smoking information that is skillfully and creatively imparted can go a long way toward assisting children to develop positive practices and attitudes relative to the smoking of tobacco. The challenge is to motivate children to consider smoking as an "out" thing to do. The earlier one starts with such a program, the more likely one is to be successful in assisting youngsters to adopt such an ideal. We must begin to realize that much of the health information once considered appropriate for the high school level is now more appropriate at the intermediate level. Smoking and its relationship to health is one of these content areas.

The lesson plans on smoking and health that follow were designed to provide you with some basic lesson plan ideas. Obviously the included lesson plans could be utilized in their present form if one so desired. However, it is intended that they provide the framework for what should be a more comprehensive and all-inclusive unit on smoking and health.

TOPIC: EFFECTS OF CIGARETTE SMOKING ON THE BODY

Grade Level: Intermediate, junior high

Outcome: The student will be able to describe how cigarette smoke affects all bodily systems.

Concept: Cigarette smoke affects all systems of the body.

Content: Effects on each body system are:

1. Respiratory system:
   a) Anesthetizes cilia and eventually destroys them.
   b) Stimulates overproduction of mucus.
   c) Uses up vitamin A and causes irritation of trachea, causing coughing.
   d) Increases susceptibility of bronchial tube to infection.
   e) Puts carbon monoxide into blood, decreasing oxygen in blood, thereby making it difficult to breathe.
   f) Reduces circulation in lung.
   g) Enhances destruction of alveoli.
   h) Greatly increases the chances of contracting lung cancer, emphysema, and chronic bronchitis (see Fig. 18.2).
2. Cardiovascular system:
   a) Nicotine increases heart rate.
   b) Constricts superficial blood vessels.
   c) Raises blood pressure.
   d) Accelerates atherosclerosis.
   e) Decreases clotting time.

Learning Experiences

1. Demonstration of the effect of cigarette smoke on the cilia of a fresh chicken's trachea or on a salamander. (Directions for conducting this demonstration are included in accompanying section on experiments and demonstrations.)
2. Demonstration of the effect of nicotine on the heart of a live frog. (For directions on how to conduct this experiment, see the accompanying section on experiments and demonstrations.)
3. Demonstration of the effect of nicotine on a live fish in a bowl. (See accompanying section for details.)
4. Tic-tac-toe game to reinforce facts.

HOW MUCH DO YOU SMOKE?

None?

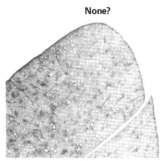

The bronchi and blood vessels appear as small round holes in this normal lung.

½ pack?

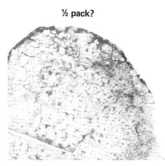

Small holes in upper lung typical of early emphysema.

1 pack?

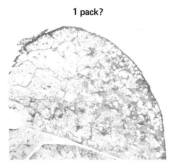

A later stage showing larger holes in the lung.

2 or more?

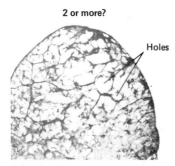

Holes

Many large holes representing far advanced emphysema.

Fig. 18.2 Photographs of whole lung sections showing changes of pulmonary emphysema as related to smoking habits. (O. Auerbach *et al.*, "Relation of Smoking and Age to Emphysema," *New England Journal of Medicine* **286** (1972): 853-857. Photographs courtesy of Smoking Research/San Diego.)

3. Nervous system:
   a) After a short period of stimulation, nicotine depresses the sympathetic and parasympathetic nerves.
   b) Nicotine depresses the functions of taste and smell.
4. Other systems:
   a) Smoking reduces appetite and stimulates peristalsis.
   b) Nicotine is actively and rapidly metabolized. The resulting metabolites are excreted in the urine and may cause irritation and bladder cancer.

c) Ulcers are greatly irritated by smoking.

d) Your risk of death from cirrhosis is doubled.

e) Nicotine causes stress to the liver and destroys vitamins B_6, C, and E. One cigarette destroys about 25 mg of vitamin C, or about one-half the recommended minimum daily allowance. Smoking jeopardizes the liver's ability to function.

f) Smoking one pack of cigarettes depletes 500 mg of vitamin C.

g) Smoking causes facial wrinkling at early age; it speeds up the aging process.

Key Questions

1. How does tobacco smoke physiologically affect the respiratory, cardiovascular, and nervous systems?

2. Does smoking affect your appetite? If so, how?

3. How is smoking a major factor in heart disease?

4. Does smoking cause lung cancer?

5. What is the relationship between smoking and such diseases as emphysema and chronic bronchitis?

TOPIC: THE CHEMICAL COMPOSITION OF CIGARETTE SMOKE

Grade Level: Intermediate, junior high school

Outcome I: The student will be able to describe the general composition of cigarette smoke.

Concept I: Cigarette smoke contains many substances.

Content	*Learning Experience*
1. Cigarette smoke is an aerosol. 2. Cigarette smoke contains 500 chemicals. 3. Cigarette smoke contains gases. 4. Cigarette smoke contains vaporized tars and nicotine.	1. Chart showing components of cigarette smoke.

Concept II: Cigarette smoke contains harmful gases.

Content

1. Carbon monoxide gas is present in cigarette smoke at 400 times the industrial safe (I. S.) level. Carbon monoxide replaces oxygen in the blood.
2. Cigarette smoke contains hydrogen cyanide gas, a powerful poison, at 160 times I. S. level.
3. Nitrogen dioxide gas, an acute irritant, is present in cigarette smoke at 50 times I. S. level.

Learning Experiences

1. Chart
2. *Demonstration:* Smoking Sam. Observe smoke in "Sam's" lungs to see gaseous nature of smoke. (See Fig. 18.3.)

Concept III: The nicotine in cigarette smoke is poisonous.

Content

1. Nicotine is a powerful poison and is used as an insecticide called "Black Leaf 40."
2. Cigarette smoke contains ½-2 mg of nicotine per cigarette.
3. 70 mg of nicotine injected will kill a person.
4. Nicotine from smoking one cigarette destroys about 25 mg of vitamin C, as well as vitamins B_6 and E.

Learning Experiences

1. Chart
2. Show prints of exhaled smoke on tissue paper (see Fig. 18.4).

Concept IV: Tobacco tar contains cancer-producing facilitating chemicals.

Content

1. Cigarette tars contain 16 cancer-producing chemicals.
2. Several chemicals in tar make the cancer producers more powerful.
3. These chemicals increase the strength of the cancer producers 40 times.

Learning Experiences

1. Smoke print tissues.
2. See tar in "Sam."

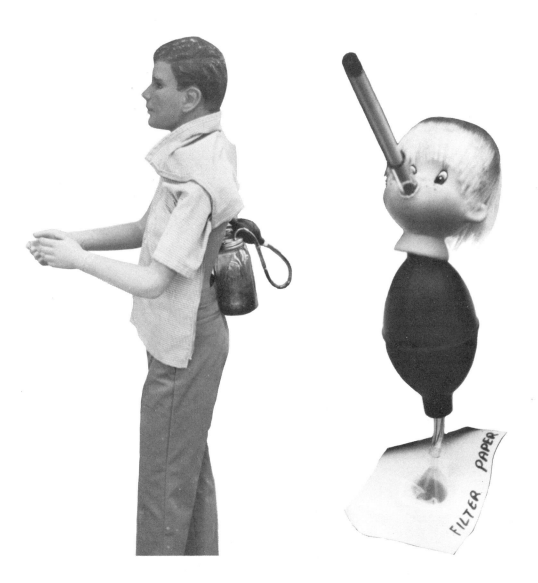

Fig. 18.3 Illustration of "Smoking Sam" and how cigarette smoke settles inside the "lungs," which have been fabricated from asbestos wool inside glass jars.

Fig. 18.4 Demonstration of composition of cigarette smoke by using "Nicotina" to smoke. Substances in cigarette smoke leave an imprint on filter paper.

Outcome II: The student will be able to identify the distasteful elements of cigarette smoke.

Concept: Cigarette smoke leaves a distasteful residue of tar and nicotine.

Content	*Learning Experiences*
1. Cooled smoke vapors turn into liquid tars and nicotine.	1. Examine and taste tars in "Sam's lungs."
2. Liquid tars and nicotine form a brown residue.	2. Smell "Sam's breath" by squeezing air from the rubber bulb.
3. Liquid tars and nicotine smell bad.	
4. Liquid tars and nicotine taste bad.	

Key Questions (Verbal quiz)

1. What are three major substances contained in cigarette smoke?
2. Why are tobacco tars harmful?
3. What does "Sam's breath" smell like?
4. What happened to the tars in Sam's cigarettes?

Teaching Aids

1. "Smoking Sam"
2. Smoking elements chart
3. Smoke print tissues

. . . .

TOPIC: WHY DO PEOPLE SMOKE?

Grade Level: Intermediate

Outcome: The student will be able to state why people smoke.

Concept: People smoke for many reasons.

Content: Reasons for smoking:

1. Curiosity and desire to explore
2. Copying smokers—monkey see, monkey do
3. Peer conformity
4. Identity
5. Immediate gratification
6. Rebellion
7. Simple experiment—to find out for self what something is like

Learning Experiences

1. Role playing

   a) *Situation 1.* Three students are off in a corner playing. A fourth student is playing alone, but decides to play with the others. The child walks over to the group, sees that they are smoking, and decides to join them.

Key Questions

1. Why do you think that the fourth student decided to smoke?
2. Does one have to smoke if his or her friends smoke?

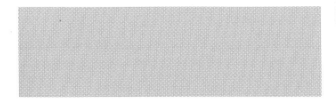

   b) *Situation 2.* Bob's mother is furious with Bob because he never obeys her. He is fed up with hearing her nag and scream at him all the time. He goes off to a place where she won't see him. He starts to smoke.

Key Questions

1. Why do you think Bob was smoking?
2. What else could Bob have done to release his anger?

   c) *Situation 3.* Dad comes home after a long day of work and sits down in his favorite chair. He takes off his shoes and reads the newspaper. His daughter sits near his chair and watches television. After reading for a while, Dad lights up a cigarette and smokes for a while. He then gets up to get something from the other room. The daughter goes to the chair, picks up a cigarette, and takes a few drags from it.

Key Questions

1. Why did the daughter decide to smoke?
2. Does smoking mean that one is grown up?

. . . .

Alternative Experiments and Demonstrations

The following experiments may help teachers to demonstrate the effects of cigarette smoke on living things and particularly on the human body. These may be used as alternatives to those suggested in the lesson plans. Teachers should select experiments that are feasible for their teaching situations. Experiments and demonstrations should be tried out by the teacher first before they are conducted with children. Such an approach helps the teacher to anticipate "hang-ups" as well as to avoid them.

Effects of cigarette smoke on living things

1. Wipe a cotton pellet that has been saturated with tobacco tars on the tongue of a live frog and observe temporary collapse.

2. Using a cotton pellet that has been saturated with tars from the smoking machine, wipe the stems of several growing plants. Keep some plants as controls to observe the differences.

3. Place a drop of solution contining paramecia on a microscope slide. With the low power of a microscope, observe the movement of these one-celled organisms. Blow smoke from collection flask on the preparation and note the effects on the paramecia.

4. Make a nicotine insecticide by soaking cotton pellets from the smoking machine or cigarette tobacco in water. Test and use as a spray on insects.

5. *Purpose:* To demonstrate the effect of the toxic compounds in cigarette smoke on fish.

    Procedure: Set up a smoking machine (Fig. 18.5). As the vacuum is applied, the smoke from the cigarette will bubble through the water. By the time three to ten cigarettes have been consumed, the toxic agents in the smoke, primarily nicotine, should begin to affect the fish, causing them to lose their equilibrium. As soon as the fish lose their equilibrium and begin to roll to one side, they should be removed from the water and placed immediately in fresh water. If fish are not transplanted into fresh water immediately, they will die.

6. *Purpose:* To observe the biological effects of cigarette tars on white mice.

    Procedure: Hook a vacuum line (from an aspirator or water pump) to a burning cigarette in such a manner that the cigarette is consumed in about four to six minutes. In the line attach a trap containing glass wool moistened with acetone. This will collect most of the tobacco tars. The distillation of the tar can be facilitated by placing the bottle in an ice water bath during the course of the experiment.

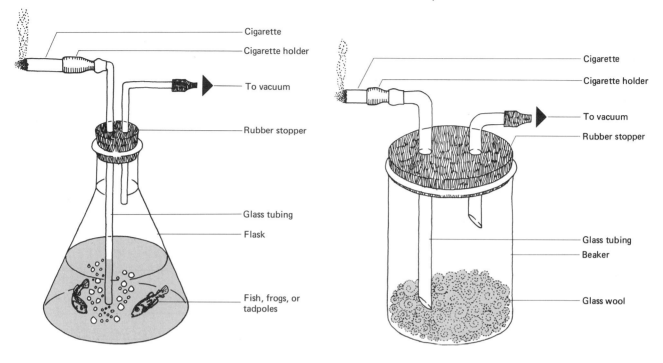

Fig. 18.5 How to set up equipment to show effects of cigarette smoke on fish.

Fig. 18.6 How to set up equipment to collect coal tar.

After the cigarettes (about 40 per day) have been smoked, the tar can be removed with additional acetone—using as little as possible to dissolve the tar. This solution should be allowed to stand for several hours in a fume hood to concentrate the tar. A vacuum distillation method in a warm water bath without flame is effective.

The backs of six to ten mice should be trimmed with electric clippers to remove heavy hair growth. The tars from about three cigarettes can be applied by eye dropper twice daily to the clipped area, five days a week.

Tumors can be expected to appear in about 40 percent of the mice in six to nine months. The tumors will be both benign and malignant.

To demonstrate effects of cigarette smoke on the respiratory system

1. *Purpose:* To demonstrate the tars that are inhaled into the mouth and lungs of a cigarette smoker. Of particular interest will be the difference in the amounts of tar in the inhaled smoke and in that which is exhaled.

    Equipment: 1 white handerchief, 1 smoker

    Procedure: Have the smoker inhale from a lighted cigarette, making every attempt to hold the smoke in his or her mouth without allowing it to go into the lungs. As rapidly as possible, after inhaling from the cigarette, stretch a handkerchief over the mouth as firmly as possible and blow the smoke back through the handkerchief. This will cause quite a dark stain.

    Now have the smoker inhale once more from the cigarette, this time allowing the smoke to go well into the lungs. Now place a different area of the handkerchief firmly over the mouth and exhale back through the handkerchief. The second stain will be much lighter than the first stain. Theoretically, the difference between the two stains represents the amount of tar that remains in the lungs with each puff of the cigarette.

2. *Purpose:* To demonstrate the effect of cigarette smoke on ciliary action.

    a) This may be demonstrated on the trachea of a chicken or salamander lung. Slit two fresh chicken tracheas upward from below and pin them on two separate stiff cardboards or plywood, so that the inside of the trachea, with cilia, may be viewed.

    Put a small drop of India ink or dye in the middle of the trachea. Lay the tracheas flat. Place one near a source of fresh air. Place the second trachea far away from the first and blow smoke on it. In both samples of trachea observe to see how far the ink has moved. The ink on the trachea that received cigarette smoke has not moved (see Fig. 18.7). This may be explained by noting that nicotine in the smoke paralyzed the cilia. An analogy can be made with the effect cigarette smoke has on the cilia in the human respiratory tract. When the cilia are inactivated, the mucus collects and becomes a fertile place for numerous pathogens. Hence a smoker becomes much more susceptible to respiratory infections than does a nonsmoker.

    b) Put a salamander to sleep by soaking it in (1) a solution of saturated chloretone diluted by adding nine parts of water, or (2) a one-percent aqueous solution of tricaine methanesulphonate. As soon as the salamander is asleep, cut off the head, open the chest and abdominal cavity, slit the lung longitudinally, and snip it off. Keep the specimen wet with Ringer's solution. Examine the lung surface under the microscope to study the cilia beating. Blow a little smoke from the collection flask over the tissue and observe the effect it has on the cilia.

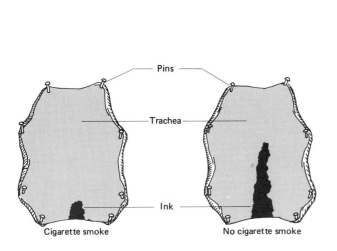

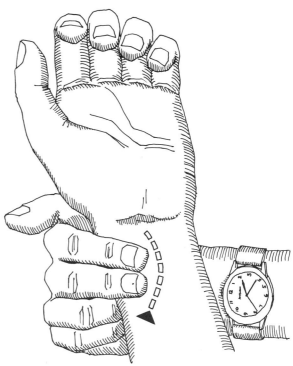

Fig. 18.7 The effects of cigarette smoke (nicotine) on fresh chicken trachea that have been slit and pinned to a board. Ink was placed in the lower end of the trachea (nearest the lung). Smoke was blown over the entire area surrounding the ink.

Fig. 18.8 How to take pulse.

To demonstrate the effect of cigarette smoke on the cardiovascular system

1. *Purpose:* To demonstrate the effect of smoking on the heart and the circulatory system.

   Procedure: It is recommended that students do this experiment on their parents at home and record their findings. The arterial pulse, taken at the wrist, is an accurate indication of the heart rate. One can take the pulse of a subject by placing two middle fingers of the right hand on the thumb side of the wrist of the patient (see Fig. 18.8).

   The subject's pulse should be taken two or three times to establish a baseline accuracy. In each instance record your pulse rate as the number of pulsations felt per minute.

   Have your subject light a cigarette, then take the pulse after he or she has concluded the third or fourth puff. When the cigarette is finished, take the

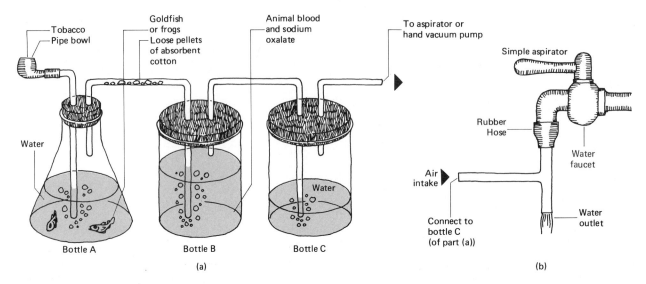

Fig. 18.9 How to set up an experiment to study the effects of cigarette smoke on animal blood. (From *Smoking and Health*, Washington, D.C.: U.S. Department of Health, Education and Welfare, 1964.)

pulse every 15 minutes until the pulse rate returns to normal. Chart your findings on a graph and determine how many extra beats one pack of cigarettes causes the subject. Since with each beat, the heart pumps approximately 70 cc of blood, calculate the extra volume of blood that is pumped by the heart induced by smoking one package of cigarettes.

2. The slowing down of blood circulation can be tested with a clinical thermometer. Have the nonsmoker, or someone who has not smoked for several hours, hold the thermometer. Then have a smoker hold the thermometer. Smokers show a drop of about six degrees or more, even when using filter cigarettes.

3. *Purpose:* To test the effects of carbon monoxide in tobacco smoke on animal blood. (The blood can be obtained from a butcher shop. Keep the blood from coagulating by adding one part of sodium oxalate solution to nine parts of blood. Place in bottle.)

   Procedure: Smoke a cigarette or tobacco in the manner described for smoking machines (see Fig. 18.9). Smoke coming through the tube from bottle A to bottle B will cause the blood to turn a deeper red as the hemoglobin takes on carbon monoxide. As a result carboxy-hemoglobin is formed. This is what happens in carbon monoxide poisoning. The hemoglobin loses its ability to release oxygen.

Add a fresh yeast culture to the blood. Also add a yeast culture to a control batch of blood. In the control, yeast enzymes cause the hemoglobin to release oxygen, which comes off as bubbles in a foam at the surface. In the experimental bottle, this oxygen release is impaired. (Bottle C is simply a trap, to keep blood from frothing into the pump or aspirator.)

4. *Purpose:* To demonstrate the effect of smoke on the circulatory system.

    Procedure: Pith a frog and place it on its back on a frog board. Spread and pin the web of a foot over an opening in the board and examine the blood vessels under low power on a microscope. Keep the specimen moist with Ringer's solution. Place a tube from the smoke bottle in the frog's mouth and blow smoke in while someone is watching the rate of blood flow. If it is possible to count the blood cells going past a given point, you may notice several rate changes; faster, then back to normal, perhaps faster again, and back to normal a second time.

5. *Purpose:* To demonstrate the effect of cigarette smoke on the heart.

    Procedure: Pith a frog and place the frog on its back on a frog board. Spread and stretch the legs and pin them rigidly to the frog board. With a scalpel, open up the chest cavity, and carefully expose the heart. Carefully remove the pericardium, or protective sac, around the heart. Observe the heart rate, time it, and record. Place a drop of pure nicotine solution on the heart. Observe, time the heart rate, and record. Compare the pre- and postrates.

    The frog's heart may be attached to a kymograph and the heart rates recorded as a kymograph.

Smoking machines

Numerous smoking machines are sold commercially. The two most popular ones are "Nicotina" and "Smoking Sam." The kind of smoking machine to be used should be relevant to the purpose of the demonstration or experiment. "Nicotina" is excellent for demonstrating that tar is part of cigarette smoke and that it is inhaled. "Smoking Sam" does much the same thing, except that the two glass jars, filled with white angel hair, simulate human lungs. When these commercial machines are not available, the amount of tar in one or more cigarettes may be demonstrated by collecting tar on cotton pellets, angel hair, or filter paper placed in the tubing of a teacher-made machine. Tar can also be observed as a residue on the tubing and containers and as a discoloration of water through which cigarette

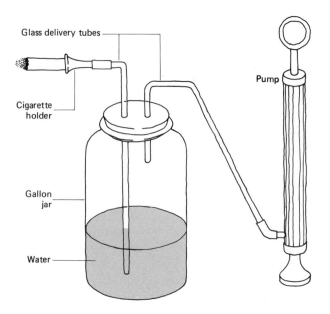

Glass delivery tubes

Pump

Cigarette holder

Gallon jar

Water

Fig. 18.10 How to design a classroom smoking machine.

smoke has been filtered. Smoking machines may be adapted to a variety of demonstrations. The following machine may be constructed for classroom demonstrations and experiments.

Equipment: A large gallon jar with a two-hole stopper, cigarettes, delivery tubes (glass), cigarette holder, vacuum pump.

Procedure: Assemble cigarette tar separating apparatus, as shown in Fig. 18.10. Fill the gallon jar half full of water. Place cigarette in intake and light. Pump vacuum pump so as to draw smoke from cigarette into gallon jar and water. Pump until cigarette is burned completely. Replace with additional cigarettes until tars can be seen in water. Examine color of water; smell and taste the liquid.

REFERENCES AND BIBLIOGRAPHY

Diehl, Harold S. *Tobacco and Your Health: The Smoking Controversy* (New York: McGraw-Hill, 1969).

Fodor, John T., and Lennin Glass. *Cigarette Smoking and Health: A Teacher's Guide—Grade Six* (Granada Hills, Calif.: HRA, 1971).

———— . *Cigarette Smoking and Health: A Teacher's Guide—Grade Eight* (Granada Hills, Calif.: HRA, 1971).

Passwater, Richard A. *Supernutrition* (New York: Pocket Books, 1976), pp. 127-128, 136, 146-149.

Smoking and Health (Washington, D.C.: U.S. Department of Health, Education and Welfare, 1964).

Smoking Research/San Diego. *Smoking and Health—A Guide For School Action Grades 1-12* (San Diego: Smoking Research, 1968).

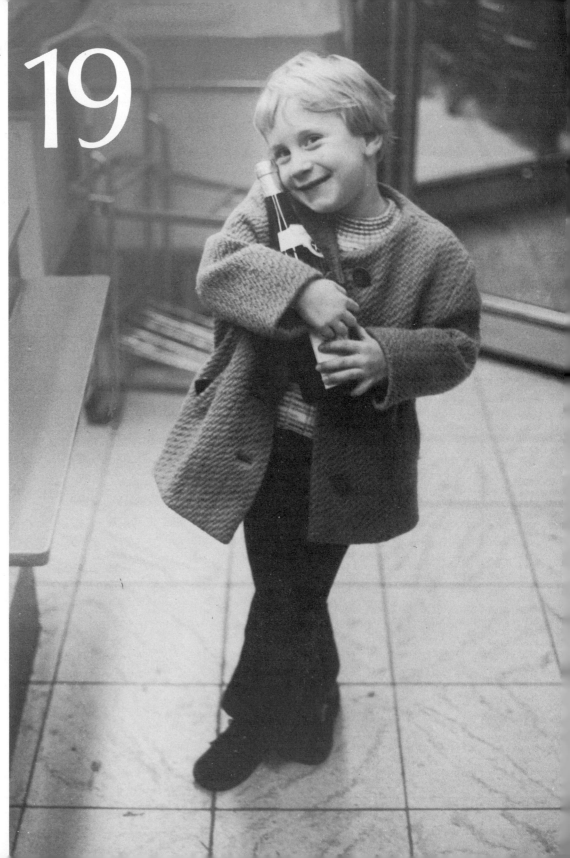

teaching about alcohol

INTRODUCTION

The consumption of alcoholic beverages is an age-old American custom. Except for some uncertain times during Prohibition, alcoholic beverages have enjoyed immense popularity with the American public. This is evidenced by the fact that approximately 71 percent of the total adult population in the United States consumes alcohol with regularity. In more meaningful terms, the yearly per capita consumption of alcoholic beverages by adults 21 and older averages approximately 26 gallons.

In addition to being a popular activity, drinking supports a most lucrative industry. Production of alcoholic beverages is presently a $13 billion industry in the United States, and approximately one-half of the total revenues go to state, federal, and local taxes.

Without reservation, alcohol is the most widely used and accepted *drug* in our society today. Alcoholic beverages can and should be classified as addicting drugs. Over a period of time, the drinker will develop a tolerance to alcohol, can become psychologically dependent on alcohol, and may even become physiologically addicted to the point of suffering withdrawal symptoms when and if he or she attempts to give up drinking. However, only one-tenth of those who choose to drink are, or will be, adversely affected by their drinking habits. The overwhelming majority of those who indulge do so in moderation. Unfortunate as it may seem, it is the small minority of problem drinkers that creates a social dilemma that has literally become an American nightmare.

For example, there are some nine to ten million chronic alcoholics in this country. They cause untold harm to their loved ones and to society in general. They are responsible for countless lost hours in business and industry, not to mention their burden on the taxpayer in the form of court costs, hospitalization, and rehabilitation. Alcoholism is a very serious affliction, as anyone who has been touched by it knows so very well. In addition to the alcoholic, the problem drinker and the overzealous occasional drinker also present a serious problem to society. For example, nearly 60,000 people are killed every year on the highway, and of this number, approximately half were involved in alcohol-related accidents in which one or both of the drivers were under the influence of alcohol.

Alcohol consumption, at high levels, affects the physiology of the body in numerous destructive ways. The depressant effects on the brain and central nervous system are well documented elsewhere. But the disruption of metabolic processes in the liver and the killing of brain cells are not too well reported. These are of greater physiological importance to the survival of the alcoholic than the affects of alcohol on other parts of the body. Small blood vessels all over the body become clogged when the blood alcohol level becomes too high (Williams, 1973). This results in partial deprivation of oxygen and food in the nerve cells of the brain. Brain cells apparently also lose their ability to use glucose as a fuel, become impaired, and die off with greater rapidity than normal (Williams, 1973). Alcohol inhibits metabolic conversions in the liver, causing a deficiency of vitamins B_1 (thiamine), B_2 (riboflavin), B_3 (nicotinic acid), B_6 (pyridoxine), B_c (folic acid), B_{12} (cobalamin), biotin, vitamins C and E, and the minerals magnesium, potassium, and zinc (see Di Cyan, 1974, pp. 36, 59; Williams, 1973, pp. 169-180). Vitamins B_1, B_6, and biotin support the oxidation-inducing enzymes; nicotinic acid and B_2 are needed to overcome the inhibition of metabolic conversion caused by alcohol; vitamin E is needed to prevent the increased peroxidation of fats in the liver; more folic acid and vitamins B_6 and B_{12} are needed to repair the damage that alcohol causes; and vitamin C is needed to keep connective tissue in healthy condition (Di Cyan, 1974, p. 36). Thus consumption of alcohol at high levels undoubtedly damages brain cells and inhibits liver function. See Fig. 19.1.

The facts are obvious. Alcohol is a powerful depressant drug with addicting qualities. It is legal, and its consumption constitutes a monumental personal and social problem. What can we do? What alternatives are available? How about declaring it illegal to possess, produce, and sell alcoholic beverages? History has already proved that such an approach is fruitless. Besides, a $13 billion industry that contributes some $6.5 billion in taxes each year does not die easily. Alcohol is very much a part of the American scene.

One viable alternative is the presentation of scientifically sound, up-to-date, and relevant information concerning alcohol and its effects to young people. There is quite a fine line between alcohol use and alcohol abuse. If one is apprised of a few basic principles regarding the use of alcohol, one is far more likely to control his or her drinking and to avoid taking that critical step which transforms casual consumption into habitual. The point to be made is that alcohol alone does not create problems; human beings create the problems, often with its assistance.

The material that follows is merely meant to be exemplary in nature. The decision concerning when to initiate alcohol education is critical, as is the case in many other controversial health education content areas today. It is imperative that children be made aware of the effects of poor health behavior with relation to these controversial health content areas at an earlier age than ever.

Note that particular attention has been paid to the druglike qualities of alcohol, its effects on the body, the reasons why one might abuse alcohol, and the chronic condition of alcoholism. It is suggested that these areas be strongly considered for inclusion in an alcohol unit at the intermediate and junior high levels.

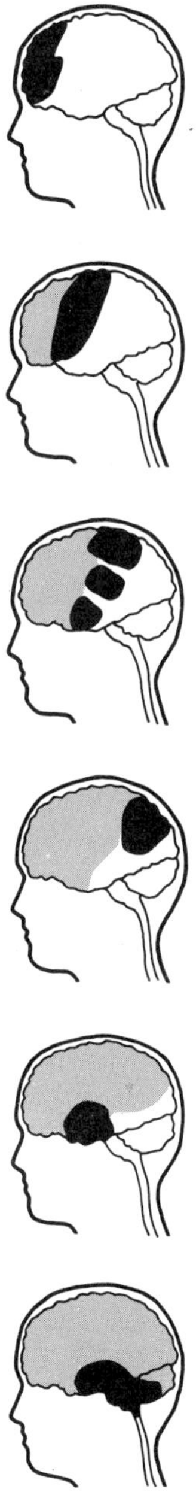

Alcohol concentration in blood stream	No. drinks* per hour	Part of brain affected	Area of brain affected
0.03%	1 bottle beer (12 oz.) 1 cocktail (whiskey) (90% proof)		1 reason/judgment (minor)
0.05%	2 bottles beer 2 cocktails		2 coordination 3 self-control
0.10%	4 bottles beer 4 cocktails		4 vision 5 speech 6 hearing 7 reaction time
0.15%	6 bottles beer 6 cocktails		8 balance 9 coordination 10 judgment
0.30%	12 bottles beer 22 cocktails		11 memory 12 unconsciousness
0.60%	24 + bottles beer 24 + cocktails		13 respiratory center inhibited 14 DEATH possible

* 4% alcohol in beer; 90% proof distilled beverage

Fig. 19.1 Effects of alcohol on the central nervous system of a person weighing 150–160 pounds.

. . . .

TOPIC: EFFECTS OF ALCOHOL ON THE BODY

Grade Level: Intermediate

Outcome: The student will be able to summarize how alcohol depresses bodily functions.

Concept: Alcohol depresses the body.

Content: Alcohol depresses various systems of the body:

Learning Experiences

1. Central nervous system

   a) *Brain:*

	Quantity
reasoning, memory	1-2 drinks
judgment, self-control	3-4 drinks
speech	5-6 drinks
hearing	5-6 drinks
sight	5-6 drinks
touch	5-6 drinks
coordination	5-6 drinks
balance	7-8 drinks
breathing	10+ drinks

2. Cardiovascular system

   a) heart beat affected

   b) white blood cells destroyed? function?

   c) vitamins C and E destroyed; vitamin C is essential for building and maintaining collagen, the body cement that holds cells together; vitamin E deficiency results in abnormal collagen, which constricts blood vessels and chokes off adequate blood supply to the tissues, eventuating in cell death.

3. Respiratory system

   a) rate reduced

1. *Rat Demonstration*

   Material

   1. One or two rats weighing about 200 grams and not fed for about six hours

   2. A mixture of .5 ml (cc) 190-proof pure grain alcohol and .5 ml distilled water

   3. Hypodermic syringe marked off in cc

   4. Hypodermic needle (Yale B-D 26 gauge, $\frac{3}{8}$ in.)

   5. Several cotton balls

   6. A small bottle of rubbing alcohol

   7. Boiling water

   8. A small saucepan

   Procedures

   1. For each 18 grams of body weight, inject 0.1 cc of the distilled water–alcohol solution into the peritoneal (abdominal) cavity of the rat. The rat will probably die from an injection that is too large.

      a) Secure the rat by either tying its hind legs to a table or a board or having someone hold its legs.

4. Digestive system

  a) interferes with absorption of food

  b) stimulates gastric secretions?

  c) stimulates flow of saliva

5. Liver

  a) vitamins B_6, C, and E destroyed, thereby impairing liver function

  b) may become inflamed

6. Skin

  a) rosy glow

  b) increased perspiration

7. Other:

  a) increased cholesterol in the body

  b) increased triglycerides, which are associated with heart disease

  b) Support the rat in one hand and place your thumb and forefinger about its neck and against its lower jaw.

  c) The needle should not be injected any deeper than ¼ of an inch; the needle should not enter straight into the rat's body, but rather at an angle such as one would use when removing a splinter from the hand. The object of the injection is to get just beneath the outer layer of the skin.

  d) Care should be taken not to puncture the viscera by going too deep or the diaphragm by going too near to the rib cage.

  e) Two to three minutes after the injection, the rat behavior tests may be tried. If the rat has been fed sooner than the six hours recommended, it will take longer for the behavior to be affected.

Observation

1. Normal rat behavior:

  a) If held by the tail and brought near an object, the rat will reach for the object.

  b) If placed on its back, the rat will right itself immediately.

  c) Place your finger near the rat's eye, and it will blink.

  d) If held several inches above a table and spun around, the rat will, when released, land on its feet, like a cat.

  e) After a few trials, the rat will be able to find its own way out of a maze without difficulty.

  f) If placed on a balancing pole (any round pole) above the table, a rat will balance itself.

2. Alcoholic rat behavior: An alcohol-injected rat will be unable to duplicate the actions performed in the previous tests. The rat may be able to duplicate the actions after a considerable lapse in time and much effort.

Conclusion

This experiment will show the students of various grade levels the effect that alcohol has on the human body. The rat is like a miniature human. Both eat and drink similar things, and one day in the growth pattern of the rat is equivalent to about one month of human growth (12 days is equal to one year). It is important to establish this analogy successfully so that the student will be readily able to relate the effect he or she observes the alcohol to produce in the rat to the effect of alcohol on the human being.

TOPIC: WHY PEOPLE DRINK

Grade Level: Intermediate

Outcome: The student will be able to discuss the many reasons why people drink alcohol.

Concept: People drink for many reasons.

Content: Reasons people drink are:

1. To get a high—enjoy aftereffects
2. To overcome unhappiness
3. To imitate others
4. To get a feeling of importance
5. To escape from worry or self-pity
6. To be more sociable, to break the ice
7. To satisfy curiosity and adventure
8. To escape frustration
9. To feel grown up
10. To seek social status and social approval for indulging in a customary activity

Learning Experiences

1. *Role playing:* Pupils act out three or four situations, with follow-up after each one:
   a) *Situation 1:* Dad and his friends gather around the TV to watch a football game and drink beer.
   b) *Situation 2:* Each member of a group in a party situation begins to drink for different reasons: John to feel grown up, Mary to escape feeling inadequate, and Rusty to conform, etc.
   c) *Situation 3:* Sam, a married man with three children, is in debt and is badgered by his wife. On the way home, he stops at the local bar and gets drunk with friend Don.
2. Have class suggest other reasons; teacher uses these suggestions to initiate class discussion (list on blackboard).

Key Questions (to be used during follow-up after each role-play situation):

Situation 1

1. Why did Dad and his friends choose to drink beer rather than some other beverage?
2. Why did they drink beer?
3. If you were old enough, would you also drink beer like Dad did?

Situation 2

1. Did you like this role play and the acting?
2. Can you suggest why these people decided to drink alcoholic beverages in this party situation?
3. Are there any other reasons that you can think of that would cause a person to feel the need to drink alcoholic beverages?
4. What could they drink instead of alcohol?
5. Are parties good or bad?

Situation 3

1. Why did Sam stop at the bar before going home to his wife?
2. Why did Don stop at the bar before going home?
3. Did drinking help Sam and Don to solve their problems?
4. What other alternatives did they have to getting drunk?

Review Questions:

1. Is there one major reason why people drink?
2. What kind of situations lend themselves easily to drinking?
3. Do all people drink for the same reason?

REFERENCES AND BIBLIOGRAPHY

Atkins, A. J. *Teaching Alcohol Education in the Schools* (New York: Macmillan, 1959).

Block, Marvin A. *Alcohol and Alcoholism* (Belmont, Calif.: Wadsworth, 1970).

Bozeman, Estelle. *Lessons About Alcohol* (Columbus, Ohio: School and College Service, 1961).

Carroll, Charles R. *Alcohol: Use, Nonuse and Abuse* (Dubuque, Iowa: Wm. C. Brown, 1970).

Di Cyan, Erwin. *Vitamins in Your Life* (New York: Simon and Schuster, 1974).

Hirsh, Joseph. *Alcohol Education* (New York: Henry Schuman, 1959).

McCarthy, Raymond. *Alcohol Education for the Classroom and Community* (New York: McGraw-Hill, 1964).

Passwater, Richard A. *Supernutrition* (New York: Pocket Book, 1976).

Todd, Frances. *Teaching About Alcohol* (New York: McGraw-Hill, 1964).

Williams, Roger J. *Nutrition Against Disease* (New York: Bantam, 1973), pp. 169-189.

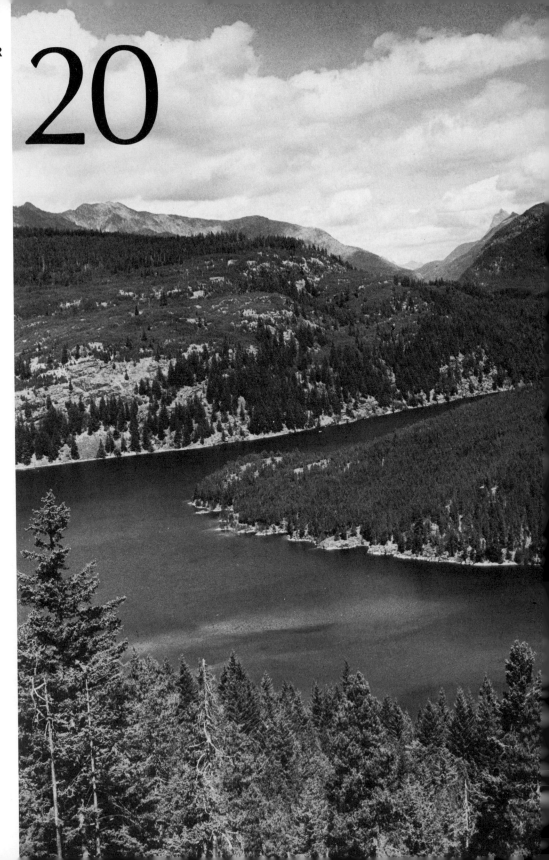

teaching about environmental conservation

INTRODUCTION

The concern for our environment is mounting. Best that it should, because there is precious little time left to atone for past ecological sins. Nature is very forgiving, as history has proved, but our senseless disregard for the environment has reached such proportions that the damage done is just now beginning to have catastrophic consequences. The inevitable is obvious. People simply cannot continue to rape their environment. If they do, human existence will be threatened in the near future.

The entire environmental dilemma is a paradoxical calamity. On the one hand, humans have been tremendously successful in dealing with the restraints that their environment and competing organisms have imposed on them throughout history. Modern technological advances have turned science fiction into reality. On the other hand, however, humans have also had the unique capacity for creating ecological mires which may be instrumental in human destruction.

It is difficult to comprehend why people continue to abuse their ecosystem. Perhaps the answer lies in the fact that humans have never really been anything but polluters. At no time have men and women ever learned to effectively deal with their overzealous needs and overwhelming amount of waste materials.

Such rationale makes sense when you consider that early humans were somewhat kept in check by nature's own selection process. The environment was able to assimilate humans and to accept their thoughtless acts because they were few in number. As time passed and humans became more effective in overcoming the many restraints imposed by the environment, the population increased rapidly. Logically, it follows that as the population increased, so did demands on the environment. These unchecked abusive demands have taken their toll and are now at an intolerable level. To even the most naive, it should be obvious that the environment can no longer continue to meet human needs if our present practices are continued.

In reality, there are too many people. The relationship between population growth and the present environmental nightmare is direct. All ecological problems are closely related to population levels. If we continue to populate the earth at our present rate, there will be 1000 people per square foot of the earth's surface some 900 years from now. Even more startling is the fact that in just 1000 years, the world's population will equal the weight of the earth. More people require more goods and services. Increased demand for goods and services prompts even more waste material. The by-products of this vicious cycle are unnatural environmental conditions in the form of air, water, noise, pesticide, and radiation pollution.

The term *pollution* can best be described as any human-caused change in the ecosystem that renders the environment less desirable for sustaining life. Beyond a shadow of a doubt, our countless ecological atrocities are the cause of the major pollutants as we know them today. These pollutants inhibit the natural functions of the highly interdependent ecosystem. Once one aspect is set askew, one or more other phases are also affected. In essence, nature's system of checks and balances has been usurped.

The answer is simple; people must quickly learn to live within the natural limitations of the environment. To accomplish such a goal requires that each person realize and accept the fact that the environment does *not* belong to humans, but rather that they belong to the environment. The human organism is simply not *independent* of the environment, but in the truest sense of the word is *interdependent* with all other forms of life on our planet. Like all organisms, a person is the product of both heredity and environment, and needs to be aware that all organisms and environments are continually changing. Indeed, the social and physical environments in the last hundred years have changed dramatically. In trying to cope with many rapid changes, people have been progressively degrading their environment. Unfortunately, the world has not fully committed itself to fostering a sensible program of global environmental conservation. The impending consequences will be catastrophic unless there is positive and productive action in the near future. Education at an early age is obviously the approach that answers such an urgent call for conservation.

The basic goal of environmental education should be to make everyone aware that although one is absolutely dependent on, and hence is affected by, the environment, he or she, in turn, simultaneously affects it. At the primary level, the emphasis should be on the environment in the school and neighborhood. At the intermediate grades, the teacher should progress to the community and region. The teacher should guide the children to discover problems by forcing them to examine their interaction with the environment. How do we use the environment to satisfy our needs? These and other questions should be answered during the discovery process. In lieu of these learning experiences, there should be a twofold environmental program in the elementary schools. The indirect approach would have the teacher planning and facilitating a physical environment in the classroom, and in the school generally, which is conducive to positive learning and sound personality development. It would reinforce the second, or direct, teaching approach. The lesson plans that follow are suggestions for initiating this latter approach. In keeping with the format established in the preceding chapters, the following lesson plans are offered as the basis for what could be a unit of instruction dealing with environmental conservation.

TOPIC: ECOLOGY

Grade Level: Intermediate, junior high

Outcome: The student will be able to describe how ecology is a way of keeping the human web of life in balance with nature.

Concept: We need to live within the limitations of our environment.

Content: Ways people keep a balance with nature, thereby not polluting the environment:

1. *Food* chains:
   a) animals
   b) insects
   c) birds   Consumers—original
   d) fish   sources need to be in state
   e) plants   of balance for food chain to
                    continue.
   f) human—a polluter, a destroyer, and consumer
   g) microscopic bacteria, fungi (decomposers)
2. *Soil:* food crops versus soil nutrients
3. *Water:* drinking and industrial uses versus availability of natural supplies
4. *Gases:* (air) CO_2-O_2 balance and human needs

Learning Experiences

1. *Stimulate* with pictures and flannel board the ecosystem of a pond. (See Fig. 20.1.)
2. *Suggested alternative experiences*
   a) *Which America do you choose?* Pupils identify what people have done right and wrong in their environment. (See Fig. 20.2.)
   b) *Film: Ecology,* 22 min, 16mm, B & W. Relationships of people, plants, and animals to their environments. Order from: Academy Films, 748 North Seward St., Hollywood, Calif.
   c) *Sound filmstrip set: Ecology; Interaction Environments:* set of seven to study the interaction of living things with one another and with their environments. Order from Scott Educational Division, Holyoke, Mass. 01040.
   d) *Filmstrips & record/cassette:* Series of filmstrips identifying and describing current ecological-pollution problems from a biological viewpoint. Order from: Holt, Rinehart and Winston Inc., 383 Madison Ave., New York, N.Y. 10017
   e) *Filmstrips: Man is the Biosphere. Introduction to Human Ecology,* plus Teacher's Guide

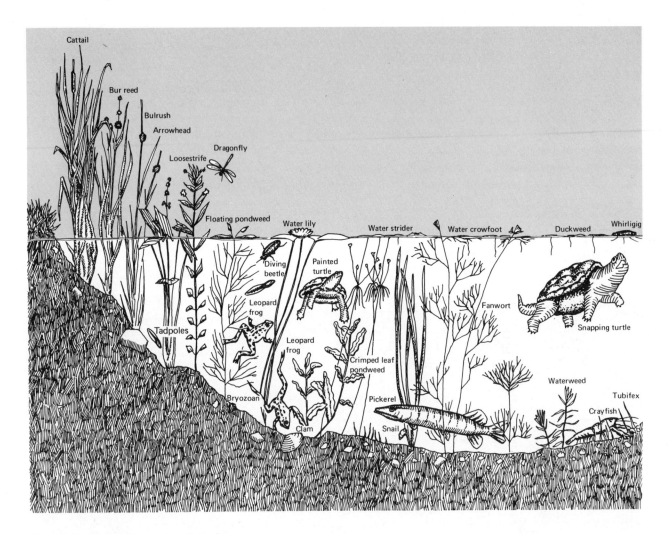

Cattail
Bur reed
Bulrush
Arrowhead
Loosestrife
Dragonfly
Floating pondweed
Water lily
Water strider
Water crowfoot
Duckweed
Whirligig
Diving beetle
Painted turtle
Leopard frog
Fanwort
Snapping turtle
Tadpoles
Leopard frog
Crimped leaf pondweed
Waterweed
Tubifex
Bryozoan
Pickerel
Crayfish
Clam
Snail

Fig. 20.1   Illustrative suggestions for a pond ecosystem, demonstration, or field trip. Can you evolve food chains in this pond?

Fig. 20.2   Which America do you ▶ choose? (a) A poor place to live—why? (b) A good place to live—why? (From *Conservation Chart: Which America Do You Choose?* Washington, D.C.: U.S. Department of the Interior.)

WHICH AMERICA DO YOU CHOOSE?

A POOR PLACE TO LIVE

Abuse of land, air, and water create problems that turn appealing areas into ghettos of ugliness and decay. The illustration immediately to the right tells the story of a watershed area where users of resources have sacrificed their environment for the quick profit—the short-term gain. Follow the keys below to conditions depicted by related keys in the illustration.

1. Lack of Water Control

A rampant stream destroys valuable land, fails to recharge ground water supplies, and jeopardizes lives. Usually it goes through periodic low-water cycles that make it an unreliable source of supply for cities. Not all streams should be dammed, of course, but some must be.

2. Ruinous Forestry Practices

Here, cut-and-get-out logging operations, inadequate fire protection, and other short-sighted actions have led to watershed soil erosion, downstream flooding, and loss of habitat for wildlife. Recreation opportunities are destroyed.

3. Poor Farming Methods

Overuse of land and repeated planting of the same crops, have exhausted the soil's fertility. The absence of contour farming leads to rapid runoff and results in erosion by wind and water.

4. Uncontrolled Growth of Suburbs

Lack of effective zoning and building regulations speeds decay. Open green space is chopped up into inadequate patches. "Bedroom" suburbs like this produce monotony, blight, and high crime rates.

5. Upstream Industrial Pollution

Industries that disregard downstream and downwind pollution degrade the entire watershed. Rural areas often encourage industrial parks without requiring adequate pollution controls.

6. Pollution from Mines

Mining companies abandon underground working without a thought that eventually they will cave in and create surface pockets or feed deadly acid water into streams. Others strip off valuable topsoil and leave ugly scars which add to stream pollution and deterioration of the area.

7. & 9. Faulty Industrial Zoning

Unregulated placing of industry pollutes city's air and water and downgrades value of adjacent property.

8. Improper Waste Disposal

Sewage treatment and waste disposal facilities lag behind population growth, hastening the poisonous suicide of the city.

10. The Polluted River

Pollution the full length of the river has made it an open sewer. Fish cannot live in it, people dislike drinking it even after costly purification. Swimming is impossible, and boating unpleasant.

11. Poorly Managed Traffic

A source of air pollution, frustration, and sudden death, poorly planned traffic facilities—added to substandard mass transportation—strangle the Central City.

12. Trapped by Towers

As the population grows and open space is lost to monstrous high-rise apartments, city dwellers become imprisoned by their own "progress." They live an elbow-to-elbow existence. The more fortunate breathe filtered air at home and at work. Others sneeze and snuffle through smog-filled days and nights.

A GOOD PLACE TO LIVE

The balance of Nature and the quality of man's environment can be maintained in an increasingly popular watershed if sound conservation practices are followed. Some of the benefits are listed below and are keyed to the right half of the illustration.

1. Proper Forestry and Mining

Good forest management means selective cutting, fire protection, and planting new trees. Such practices promote continuing yields of forest products. Stripmined areas have been recovered with topsoil. Planting holds the soil in place and keeps streams silt-free.

2. Space to Roam

Wilderness areas are protected, providing assured wildlife habitat, a healthy forest base for the watershed, and outdoor recreation for all.

3. Multipurpose Reservoir

Flood control, power generation, municipal and industrial water supply source, and outdoor recreation facilities are some of the benefits of this reservoir.

4. Farm Land Management

Rotation of crops and grasslands, contour strip planting, wildlife hedgerows, all make this farm flourish while protecting the health and quality of the land.

5. Irrigation

Water provided by a diversion dam and a high-line canal turns normally non-productive land into fertile farms.

6. Industrial Parks

Planning and zoning provide attractive and efficient clustering of industry, to the benefit of both industry and city. Sources of industrial water and air pollution are controlled within the regulated industrial park complex.

7. Fish Hatchery

Hatcheries provide fish to supplement stocks in reservoirs, streams, and lakes.

8. Satellite Communities

Self-contained communities like this offer the services and advantages of close-in suburban living. The beauty of the natural terrain and setting is carefully preserved.

9. Waste Disposal

Efficient sewage plants treat effluents from city systems, keeping the river clean. Refuse is burned to generate power in plants equipped with air pollution abatement devices.

10. The Beautiful City

Careful planning and development provide a beautiful, livable Central City environment. Area-wide master plans control the city's growth, provide a smooth traffic flow, and promote work and living patterns oriented not to technology but to people.

11. & 13. Highways and Rapid Transit

Recessed and underground superhighways, combined with a rapid transit system that extends to the suburban satellite communities, provide efficient movement of people and goods to and from the Central City. With home-to-work rapid transit, private car use is reduced. Combining highway and rapid transit operations uses less open space and requires fewer river crossings.

12. City Park and Recreation Areas

Planned parks like this provide the Central City with large wedges of open space and afford many forms of recreation and cultural facilities for the city dweller.

14. Footpaths and Bicycle Trails

Trails follow the natural terrain of the river banks from city to headwaters.

15. Green Spaces

Through proper planning and zoning, abundant open space in and around the city is preserved. This green space provides a natural source of beauty and recreation opportunities.

16. The Clean River

Pollution control and good watershed management keep the river clean, making it a recreational delight.

17. Scenic Easements

Scenic easements along river banks protect the natural beauty of the river. Pollution control is made easier and bank erosion prevented. Outdoor recreation opportunities abound in the natural areas preserved.

(70w4100). Order from: Ward's Natural Science Establishment, P.O. Box 1749, Monterey, Calif., 93940.

f) *AEP Ecology Program:* Weekly reader practice books to make students aware of delicate balances between all forms of life and their supportive habitats. Four ecological concepts stressed: diversity, adaptations, interrelationships, and change. Order from: *My Weekly Reader,* Education Center, Columbus, Ohio, 43216.

g) *Filmstrips:* Order from Life Filmstrips

(1) *Water Pollution, Part 1: The Great Lakes—History and Ecology.* Pollution problems of the Great Lakes.

(2) *Water Pollution, Part II: The Causes of Pollution.* Shipping pollution, municipal sewage landfill, agricultural pesticides, detergents, industrial wastes, and new pollutants.

(3) *Water Pollution, Part III: The Results of Pollution.* Closed beaches, ruination of fishing, decline in tourism, stinking marshes, threatened dunes, endangered health and what can be done about it.

Key Questions

1. What is ecology?
2. How do food chains keep a balance of all living things?
3. What basic kinds of environments are there?
4. How do people disrupt their food chain?
5. How does nature get rid of wastes?
6. Who are nature's scavengers?
7. Can you trace your own food chain?
8. How can you keep in ecological balance with nature?

TOPIC: ECOSYSTEMS

Grade Level: Intermediate

Outcome: The student will be able to describe how pollution results when ecosystems are disturbed.

Concept: Pollution results when ecosystems are disturbed or disrupted.

Content: Ecosystems are dependent on food chains:

Learning Experiences

1. First-order consumers, e.g., plankton, tadpoles, feed on plants.
2. Second-order consumers, e.g., bass, feed on tadpoles.
3. Third-order consumers, e.g., those living things that feed on bass, plankton, and tadpoles; humans.
4. Examples of ecosystems:
    a) grass → zebra → lion
    b) grass → cattle → person
    c) meadow → grass → cricket → frog → hawk
    d) pond algae → protozoa → insects → larger insects → black bass → pickerel → person

1. *Games:* Bass Ecosystem (see Fig. 20.3).

Bass Ecosystem Game

Objective: To have each pupil evolve a balanced pond ecosystem and avoid a polluted pond.

Description: This game allows each pupil to play. Teacher has pupils duplicate the original board and makes enough organism-exchange pieces and pollution-result cards for all in class to participate. Pupils can also make their own die. For best results, have four or five players per card and a banker or a card for each pupil and a banker. (An adaptation of an Urban Systems ecological game.)

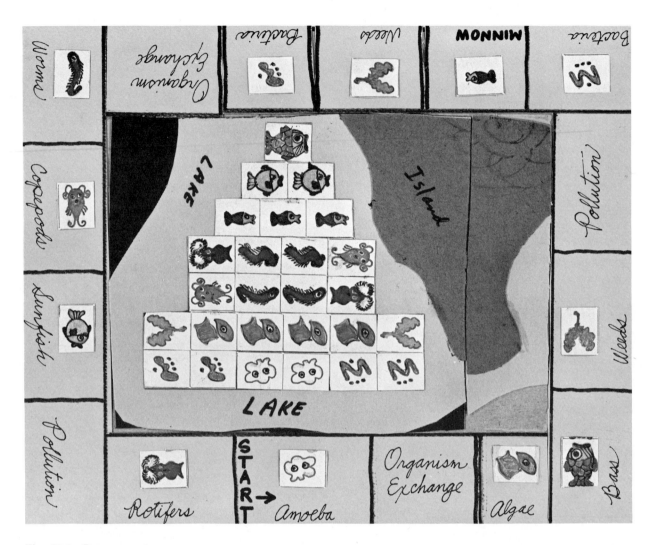

Fig. 20.3   Bass ecosystem game.

Game Rules

1. High throw of die determines starting player.
2. All players place token in the START space on the board.
3. Each player throws die to determine number of spaces to move on board.
4. Each player interprets the consequence of his or her move:

a) If a player lands on an ORGANISM space (e.g., sunfish, rotifers, algae, bass, weeds, bacteria, minnows, worms, and copepods), he or she takes an organism of the species and places it in his or her lake.

b) If a player lands on an ORGANISM EXCHANGE space, he or she may exchange extra pieces for others that are equal to or higher than his or her original organism. The player may exchange one piece for an organism (from the banker).

c) If a player lands on a POLLUTION space, he or she throws the die to determine the source of pollution and suffers the consequences outlined on the POLLUTION RESULT card (teacher can draft own cards).

5. Overpopulation occurs when the player gains more than the number provided for in the lake. For example, there are three minnows in the lake, so although the player may keep more than three minnows, he or she may not make an exchange for any more than three. If the lake becomes overpopulated, the player returns all the extras of that species and pays the penalty (series of consequences of overpopulation, which the teacher can draft).

6. A player wins by covering each organism in his or her lake with an organism-exchange card. He or she has then constructed his or her own ecosystem.

2. *Demonstration:* Evolve an ecosystem in two identical *aquariums* over a period of several months. Keep one healthy and balanced. Disrupt the ecological balance of the other and compare the consequences.

An Ecosystem Aquarium

Purpose: To learn about the balance of life in an aquatic ecosystem.

Procedure: The teacher and pupils may plan their own aquarium. Help may be obtained by referring to "Life in the Water" kit and conducting suggested experiments on food sources of brine shrimp and plankton (algae). Kit No. 71354 may be ordered from Edmund Scientific Co., 100 Edscorp Building, Barrington, New Jersey, 08007.

A filmstrip, *Keeping An Aquarium*, may be obtained from Scott Education Division, Holyoke, Mass., 01040.

3. Study the history of Lake Erie and identify how the ecosystems were disrupted by human activity.

4. Field trip to a nearby lake or pond.

5. *Alternative learning experiences*

a) *Pupil Project:* Making a Jam Jar Aquarium.

b) Making an aquarium for larger water animals.

An Aquarium for Larger Water Animals

A glass aquarium 50 cm by 25 cm is of useful size. Old accumulator cells are suitable, but the glass is not very clear.

To prepare such an aquarium, get some fine silt from the bottom of a clear stream or pond and wash it carefully in running water. Cover the floor of the aquarium with it to a depth of about 2 cm. Plant a few reeds in this, weighting the roots with a stone or lead ring. Then put in a layer of coarse sand or gravel and some large stones to serve as hiding places for the water insects. Fill with a slow stream of water and allow to stand for a day or two until clear. Clean water plants should be introduced. There is no need for elaborate aerating arrangements if plenty of water weeds are present. If tap water is used, some live food such as daphnia should preferably be added.

The animals can now be introduced with a few snails to keep the glass clean. Very little feeding will be necessary. Fish will eat the snails' eggs, and enough small water organisms can be found in the average pond to supply other needs. If

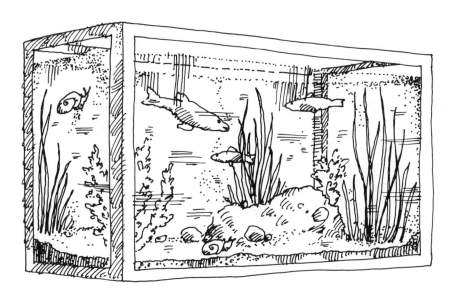

Fig. 20.4 Water aquarium.

worms are used as food, they should be given only once a week, at which time they should be cut into pieces small enough to be eaten. Unless unconsumed food is removed immediately, fungi will grow and will infect the fish.

The aquarium must be covered with a glass plate or perforated zinc lid to keep out dust. If frogs or newts are kept, a floating piece of cork must be provided for them to sit on; the glass or zinc cover will then prevent their escape.

c) *Film: Lakes—Aging and Pollution;* 15 min, color, 1971; Underwater photography to show aging of lakes, life cycles, and changes of water quality with emphasis on human input. Order from: Centron Educational Films, 1621 West Ninth St., Lawrence, Kansas, 66044.

d) *Film: Energy and Living Things;* 11 min, color, 1972. The relationship of energy and matter is brought out by tracing solar energy through plants, herbivores, and carnivores to fossil fuels. Order from: Centron Educational Films.

Key Questions

1. What is an ecosystem?
2. What is the food chain that supplies support for the bass?
2. How can the ecosystem of the bass be thrown out of balance?
4. What kind of environment does the bass need to survive?
5. How does the bass get rid of its wastes?
6. How can you keep your human ecosystem in balance?

. . . .

TOPIC: PREVENTION OF AIR POLLUTION

Grade Level: Intermediate

Outcome: The student will be able to identify ways in which air pollution may be reduced or eliminated.

Concept: Air pollution can be reduced.

Content: Ways of reducing air pollution are (alternatives):

1. To reduce pollution from autos:
   a) Have your mom or dad get regular engine tune-up.
   b) Use lead-free gasoline.
   c) Walk to and from school.
   d) Use bicycle instead of car.
   e) Use buses more often.
   f) Impose high taxes or fines on polluters.
2. To reduce pollution from factories:
   a) Write letters of complaint to politicians.
   b) Write letters of complaint to industries.
   c) Boycott products of industries that pollute air.
   d) Support strong legislation to force offenders to eliminate pollution.
3. To reduce pollution from airplanes:
   a) Support legislation to force airlines to develop an improved airplane engine which will be pollution-free.
   b) Relocate airports.
   c) Fine airlines on basis of pollutants emitted.
4. To reduce pollution from power plants:
   a) Turn off lights when not needed.

Learning Experiences

1. *Game: SMOG*
   Description: SMOG illustrates the complex problem of air pollution. Each of the two to four players is the "Air Quality Manager" in his or her city and learns about actual abatement (air pollution control) techniques. The player who first earns 2000 management credits is the best manager of his or her city's resources and aims.
   SMOG includes: 19½" square gameboard, hundreds of pegs, smoke plumes, rings, outrageous fortune cards, play money, die, pad, and an 11-page informative instruction booklet. Ages 12+.
   Order from either: (1) Edmund Scientific Co., 100 Edscorp Building, Barrington, New Jersey, 08007, or (2) Damon/Educational Division, 80 Wilson Way, Westwood, Mass. 02090.
2. *Buzz sessions:* Break class into small groups and have pupils discuss ways of reducing air pollution.
3. *Role-playing simulation:* An open town council meeting to resolve smog. Represented are: mayor, town council, presidents of a meat-packing plant, a large chemical factory, an oil refinery, gas and electric power company, anti-air pollution council chairperson, students, parents, etc.

b) Use less electricity.

c) Do not use electrical gadgets.

d) Support implementation by nuclear power plants.

5. To reduce overpopulation:

a) Stress the concept of zero population.

b) Limit each family to a total of two offspring, and in approximately 70 years the number of deaths will equal the number of births.

Individuals present their points of view and indicate how they will reduce pollution. Members may criticize one another, or teacher may conduct meeting as she or he wishes.

Objective: To make pupils aware of air pollution control.

Key Questions

1. How can your mom or dad help reduce car pollution?

2. What can you do to reduce air pollution?

3. Which should you do to reduce pollution—have mom or dad drive the car to work or take a bus? Why?

4. How can you get factories to reduce air pollution?

5. How can we get jets to reduce air pollution?

6. Can we reduce air pollution?

7. Can we eliminate it completely?

. . . .

TOPIC: PROPER GARBAGE DISPOSAL

Grade Level: Primary

Outcome: The student will demonstrate ability to dispose of garbage properly.

Concept: Proper disposal of garbage makes a healthier world for us to live in.

Content: Proper ways of disposing of garbage are:

1. Wrap garbage in a paper or plastic bag.
2. Wash garbage can once a week.
3. Elevate can six inches above the ground.
4. Use a tight-fitting lid.
5. Have frequent pick-up (twice a week).
6. No dirt or rocks in garbage can.

Learning Experiences

1. *Demonstration:* Teacher invites custodian to bring a garbage can and some actual trash and garbage, which they spread around classroom. Children take turns disposing of various items of garbage, wtih class expressing approval or disapproval.
2. *Alternative learning experiences*
   a) *Ditto work sheets* illustrating proper and improper disposal of garbage. (See Fig. 20.5.)
   b) *Student report* on county/city garbage disposal ordinances.
   c) Role-play situations depicting right and wrong ways of garbage disposal.
   d) Make a weekly chart of how your family disposes of garbage. (See Fig. 20.6.)

Key Questions
1. What is garbage?
2. How should we dispose of vegetable wastes?
3. What should you do before using the trash can?
4. Why should the lid be put over the trash can?
5. Can we get sick from improper garbage disposal?
6. Can garbage pollute the environment?

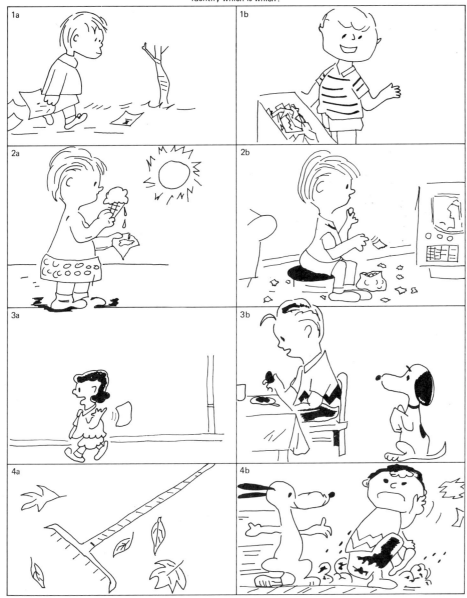

WORK SHEET
Ways of getting rid of garbage
Directions:
Two pictures across have the same theme. In one, the boy
disposes of garbage properly, and in the other improperly.
Identify which is which!

Fig. 20.5 A work sheet illustrating proper and improper disposal of garbage.

GARBAGE		Sun.	Mon.	Tues.	Wed.	Thur.	Fri.	Sat.	Total
Glass bottles									
Organic waste									
Tin cans									
Paperbags, wrappers, and towels									
Plastic boxes and containers									
Newspapers, magazines, writing paper, and envelopes									
Cardboard boxes and wrappings									
Aluminum									
Plastic or cellophane wrappings and bags									
Discarded furniture and toys									

Fig. 20.6   A weekly chart to help record family disposal of garbage.

TOPIC: COMPONENTS OF AIR POLLUTION

Grade Level: Intermediate

Outcome: The student will be able to describe how air is polluted by gases and solid particles.

Concept: Air is contaminated by an overabundance of gases and solid particles.

Content: Polluted air is made up of:

1. Gases
   a) carbon monoxide—autos
   b) carbon dioxide—autos
   c) sulfur oxides—coal-burning plants
   d) hydrocarbons—autos
   e) nitrogen oxides—power plants

Learning Experiences

1. Obtain air samples from various sources of city or community and test for gaseous concentrations. Record.
   a) *Air Pollution Tester Kit For Gases*
      Gases: CO_2, CO, NO_2
      Purpose: To demonstrate the degree of air pollution in the community.

f) ozone and oxidants—general indicators of smog

2. Solid particles

   a) dust—construction, autos

   b) smoke and ashes—industry, homes

   c) lead—cars

   d) pollen and plant spores

   e) pesticides—agriculture, homes

Description: Sample and test pollutant gases in the threshold limit ranges set up by the American Conference of Governmental Industrial Hygienists. Kit is portable and lightweight.

Kit contains a plastic sampling pump; coupling tube; ten ready-to-use, break-tip test ampules (two each for CO_2, CO, H_2S, NO_2, SO_2), and complete instructions with scales for interpreting results.

Pump draws air through ampule containing impregnated chemical specific for a pollutant gas. The length of the stain that appears indicates the concentration of the gas in the air. It only takes a few minutes to test for: carbon dioxide (CO_2), 01-10% by volume; carbon monoxide (CO), 10-3000 ppm; and nitrogen dioxide (NO_2), 1-50 ppm. Kit includes enough ampules for two to four tests for each gas. Replacement ampules are available.

Order kit from: Edmund Scientific Co., 100 Edscorp Building, Barrington, New Jersey, 08007.

2. *Pollution map:* Plot concentrations of gaseous pollution on a city map.

3. Take pictures of local polluters.

4. Test air for dust and solid particles.

   a) *Dust Collection.* A jar to collect solid (dust) particles in the air. A glass jar having a mouth diameter of about four inches is satisfactory. Pour one quart of distilled water in the jar. Place a wire screen over the top to keep insects out. Set the jar on top of roof for 30 days. At this time, remove contents with distilled water, then with .025% sodium lauryl sulfate solution to loosen any tarlike substances. Pour washings through the 20-mesh screen or filter paper. Weigh residue and interpret. (See Fig. 20.7.)

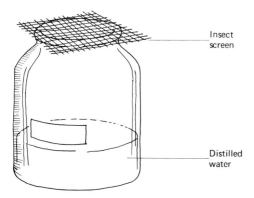

Insect screen

Distilled water

Fig. 20.7 Design for collecting dust sample.

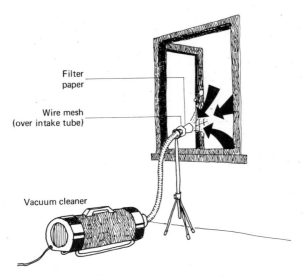

Filter paper

Wire mesh (over intake tube)

Vacuum cleaner

b) *Vacuum cleaner filter paper:* This alternative to analyzing solid particles in the air is a rapid way of drawing air through filter paper. Set equipment on top of flat roof or test area and allow air to be drawn through for 45 minutes. (A model may be constructed as suggested in Fig. 20.8.)

5. Other ecology kits to chemically analyze air and water. Teachers should seek guidance of high school chemistry teachers. Order from: (1) Macalaster Scientific Co., Rt. 111 and Everett Turnpike, Nashua, New Hampshire, 03060; (2) Pawnee Publishing Co. Inc., P.O. Box 3435, Boulder, Colorado, 80303; (3) Damon/ Educational Division.

Fig. 20.8 Vacuum cleaner assembly for sampling air for its soiling properties.

Key Questions

1. What makes up clean air?
2. What makes up polluted air?
3. What gases increase air pollution?
4. What gases do cars give off?
5. Is the air you live in polluted?
6. Does the air you live in contain more pollutant gases or more solid particles? or both?

TOPIC: SOURCES OF NOISE POLLUTION

Grade Level: Intermediate

Outcome: The student will be able to identify sources of noise pollution.

Concept: There are many human-made sources of noise.

Content: Sources of noise pollution are:

1. Automobiles
2. Airplanes
3. Industrial machines
4. Crowds
5. Home appliances, e.g., radios, TVs, vacuum cleaners, can openers

Learning Experiences

1. *Demonstration survey:* Have several pupils assist in recording different sound sources in the community on a tape recorder and simultaneously monitoring noise levels with a noise meter. Replay the tape in the classroom.

   Have pupils monitor various noise levels in the classroom with a noise meter.
2. Plot a noise contour map of the community.

Key Questions

1. Who makes noise pollution?
2. Who makes the loudest noises?
3. In what ways do you create noise pollution in school? at home?
4. When is sound humanly comfortable?
5. When does sound become irritable to humans?
6. Can we adjust to sound? to noise?

TOPIC: KEEPING OUR ENVIRONMENT CLEAN

Grade Level: Primary

Outcome: The student will be able to state ways to help keep our environment healthy.

Concept: There are many ways of keeping our environment healthy and safe.

Content: Ways of conserving our equipment are:

1. Throw trash into garbage can.
2. Collect newspapers and bottles for recycling.
3. Replant trees in forest.
4. Clean beaches.
5. Use bike instead of car.
6. Keep house clean.
7. Clean up backyard.
8. Don't throw cans into lakes and rivers.
9. Eat up all your food.
10. Don't burn trash.
11. Turn off lights when not using them.
12. Shower instead of taking a bath.
13. Keep radio noise down.
14. Clean your own room regularly.
15. Use nondetergent soaps.
16. Encourage recycling of bottles, cans, papers, oils, etc.

Learning Experiences

1. *Board game: S.O.D.E.*—Save Our Doomed Earth. The game makes children aware of ways to conserve and destroy our environment.
2. *Alternative experiences*
   a) *Role playing:* to depict various environmental situations and ways of practicing conservation
   b) Buzz sessions
   c) *Poster:* "How Man Pollutes His World," *National Geographic Magazine,* Washington, D.C., 1970.
   d) *Games:* Litterbug or clean-up
      Litterbug: An antilitter campaign to teach children the evil of littering and the importance of picking up trash. The player who does the best job cleaning up the streets and sidewalks by collecting litter in his or her trash can wins. For ages 4-10.
      Clean-Up: An antilitter game to develop an antilitter consciousness. Each player spins the arrow to find out what to do. Then he or she hops from block to block, removing trash, planting trees, grass, and flowers in his or her neighborhood. The player who

does the most to beautify the town without falling down on the job, wins. Ages 4-10.

Order both games from: Damon/ Educational Division.

Key Questions

1. Did you enjoy playing the game?
2. What can you do to keep your environment safe and healthy?

e) *Teacher demonstration:* Effect of sulfur dioxide on plant life. Using a controlled environment and a common air pollutant, sulfur dioxide, have students observe effects of the gas on plant seedlings (see Fig. 20.9). Effects can be observed in a few days. Directions for conducting this experiment, including the "Environmental" transparent plastic chamber and materials, may be ordered from: Educational Aids Dept., Union Carbide Corporation, Sterling Forest Research Center, P.O. Box 363, Tuxedo, N.Y., 10987.

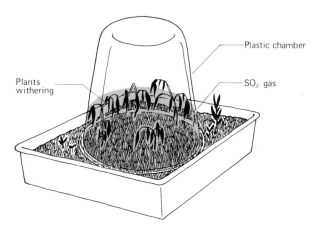

Fig. 20.9 Use of transparent plastic chamber to study the effect of sulfur dioxide on plant life.

Key Questions

1. How can we keep our school clean?
2. How can we keep our playgrounds clean?
3. How can we keep our homes clean?
4. How can we keep our beaches clean?
5. What should you do with an empty soft drink can?
6. What should you do with a chocolate bar wrapper?
7. Where should you throw away your gum?
8. Where should you throw away old newspapers?

. . . .

TOPIC: SYMPTOMS OF AIR POLLUTION

Grade Level: Intermediate

Outcome: The student will be able to identify the symptoms of air pollution.

Concept: Air pollutants cause physical stress on living things. Air pollution is hazardous to our well-being.

Content: Symptoms of air pollution are:

1. Physiological human responses:

   a) irritation and burning of eyes

   b) itchy irritating skin

   c) throat irritation

   d) coughing

   e) difficulty in breathing

   f) more frequent allergies and asthma attacks

   g) emotional stress

   h) susceptibility to respiratory infections

   i) chronic diseases from lung exposure: emphysema, lung cancer

Learning Experiences

1. *Film:* Contact your local or state public health department for an appropriate film.

2. a) *Demonstration:* Place several greenhouse plants (in pots) alongside a freeway for a week. Water the plants during this time. Observe plants after one to three weeks.

   b) *Pictures:* of plants dying, e.g., pines.

3. a) Pictures

   b) Compare bird habitats in polluted regions with those in nonpolluted regions.

4. a) Pictures of photographs of this haze.

   b) Pictures of severe smog.

2. Plants
   a) growth stops
   b) leaves become discolored
   c) flowers do not bloom
   d) plants die
3. Birds and fish
   a) migrations
   b) fewer births
   c) death
4. Physical description and chemical property
   a) yellowish-brown haze (nitrogen-oxide haze)
   b) smog—dimming out of the sunlight
   c) nylon becomes degraded
   d) rubber deteriorates

c) Experiments:
   (1) Effect of air pollution on nylon
       Purpose: The usable life of nylon goods is shortened by air pollution. The agents probably responsible for the destruction of nylon have been identified. Among them are: hot particles contained in smoke, soot laden with sulphuric acid, aerosols, nitrogen oxides, aldehydes from internal combustion engines, and solvent vapors and droplets.

       Procedure: Get good quality (15 denier) nylon hose. Prepare three 3¼" × 4" slides and mount square pieces of nylon hose on each slide. Place two slides on the school roof so that the nylon is held in a horizontal position and so that the air can come in contact with both sides of the nylon. Leave one sample exposed for 30 days, the second for 90 days. At the end of its exposure period, check each sample and examine it for broken threads. A sample stored inside for the same period of time may be used as a control for comparison.

   (2) Effect of ozone on rubber
       Purpose: To demonstrate the effect of ozone in the air on rubber (car tires).

       Procedure: Ozone, an oxidizing agent in the atmosphere, vigorously attacks rubber. The attack is most serious when the rubber is exposed while stretched, folded, or otherwise subjected to stress. The physical effect is readily visible as cracking and checking of the rubber. At the same time, its ability to be stretched and then return to its original shape and size is greatly reduced.

       Cut rubber strips from a 9" × 9" × 16" sheet of ozone-sensitive test-pads, Goodyear Specification No. 563-27303. This special rubber may be ordered from:

Goodyear Tire and Rubber Company, 1357 Tennessee Avenue, Cincinnati, Ohio. Mount the strips and stretch them. Place a small shelter box over the rubber and mountings to keep the sunlight out. The box should allow air to move freely. After seven days of exposure, remove the rubber strip and examine it for degree of cracking and checking. Check also for loss of elasticity. If exposure of one week is not sufficient to cause noticeable cracking or other degradation, the period of exposure should be extended.

Key Questions

1. What are the physiological symptoms of air pollution?
2. Have you ever experienced any of these symptoms?
3. What should you do when you have an air pollution crisis?
4. How do plants react to air pollution?
5. How do birds react to air pollution?
6. Can you see smog? smell it? feel it?

REFERENCES AND BIBLIOGRAPHY

Ames, William. *The Life of the Pond* (New York: McGraw-Hill, 1967).

Billington, Ely T. *Understanding Ecology* (New York: Fredrick Warne, 1968).

DeBell, Garrett. *The Environmental Handbook* (New York: Ballantine, 1969).

Ehlers, Victor, and Ernest Steel. *Municipal and Rural Sanitation* (New York: McGraw-Hill, 1965), pp. 151-182.

Ehrlich, Paul. *The Population Bomb* (New York: Ballantine, 1968).

Graham, Frank. *Since Silent Spring* (Boston: Houghton Mifflin, 1970).

Guide to Appraisal and Control of Air Pollution (New York: American Public Health Association, 1969).

Helfrich, Harold W. *The Environmental Crisis* (New Haven: Yale University Press, 1971).

Hunter, Donald C., and Henry C. Wohlers. *Air Pollution Experiments for Junior and Senior High School Science Classes* (Pittsburgh, Pa.: Air Pollution Control Association, 1968).

Kormondy, Edward J. *Concepts of Ecology* (Englewood Cliffs, N.J.: Prentice-Hall, 1969).

Local city Department of Public Works pamphlet on garbage-disposal regulations.

MacDonald, Frank, and John Trygy. *Environmental Hygiene* (New Orleans: Tulane University Press, 1963), pp. 153-162.

Mitchell, John G., and Constance C. Stallings. *Ecotactics* (New York: Pocket Books, 1970).

Navarra, John G. *Our Noisy World: The Problem of Noise Pollution* (Garden City, N.Y.: Doubleday, 1969).

Peterson, A. P. G., and E. E. Gross, Jr. *Handbook of Noise Measurement* (West Concord, Mass.: General Radio Company, 1967).

Rienow, Robert, and Leona Rienow. *Moment in the Sun* (New York: Ballantine, 1969).

Rodda, Michael. *Noise and Society* (London: Oliver and Boyd, 1972).

Rose, J. *Technological Injury* (New York: Gordon and Breach Science Publishers, 1969).

Roth, Robert E. "Fundamental Concepts for Environmental Management Education (K-16)," in *Outlines of Environmental Education*, pp. 65-74; edited by Clay Schoenfeld (Madison, Wisc.: Dembar Educational Research Services, 1971).

Storer, John. *The Web of Life* (New York: Signet Science Library, 1963).

Storin, Diane. *Investigating Air, Land, and Water Pollution* (Bronxville, N.Y.: Pawnee, 1971).

Toffler, Alvin. *Future Shock* (New York: Random House, 1970).

Weaver, Elbert C., ed. *Scientific Experiments in Environmental Pollution* (New York: Holt, Rinehart and Winston, 1968).

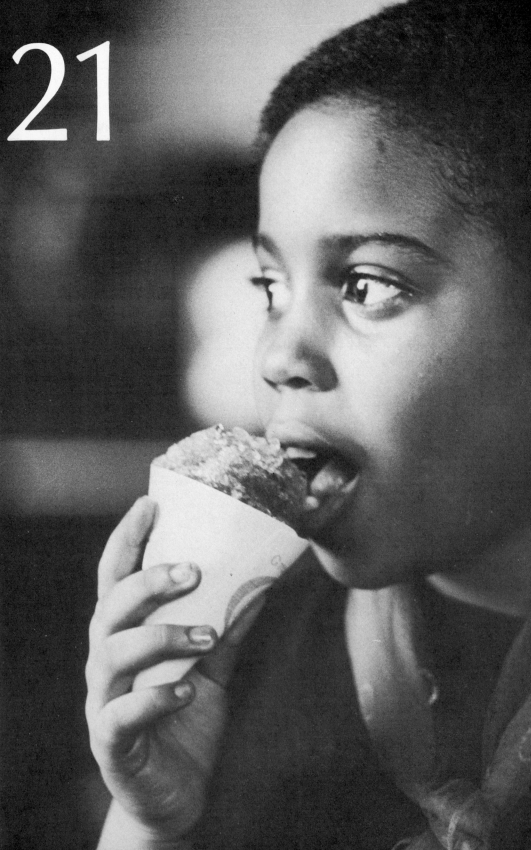

teaching about nutrition

INTRODUCTION

The consumption of food is both a vital function and a cherished experience. However, the quantity and quality of food that each American consumes vary to a great extent. Even though the United States is the wealthiest nation in the world, Americans still die from lack of food, malnutrition, and/or nutrition-created chronic deseases. In all too many cases, ignorance of the principles of nutrition prevents many people from feeding themselves effectively. This is indeed unfortunate, for the principles of nutrition are few in number and easily understood.

Food intake is essential to the building and repairing of body tissue. It is also basic to energy production in the form of heat to keep the body warm and to create strength. The challenge, then, is to match our specific food needs with the essential ingredients found in foods. This brings us to the key aspect of nutrition—balance. The well-fed person may not at all be a well-nourished person. Without the proper balance of vitamins, proteins, minerals, carbohydrates, essential fatty acids, fiber, and water, we cannot expect to be well nourished.

Theoretically, good nutrition is relatively easy to attain. Many people actually practice sound nutritional habits and maintain a good diet without ever thinking about it. In many instances the practice involves merely following the elementary principles of nutrition that were presented during one's youth, such as eating a balanced diet, eating a variety of foods, and eating regularly.

LIFESTYLE AND NUTRITION

However, what sounds so simple presents a major problem for many. Our American lifestyle is not at all conducive to sound nutritional habits and optimal well-being. Most Americans attempt to eat a variety of foods and hope that their meals are nutritionally balanced. They assume that they are getting the proper amounts of vitamins, minerals, and other essential micronutrients that their bodies need. Unfortunately, this may not always be true.

Most Americans eat a lot of convenience and snack foods (hot dogs and french fries, frozen TV dinners, potato chips, soft drinks, and beer). Such foods are usually "empty calorie" foods—rich in sugar and deficient in vitamins and minerals. Children ingesting such foods regularly not only evolve poor eating habits and problems related to overweight, but also initiate and incubate chronic diseases of related nutrient deficiencies.

There are other lifestyle circumstances that may contribute to vitamin and mineral deficiencies. Today fully 55 percent of foods found in the marketplace are convenience foods (Passwater, 1976, p. 17). Thus the possibility of poor food choice is compounded by the availability of numerous snack and convenience foods. In order to retard their spoilage and to lengthen their shelf life, convenience foods are preserved in numerous ways, thereby losing much of their nutrient values. For example, milling wheat into white flour removes vitamin E, bran, wheat germ, and most trace minerals. Although breads and cereals are often enriched, or "fortified," by the return of vitamins B_1, B_2, and niacin, 12 other essential B vitamins and most trace minerals are not returned (Passwater, 1976, p. 22).

Another lifestyle habit that may contribute to nutritional deficiencies is eating out in restaurants and cafeterias, which often keep food warm in steam tables for many hours. Although such prolonged heating keeps the food sanitary, it destroys a large proportion of the vitamin content (vitamins B and C) of most meats and vegetables. Yet we eat in such places on the assumption that cooked and preheated food does retain its original vitamins.

In addition, nutrients in the body are depleted when the liver detoxifies the more than 2000 chemicals that may find their way into our bodies (Nutrition Research, 1975, p. 161). These chemicals include food additives, preservatives, coloring agents, sweeteners, insecticides, and antibiotics. Ingesting these chemicals adds to the "normal" detoxification load of the liver. Thus the liver, in working overtime to get rid of these chemicals, utilizes extra amounts of vitamins B_6, C, and E and minerals, such as selenium. If these micronutrients are not present in sufficient quantities, one feels fatigued and functions suboptimally. Such reactions often reflect nutrient deficiency.

Another lifestyle factor adding work burden to the liver occurs when one lives in an air-polluted community. Ozone and nitrous oxide detoxification by the liver creates additional nutrient demands. Likewise, such nutrient demands are also compounded in those persons who inhale cigarette smoke; drink colas, coffee, and alcoholic beverages; and work under emotional stress.

In summary, significant losses of nutrients do occur during cooking, storage, transportation, and processing of foods. Many persons experience lifestyle episodes that further deplete vitamins and minerals in their bodies. Such nutrient losses in foods and their depletions in the body weaken one's natural body resistance to stress, diseases, and disorders. It is possible that many children, teenagers, and adults have nutrient deficiencies and do not know it. Consequently, their potentials for optimal well-being are suppressed, and they function with a lowered level of well-being.

Eating Habits

There is mounting support from scientists and physicians in this country, and especially foreign countries, that many health problems and diseases stem from vitamin and mineral deficiencies or/and eating too many of the wrong foods (see the sources cited at the end of this chapter). The causative treatment and preventive answers to heart disease, cancer, obesity, diabetes, arthritis, emotional disturbances, allergies, and other diseases may very well be found in new nutritional lifestyle approaches. This should not be too startling, as food provides the framework for everything that the body synthesizes and uses. Without food, life cannot go on! Lack of enough vitamins and minerals leads to a subsistence life. We should think of food and nutrition as helping us to attain "optimal" health and not just "average" health or freedom from diseases and illnesses. In general, we have focused on counting calories and having a diet balanced in terms of fats, carbohydrates, and proteins. Thus a person who ingests the required number of calories each day is thought of as well fed. However, such a person may not be well nourished. We appear to be eating a lot of calories, but not too many vitamins and minerals.

Are Americans nutrient-deficient? Is there a need for elementary school teachers to be concerned about this? The answer to both is *yes*. Several intensive dietary surveys were conducted in the late 1960s to determine the nutritional status of American people. The U.S. Department of Agriculture in 1965 discovered that only 50 percent of American households had diets that were rated "good" on their standards (Passwater, 1976, p. 17). A 1970 follow-up national study by the U.S. Public Health Service into Americans' eating habits revealed gross vitamin and iron deficiencies (Labuza, 1975, pp. 67, 104-105). Numerous vitamin C deficiencies were found among the 18-25 age group and the elderly.

These and other studies point out that our food and eating habits have, since 1946, been continually deteriorating. "Dietary Goals for the United States" (1977, p. 1), a recent study prepared by the Select Committee on Nutrition and Human Needs of the United States Senate, lends support to the concerns expressed in this chapter:

The simple fact is that our diets have changed radically within the last 50 years, with great and often very harmful effects on our health. These dietary changes represent as great a threat to public health as smoking. Too much fat, too much sugar or salt, can be and are linked directly to heart disease, cancer, obesity, and stroke, among other killer diseases. In all, six of the ten leading causes of death in the United States have been linked to our diet. . . .

In the early 1900's, almost 40 percent of our caloric intake came from fruit, vegetable, and grain products. Today, only a little more than 20 percent of calories comes from these sources.

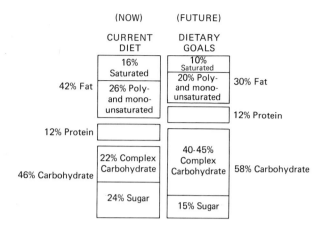

Fig. 21.1 Composition of average American diet in the 1970s as contrasted to the recommended dietary goals. (Select Committee on Nutrition and Human Needs of United States Senate, *Dietary Goals for the United States,* Washington, D.C.: U.S. Government Printing Office, 1977, pp. 12-13.)

The six recommended dietary goals and changes in food selection and preparation are summarized in Fig. 21.1. The goals are as follows:

1. Increase carbohydrate consumption to account for 55 to 60 percent of the energy (calorie) intake.

2. Reduce overall fat consumption from approximately 40 to 30 percent of energy intake.

3. Reduce saturated fat consumption to account for about 10 percent of total energy intake, and balance that with polyunsaturated and monounsaturated fats, which should account for about 10 percent of energy intake each.

4. Reduce cholesterol consumption to about 300 mg a day.

5. Reduce sugar consumption by about 40 percent to account for about 15 percent of total energy intake.

6. Reduce salt consumption by about 50 to 85 percent to approximately 3 grams a day.

These goals suggest the following changes in food selection and preparation:

1. Increase consumption of fruits, vegetables, and whole grains.

2. Decrease consumption of meat and increase consumption of poultry and fish.

3. Decrease consumption of foods high in fat, and partially substitute polyunsaturated fat for saturated fat.

4. Substitute nonfat milk for whole milk.

5. Decrease consumption of butterfat, eggs, and other high-cholesterol sources.

6. Decrease consumption of sugar and foods high in sugar content.

7. Decrease consumption of salt and foods high in salt content.

The national dietary recommendations raise the question of how much of a vitamin or mineral one needs for one day. The stock approach is to refer to the 1974 Recommended Daily Allowances (USRDA) of vitamins and minerals for the answer. Although intended to guard against disease deficiencies and to maintain an "undefined" health of most people, the RDA recommendations fail to consider the variances in lifestyle and eating habits or the destruction of nutrients in foods through storage, preservation, freezing, and cooking. Rather, RDA levels are intakes of nutrients that meet the needs of healthy adults living under *non*stressful environmental conditions; they do not take into account special needs arising from infections, metabolic disorders, chronic diseases, or other abnormalities (National Academy of Sciences, 1974, p. 3). This report states that continued use of drugs, such as antibiotics, antidepressants, insomnia and headache medications, and oral contraceptives will greatly deplete essential nutrients. The report suggests making nutrient allowances whenever such depletion episodes and lifestyle conditions exist or whenever food intake is curtailed or the diet is marginal in specific nutrients (e.g., eating refined white flour bread, cereals, and pastries). Obviously, there are many times, often on a continuous basis, when some nutrients will be depleted in a person. At other times, for many, skipping meals, eating junk foods, and/or eating food without any idea of balance is a regular lifestyle behavior that results in nutrient depletion. It should be obvious that RDA levels are only dietary guidelines at best and have definite limitations. As stated in the National Academy of Sciences report (1974, p. 19):

RDA have been established for only about one-third of the essential nutrients, that foods are ordinarily analyzed for only a small number of nutrients, and that interactions of various types between nutrients and food constituents may reduce the availability of some nutrients and, hence, the accuracy of information about food composition. . . . RDA are recommendations for the amounts of nutrients that should be consumed daily, not for the nutrient content of foods.

Moreover, Dr. Linus Pauling (1976) and Dr. Roger Williams (1973) have postulated that in many individuals the constitutional need may be ten or more times the recommended daily allowances. Biochemical individuality takes into account the genetic, metabolic, and biochemical enzyme variability that exists among individuals, that each person has his or her own physiological and nutritional "norm," and that nutritional needs must be geared for the individual and not the general public.

MYTHS ABOUT NUTRITION

Many nutritional and disease problems arise from misinformation or lack of information about food.

Some misconceptions and the facts follow.

1. *One should take vitamin/mineral supplements.* There is considerable controversy about this practice. Much of the rationale to support this practice has already been substantiated. One alternative to bolster a poor diet is to take nutrient supplements. However, one should never "pop vitamin pills" as a substitute for not eating a balanced daily diet. The best way to get your vitamins and minerals is in the food itself, not in pills or tablets.

2. *Sugar is a good source of energy and is good for us.* Although refined white sugar is an energy source, it lacks the very B vitamins and minerals necessary for its assimilation in the body. This means that the liver must leach out from other cells the needed vitamins and minerals needed in order to utilize the sugar. Sugar is the leading food additive in the United States today. It is used in almost all fruit drinks, salad dressings, many baby foods, sauces, canned and dehydrated soups, pot pies, frozen TV dinners, bacon and other cured meats, canned and frozen vegetables, fruit yogurt, and breakfast cereals. Tomato ketchup contains as much as 29 percent sugar, and coffee creamer contains 65 percent sugar ("Too Much Sugar?" 1978). Sugar is used as a preservative and to improve food appearances and taste. When ingested by itself or in other foods, it displaces natural complex starches that have essential functions in the body. A child drinking a six-ounce bottle of cola ingests about 4½ teaspoons of sugar (Airola, 1977, p. 24). Sugar masks the bitter taste of cola.

The exact effects of sugar on the biochemistry of the body are not too well understood at the present time. There is considerable controversy, for example, as to whether sugar causes hypoglycemia. Sugar is suspected of causing a condition of constantly overshooting insulin and depleting the liver of glycogen (stored sugar), causing insufficient blood sugar levels, or hypoglycemia (Duffy, 1976; Williams, 1973, p. 140). It is not how low the blood sugar level drops, but the speed at which it drops that causes the symptoms of hypoglycemia (Airola, 1977, p. 15). The sudden drop in blood sugar level sends the body into a condition of "near-shock." This condition may be further aggravated by caffeine (coffee or cola) and intensified by stress. Symptoms of hypoglycemia include anxiety, insomnia, frigidity in women and impotence in men, suicidal depression, and craving for sweets and alcoholic beverages (Fredericks, 1976, p. 58). Sugar also increases triglyceride and free fatty acid blood levels in the aorta and causes stress in the adrenal glands and liver (DiCyan, 1974, pp. 20-30; Fredericks, 1976, p. 58; Leonard, 1977, pp. 56-59; Passwater, 1976, p. 140). Sugar is also suspected of aggravating the conditions of diabetes, dental decay, mental depression, hormonal disorders, overweight, cancer, heart disease, immobilizing natural body defenses, and causing a general inability to function optimally in life (Airola, 1977, p. 55; Cheraskin, 1976, p. 22; Leonard, Hofer, and Pritikin, 1977, pp. 55-59; Passwater, 1976, pp. 142-145; Williams, 1973, pp. 38-144). The number of persons suspected of suffering from hypoglycemia is in the unknown millions. Many children drink soft drinks, eat chocolate bars and sweets, and unknowingly have become "sugar addicts." Sugar has also been linked to autism and hyperkinetic children with learning difficulties. Incidentally, numerous biochemists have suggested eliminating or reducing the intake of refined sugar, nicotine, and alcohol as a way of controlling hypoglycemia and its related symptoms.

The amount of sugar used in this country averages out to 125 pounds per person per year (Select Committee, 1977; "Too Much Sugar?" 1978). Eating refined sugar is our worst food/health habit.

3. *Vitamins regulate specific parts of the body* (e.g., vitamin A regulates eyes, and vitamin E is for reproduction). This misconception stems from the outdated medical version of "there is a specific

cause for a specific disease." Although still not clearly understood, there is ample evidence that vitamins, minerals, and amino acids work collectively with one another on a shotgun approach, as a team, and together have a "splattered" effect on the body as a whole. Vitamins and minerals need each other in order to be absorbed and utilized in the body. For example, in order for a cell to build a particular protein molecule, all of the eight essential amino acids that make up that protein have to be available at the same time. If they are not present simultaneously, the protein cannot be built. The same is true for the B vitamins, all of which are complementary in their action and must be taken together. Although probably an incomplete scenario, vitamins A, B_6, C, and E and selenium have been identified as essential for the liver to detoxify polluted air and cigarette smoke in affected persons. Vitamins A, B, C, D, and E have all been found to be essential for good eye health. Although vitamin C has been characterized as an "all-around" vitamin affecting almost all body functions, it is probably aided in its functions by the presence of other vitamins and minerals. Although these few examples do not paint a complete picture, they should reinforce the concept that nutrients work together. Perhaps these examples will also help you to understand that a balanced diet helps to provide a balance of the essential nutrients.

4. *We can substitute soft drinks and beer/wine for water.* We need water to replace water lost in normal body functions and physical activities. Soft drinks contain the addictive chemicals caffeine and sugar. Both rob the body of essential vitamins and minerals. It is possible that sugar and caffeine both destroy or distort the ability to taste. Hence water does not appear to taste very good to those ingesting lots of sugar and caffeine. Soft drinks and alcoholic beverages are no substitutes for water.

5. *We should not eat cholesterol foods, because they cause heart disease.* Cholesterol foods do not cause heart disease (Williams, 1973, pp. 88-109). The early statistical and medical evidence linking heart disease to cholesterol was misleading, but nonetheless the question of cholesterol continues to be a controversy.

Whole milk is related to the cholesterol controversy. Whole milk has a chemical balance of nutrients essential for human well-being. Whole milk, containing about four percent fat, supplies fat-soluble vitamins A, D, E, and K, as well as lecithin and other nutrients. Eliminating fat from whole milk also eliminates the essential vitamins. Whole milk is too nutritious to be deleted from the diet. If one wishes to cut down cholesterol and fat intake, one should cut down the foods contributing the largest amount of fat calories—beefsteaks, hamburger, hot dogs, and cold meats.

6. *One can avoid overweight and obesity by not eating fats and carbohydrates.* The secret of avoiding obesity and maintaining desirable weight lies in not avoiding fat and/or carbohydrates, but in ingesting the nutrients necessary for optimal well-being, exercising regularly, and fulfilling one's emotional needs. Nutrients and exercise are both essential for proper functioning of the appestat mechanism (control center in the hypothalamus of the brain for regulating hunger, thirst, appetite, and emotions). Regular exercise keeps the appestat "tuned up" and maintains its balancing/regulatory function intact. Along with resetting the appestat, one should correct faulty eating habits. Counting energy calories may not be as important as ensuring a daily balanced intake of vitamins and minerals.

7. *Poor nutrition causes overweight and obesity.* Poor nutrition fosters worse nutrition. Persons experiencing poor nutrition tend to consume more starchy and sugar-rich foods. Lack of vitamin B_1, for example, disrupts and upsets the appestat mechanism, predisposing one to obesity. Poor nutrition usually reflects poor eating habits.

Summary

It should be obvious from the material presented that we are entering an era of nutrition-knowledge explosion and a nutrition revolution in this country. Indeed, there are numerous controversies among physicians, nutritionists, biochemists, and the lay public about many aspects of nutrition, weight control, and eating practices. Often the patient knows more than the physician about nutrition. With new information on nutrition surfacing daily, we can expect the revolution to gain momentum and to continue for some time. As Dr. Sheldon Margen, professor of human nutrition at the University of California at Berkeley and a major consultant to the 1977 Senate Select Committee on Nutrition and Human Needs, put it (Rice, 1978): "Can a change in the nation's diet reduce the rate of the killer diseases such as cancer, arteriosclerosis and diabetes? We don't know for sure, but can't afford to spend another 20 to 30 years finding out."

We believe in bringing the nutrition controversy out into the open. The nutrition revolution is just beginning. Dr. Richard Wurton, professor of nutrition at the Massachusetts Institute of Technology, postulates that within five to ten years, physicians will be able to use nutrition instead of drugs in the treatment of diseases and disorders of the brain ("Nutrient Approach," 1978). Nutrition therapy may even replace drug therapy and surgery as the medical mode of treating and preventing many of today's diseases and disorders. We can expect the field of nutrition to gain greater public recognition and our eating habits to change when medical schools begin to earnestly include nutrition courses in the preparation of physicians, when the medical community begins to recognize the importance of nutrition to health and in the treatment and prevention of diseases, and when the food industry stops destroying nutrients in foods. Meanwhile, teachers should continue to offer up-to-date information on nutrition and not wait for miracle changes in medicine and the food industry.

Good Eating Habits

American tradition dictates the eating of three meals a day. Such a policy becomes faulty, however, when we realize that the stomach empties every three to five hours, depending on its contents. It follows that we should actually be eating every three to five hours if the body is to be truly satisfied from a physiological standpoint.

Perhaps a more sensible approach than the "three square meals a day" theory is to eat more frequent small meals during the course of the day. The overall consumption does not have to change, just the frequency of consumption. To the individual attempting to diet, such advice probably sounds ludicrous. However, it is not at all uncommon to find oneself actually reducing overall consumption by increasing consumption frequency, assuming, of course, that the extra meals are considerably smaller. The point to be made is that there surely is nothing sacred about eating three meals a day. Five or more small meals may be more appropriate.

Contemporary society has also of late been besieged by some rather bizarre diets and other related approaches to losing weight or what some people term "cleansing the body." Such approaches include fasting, crash diets, and overzealous adherence to ill-founded health food practices. Should such nutritional behavior be misguided (and it very often is), the important nutritional concept of balance surely will be disrupted and the victim made to face the consequences. Dieting is serious business and requires the utmost of forethought and medical advice.

Another American nutritional catastrophe is the breakfast meal. Americans are notorious for their lack of regard for breakfast. How unfortunate, for breakfast is by far the most important meal of the day. After sleeping for an extended period, an individual invariably awakens with a low blood sugar level, and a good breakfast is necessary to replenish the energy supply. Failing to do so takes away from one's well-being both physically and emotionally. In reality, the attainment of short-range optimal well-being is next to impossible without the benefit of a nutritious breakfast to start the day.

(Suffice it to say that food is one of the most important bases of good health.) Our behavior relative to nutrition will have a great bearing on our potential for the attainment of optimal well-being. The justifications for nutrition education are obvious. Youngsters should be afforded the opportunity to explore the chemistry of food and its many ramifications. Their lives might depend on it.

The nutrition lesson plans that follow touch on many of the more important concepts of nutrition. By no means should they be considered as all-encompassing. They are simply intended to serve as models depicting what could be done along the lines of nutrition education.

. . . .

TOPIC: A GOOD BREAKFAST

Grade Level: Primary

Outcome I: The student will be able to state the importance of breakfast.

Concept: Breakfast is the most important meal of the day.

Content: Breakfast is important for the following reasons:

1. A long time has passed since the last meal.
2. It gives us energy to go to school.
3. It gives us energy to learn.
4. It gives us energy to work.
5. It gives us energy to play.

Learning Experiences

1. *Survey:* How many didn't eat breakfast?
2. *Picture simulation:* Pictures of different people and discussion of how they feel and possible relationship to a good breakfast.
3. Storytelling.

Outcome II: The student will be able to select a nutritionally sound breakfast.

Concept: A good breakfast has a variety of foods.

Content: A good breakfast includes such foods as:

1. A fruit
2. Cereal
3. Milk
4. Egg
5. Bread

Learning Experiences

1. *Simulation breakfast:* Pupils select a breakfast from food cutouts. Class and teacher analyze various breakfasts.
2. Filmstrip such as: *Skimpy and a Good Breakfast.*
3. Color various breakfast foods.

Key Questions

1. Do you like to eat breakfast?
2. Why should we eat a good breakfast?
3. What happens when we don't eat breakfast?
4. What foods make up a good breakfast?
5. Are you going to eat a breakfast tomorrow?

. . . .

TOPIC: EATING A VARIETY OF FOODS

Grade Level: Primary

Outcome: The student will be able to construct a meal that is composed of a variety of foods from each food group.

Concept: Eating different foods from each group keeps us healthy and strong.

Content: Foods in respective food groups are:

1. *Vegetables* (rich in carbohydrates): Eat rice, potatoes, corn, carrots on different days.

Learning Experience

1. Pupils simulate two meals by indicating concept of variety within each group.

2. *Fruits* (rich in vitamin C): Eat oranges, to-matoes, strawberries, pineapple, peaches on different days.

3. *Meats:* Eat fish, hamburger, steak, chicken, turkey, ham on different days.

4. *Dairy products:* Drink milk regularly, but alternate eggs, cheese, and ice cream.

5. *Cereals and breads:* Eat corn flakes one day, granola the next, cooked oatmeal the third, and so on. Eat a variety of bread and flour products.

Key Questions

1. What could you eat instead of apples?
2. What could you have instead of orange juice?
3. What could you eat instead of hamburger?
4. What do we mean by "variety"?

TOPIC: FUNCTIONS OF FOODS

Grade Level: Primary

Outcome: The student will be able to discuss how foods keep our bodies in good working order.

Concept I: Foods provide us with energy for doing things.

Content: Foods providing energy are:

1. Bread
2. Potatoes
3. Corn
4. Cereals
5. Butter

Learning Experience

1. *Matching bee:* Match function to various parts of body.

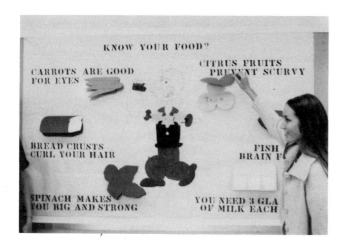

Fig. 21.2 A bulletin board idea on nutrition. Children help to build "Popeye" by correctly answering the questions. Popeye's body parts are mobile. Does this bulletin board allow children to be active or passive participants?

Concept II: Foods repair and build our bodies.

Content: Foods repairing our bodies are:

1. Hamburger
2. Fish
3. Chicken
4. Cheese
5. Eggs

Concept III: Foods regulate our bodies.

Content: Foods that regulate our bodies are:

1. Carrots—good eyesight, keep lungs healthy
2. Milk—keep all of body healthy, give us energy
3. Oranges—help heal wounds, help liver get rid of poisons, make cellular glue, prevent colds and diseases
4. Green vegetables—healthy skin, help liver get rid of poisons, prevent diseases

Key Questions

1. What kind of foods give us energy?
2. What kind of foods help us to grow big?
3. What food helps us to see better?
4. What foods help to build muscles?

. . . .

TOPIC: DIGESTIVE SYSTEM

Grade Level: Intermediate

Outcome: The student will be able to identify the parts, locations, and functions of the digestive system.

Concept: The digestive system breaks down food for use in the body.

Content: The digestive system consists of:

1. *Mouth:* location—head; function—chew and moisten food.
2. *Esophagus:* location—throat area; function—carry food from mouth to stomach.
3. *Stomach:* location—left side, lower ribs; function—churn food with digestive juices.
4. *Liver:* location—right side, lower ribs; function—produces digestive juice called bile for small intestine.
5. *Small intestine:* location—midtorso, below ribs, 20 feet long and coiled; function—completes digestion or breaking down of food and allows for food absorption into blood.
6. *Large intestine:* location—coils around outside edges of small intestine; function—absorbs water and eliminates wastes.

Learning Experiences

1. *Matching bee:* Teacher and pupil using human torso or mobile made from colored paper cutout parts.
2. Use of balloon or plastic bag to conceptualize stomach action. Put water and slice of bread in bag. Use fingers, representing stomach muscles, to churn the contents.
3. Use flour sifter or screen to conceptualize how substances pass through intestinal wall (screen).
4. *Review Quiz*

7. *Pancreas:* location—back of and below stomach; function—secretes pancreatic juice which is essential to food digestion.

Review Quiz

Part I. Match location to organ or part.

Location	*Organ*
1. Throat	_____ Esophagus
2. Back of and below stomach	_____ Mouth
3. Midtorso, below ribs	_____ Liver
4. Right side, lower ribs	_____ Small intestine, large intestine
5. Head	_____ Pancreas
6. Left side, lower ribs	_____ Stomach

Part II. Match organ with function (what it does) listed below:

Organ	*Function*
1. Esophagus	_____ Absorbs food
2. Mouth	_____ Churns
3. Liver	_____ Pancreatic juice
4. Small intestine	_____ Chews
5. Large intestine	_____ Absorbs liquids, eliminates wastes
6. Pancreas	_____ Carries food from mouth to stomach
7. Stomach	_____ Bile secretion

Key Questions

1. Where is most of the food absorbed into the blood?
2. What is the function of the stomach?
3. What is the function of the digestive system?
4. What can you do to take good care of your digestive system?

TOPIC: EATING A BALANCED DIET

Grade Level: Intermediate

Outcome: The student will be able to select a balanced diet.

Concept: A balanced diet includes foods from the four food groups, plus water.

Content: Food groups contributing to a balanced diet are:

Learning Experiences

1. Dairy products
   a) milk—3+ glasses
   b) butter
   c) eggs
   d) ice cream
2. Fruits and vegetables
   a) orange-tomato juice
   b) lettuce
   c) cabbage
   d) carrots
   e) peas
   f) potatoes
   g) celery
3. Breads and cereals
   a) bread
   b) cereals
4. Meats
   a) beef
   b) pork, ham
   c) chicken
   d) fish
5. Water

1. *Matching-bee analysis:* Pupils start out by listing foods they ate previous day.
2. Locate a pupil with a well-balanced diet and another with a poorly balanced diet. Match the picture cut-outs of foods they ate on large pie plates representing breakfast, lunch, and dinner. Let class decide which is balanced.

Are My Meals Balanced?

Directions: Using the list of foods, write in the circles the foods you ate yesterday. Do these foods form a balanced diet? To help you answer this question, regroup your foods in the bottom four food groups.

◯ Breakfast ◯ Lunch ◯ Snacks ◯ Dinner

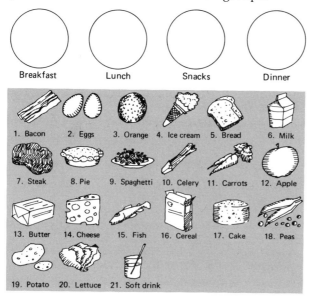

1. Bacon 2. Eggs 3. Orange 4. Ice cream 5. Bread 6. Milk

7. Steak 8. Pie 9. Spaghetti 10. Celery 11. Carrots 12. Apple

13. Butter 14. Cheese 15. Fish 16. Cereal 17. Cake 18. Peas

19. Potato 20. Lettuce 21. Soft drink

Meat	Fruits and vegetables	Milk	Breads and cereals

3. Worksheet for planning a balanced school lunch.

4. *Animal-feeding experiment:* Rat nutrition

Rat Nutrition Experiment *

Planning the Demonstration

1. Establish objectives for experiment:
   a) Demonstrate the importance of good nutrition in the growth and development of rats.
   b) Relate the growth of the rats to growth in other living things.
   c) Include as many students and groups as possible in the experiment.
   d) Create an awareness of eating habits.
   e) Create an interest in nutrition.
   f) Help students develop the ability to organize and evaluate a project from beginning to end with as little help from teacher as possible.

2. Plan the committees that will be needed:
   a) Consider the Committee for Care of Rats:
      (1) Fasten the cages securely.
      (2) Cover the floor of cages with newspaper strips, sawdust, shavings.
      (3) Water and food cups—cold cream jars.
      (4) Temperature—no drafts; even temperature—70° to 80°.
      (5) Cover the cages with blankets or newspapers at night and on weekend.
      (6) Daily care: change floor material; remove left-over meals; clean food and water cups.
      (7) Weekly routine: wash cages with soap, water, and brush.
      (8) At all times: handle the rats quietly and gently. Do not excite them with shrill, loud voices or loud noises.
   b) Committees needed:
      (1) Equipment Committee: Obtain the following equipment:
         (a) Rat cage—may be obtained through health department
         (b) Feeding cups—heavy enough so that they would not tip over
         (c) Wood shavings for covering bottom of cage (newspapers)
         (d) An old pair of gloves for handling the rats
         (e) Cloth for covering the cage at night

---

* *Reference: Animal Feeding Demonstrations for the Classroom* (pamphlet), National Dairy Council, Chicago, 1963.

(f) Container for holding the rat while he is being weighed (Oatmeal box)

(g) Gram scales for weighing rats

(h) Utensils for cutting up food

(2) Food Committee:

(a) Prepare food for feeding the rats.

(b) Feed the rats. (Food kept in cages at all times.) Follow this routine:

i) daily—fill cups with food; fill cups with liquid.

ii) weekends—provide extra cups of food and water.

iii) cage food (dry bread crumbs with salt) at all times.

iv) display the contrasting diet, in food models, near the cages.

(3) Committee for Weighing Rats:

(a) Weigh weekly.

(b) Use box for weighing—same box for each weighing.

(4) Committee for Cleaning Cages:

(a) Daily clean-up

(b) Weekly washing of cages

(5) Committee to Observe Changes in Rats:

(a) Well nourished rat

i) clean, smooth, glossy fur

ii) smooth tail, free from roughness

iii) firm nails

iv) quick, alert movements; good muscle control

v) clean and tidy habits

vi) easily handled, good natured

vii) bright pink eyes, pink nose, ears, feet, and tail

(b) Poorly nourished rat:

i) shaggy, dull, and possible thin fur

ii) rough, dry, scaly ears, feet, and tail

iii) possibly soft nails

iv) restless, irritable, and cross

v) whiskers not long and sharp, possibly dirty

vi) breathing difficult, susceptible to "sniffles"

vii) eyes not clear, pinched look in face

  (6) Publicity Committee:

    (a) Posters

    (b) Talks

    (c) Radio and newspaper articles

    (d) Photographing the demonstration

    (e) School paper and assemblies

  (7) Chart and Graph Committees:

    (a) Plot the growth of the rats.

    (b) Each pupil may keep individual weight graphs on rats, which the committee may check for accuracy.

3. Establish guidelines for each committee to follow.

4. Plan the extra activities:

  a) Puppet show—open house or assembly program

  b) Flannel-board story for second graders

  c) Diaries

  d) Rat race

  e) Poster

  f) Business places

5. Plan what other subjects you are to emphasize in demonstration:

  a) Arithmetic—graphs, bar graphs, line graphs

Compare ages of human with ages of rats:

Human in years—	2½	3	3½	4	4½	5	5½
Rats in weeks—	4	5	6	7	8	9	10

  b) Language—newspaper articles, plays, diaries, scrapbook

  c) Art—scrapbook, posters, bulletin boards

  d) Spelling

  e) Science

  f) Family life

6. Problems:
   a) Acquiring the white rats
   b) Cages
   c) Scales
   d) Local situation—water
   e) What to do with rats on weekends
   f) Pets
   g) How to dispose of animals when demonstration is completed
7. Plan your evaluation

Key Questions

   1. What do we mean by "balanced"?
   2. Does what we eat really matter?
   3. Whose daily diet was balanced? Why?
   4. Did you eat a balanced diet yesterday?
   5. How do you know if you are getting a balanced meal?

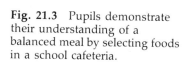

5. Pupils select a balanced diet in cafeteria.

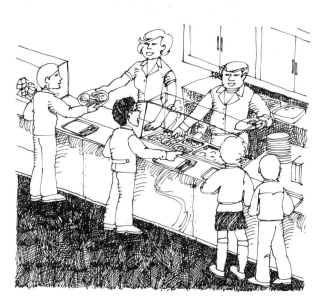

Fig. 21.3 Pupils demonstrate their understanding of a balanced meal by selecting foods in a school cafeteria.

. . . .

TOPIC: VITAMINS

Grade Level: Intermediate

Outcome: The student will be able to list the functions and sources of vitamins.

Concept: Vitamins are essential to the proper functioning of our bodies.

Content: Six major vitamins are:

1. Vitamin A
   a) source: yellow-green vegetables, carrots, milk, liver, eggs, butter, parsley, green vegetables
   b) function: improves vision, keeps skin and teeth healthy, protects against cancer, colds, and flu
2. Vitamin B—Complex
   a) source: whole grains and cereals, wheat germ, meats, eggs, nuts, green leafy vegetables, milk, sprouts, seeds
   b) function: helps with normal growth; aids in digestion; keeps eyes healthy; prevents heart disease; helps manage stress; detoxifies cigarette smoke, alcohol, sugar, coffee, polluted air
3. Vitamin C
   a) source: citrus fruits, tomatoes, potatoes, cabbage, green vegetables
   b) function: helps to heal wounds; forms bones and teeth; prevents cancer, heart disease, colds, flu, and stress; detoxifies cigarette smoke, alcohol, sugar, cola, coffee, polluted air, pesticides; builds intercellular cement (collagen)

Learning Experiences

1. *Matching Bee Game:* Match various pictures of foods as sources with various vitamins. Repeat matching vitamins with functions.

4. Vitamin D

    a) source: eggs, butter, milk, sunshine

    b) function: helps to form and protect bones and teeth, use of other vitamins

5. Vitamin E

    a) source: vegetable oils, peanuts

    b) function: energy booster, keeps reproductive system in good health, deactivates chemical poisons, prolongs life, prevents heart disease

6. Vitamin K

    a) source: green leafy vegetables, eggs, liver, cauliflower, green cabbage

    b) function: helps with clotting of blood

Directions: Match the foods below with the vitamin.

Matching Bee Chart

	Vitamins					
	A	B	C	D	E	K
Sources						
Functions						

List of foods: (Teacher lists these and provides pictures).

2. *Team Competition:* Pupils divided into teams. Teacher acts as mediator—asks a question. Team 1 member responds, and a member of Team 2 decides whether the answer is right or wrong. Scorekeeper keeps score.

Key Questions

1. What is a vitamin?
2. Which food has many vitamins in it?
3. What is the function of vitamin _____?
4. Of what value to your body are carrots?
5. Why are oranges good for you?

TOPIC: WEIGHT CONTROL

Grade Level: Intermediate

Outcome: The student will be able to describe how a healthful lifestyle helps to control body weight.

Concept: A healthful style of living contributes to the control of body weight.

Content: A good lifestyle to control body weight consists of:

Learning Experience

1. Eating a balanced diet
2. Eating a variety of foods
3. Exercising regularly
4. Enjoying good friends
5. Being happy in what you do
6. Avoiding substituting food for friends and activity
7. Having a variety of interests (hobby)
8. Caring for someone and receiving love and affection.

1. *Checklist Inventory* and analysis of lifestyle. Teacher offers guidance.

REFERENCES AND BIBLIOGRAPHY

Airola, Paavo. *Hypoglycemia* (Phoenix: Health Plus Publishers, 1977).

Altschule, Mark David. "Some Ambiguities Concerning Vitamins in Medical Practice," *Preventive Medicine* **3** (1974): 125-186.

Banks, Mary Alice, and Margaret A. Dunham. *Teaching Nutrition in the Elementary School* (Washington D.C.: American Association of Health, Physical Education and Recreation, 1966).

Berland, Theodore, *et al. Rating the Diets* (Skokie, Ill.: Consumer Guide, 1974).

Bieler, Henry G. *Food Is Your Best Medicine* (New York: Vintage Books, 1973).

Big Ideas in Nutrition Education and How to Teach Them 4-6 (Dairy Council of California, 1970).

Bogert, L. Jean. *Nutrition and Physical Fitness* (Philadelphia: Saunders, 1973).

Borsook, Henry. *Vitamins* (New York: Pyramid Books, 1977).

Cheraskin, Emanuel, and William Ringsdorf. *Psychodietetics* (New York: Bantam, 1976).

Clark, Linda. *Know Your Nutrition* (New Canaan, Conn.: Keats, 1973).

Deutch, Ronald M. *Realities of Nutrition* (Palo Alto, Calif.: Bull, 1976).

————. *The New Nuts Among the Berries* (Palo Alto, Calif.: Bull, 1977).

DiCyan, Erwin. *Vitamins in Your Life* (New York: Simon & Schuster, 1974).

Duffy, William. *Sugar Blues* (New York: Warner, 1976).

Eppright, Ercil. *Teaching Nutrition* (Ames: Iowa State University Press, 1963).

"Food Additives," *Lancet*, August 16, 1969, p. 361.

Fredericks, Carlton. *High-Fiber Way to Total Health* (New York: Pocket Books, 1976).

Labuza, Theodore P. *The Nutrition Crises: A Reader* (St. Paul, Minn.: West, 1975).

Leonard, Jon N., J. L. Hofer, and N. Pritikin. *Live Longer Now* (New York: Grosset and Dunlap, 1977).

Mayer, Jean. *A Diet for Living* (New York: Pocket Books, 1977).

National Academy of Sciences. *Recommended Daily Allowances* (Washington, D.C.: National Academy of Sciences, 1974).

"Nutrient Approach to Treat Brain Ills," *The Province* (Vancouver), March 22, 1978.

Nutrition Research Inc. *Nutrition Almanac* (New York: McGraw-Hill, 1975).

Passwater, Richard A. *Supernutrition* (New York: Pocket Books, 1976).

Pauling, Linus. *Vitamin C, the Common Cold and the Flu* (San Francisco: Freeman, 1976).

Proxmire, William. "Why Title IV—The Vitamin Title of S.988—Should be Passed," *Congressional Record* (Washington, D.C.: U.S. Printing Office, December 11, 1975).

Rice, Marjorie. "Physician Feels Diet Could KO Killer Diseases," *San Diego Union*, March 21, 1978.

Rosenberg, Harold, and A. N. Feldzaman. *The Book of Vitamin Therapy* (New York: Berkeley-Windhover, 1975).

Select Committee on Nutrition and Human Needs of the United States Senate. *Dietary Goals for the United States*, 2nd ed. (Washington, D. C.: U. S. Printing Office, December 1977).

"Too Much Sugar?" *Consumer Reports*, March 1978, pp. 136-142.

Williams, Roger J. *Nutrition Against Disease* (New York: Bantam, 1973).

Winikoff, Beverly. "Changing Public Diet," *Human Nature*, January 1978, pp. 60-65.

CHAPTER 22

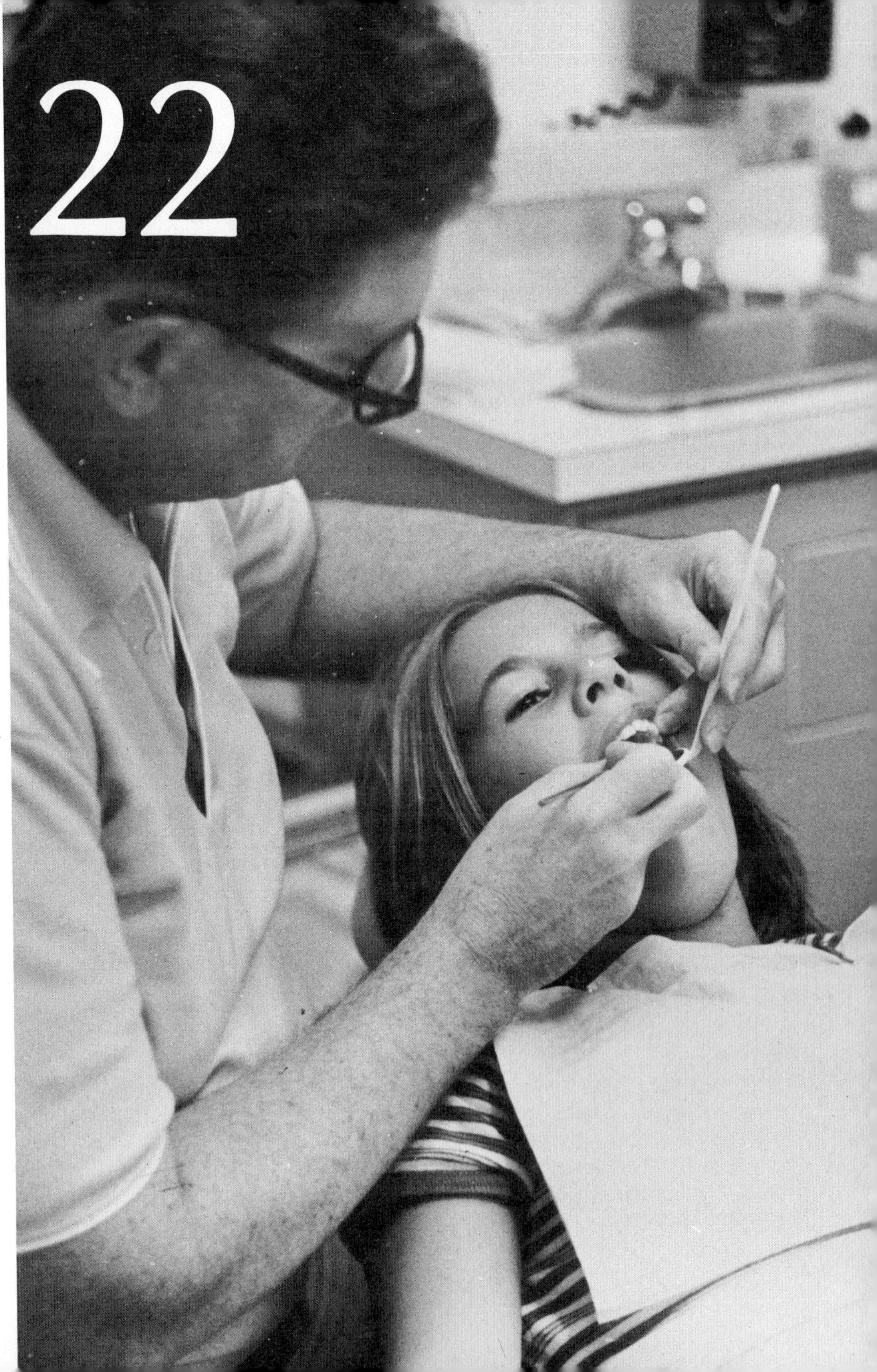

teaching about dental health

INTRODUCTION

Believe it or not, one of the more pressing health problems facing us today is dental disease. Although it does not receive the headlines that drug abuse, sex education, and some of the other behavioral health problems do, it is nevertheless a health problem that deserves a great deal of attention. This is evidenced by the fact that 95 percent of the American population lives with dental problems. Many of your students have probably never visited a dentist. The average youngster in your class will have anywhere from one to three decaying teeth, and this number will increase as the child grows older (see Fig. 22.1). In many instances it is essentially ignorance due to a lack of proper dental health education that contributes to such decay statistics.

The most common dental health-related problem in adults is periodontal disease, or pyorrhea. The word "periodontal" comes from two Greek words meaning "around the tooth." Hence diseases of the gums and other supporting structures of the teeth are known as periodontal disease. It seems logical to assume that the prevalence of such

a disease would be given instant preventive attention. Unfortunately, most people are unable to care properly for their teeth, do not know how, don't care, or simply ignore good dental hygiene. In addition, most of us have been conditioned to employ ineffective brushing techniques that were in vogue 20 to 30 years ago. We tend to transmit these outmoded practices to children.

Two major factors affecting dental caries and peridontal disease are (1) nutrition of the mother during all stages of pregnancy, and (2) nutrition of the infant and oral hygiene in control of dental plaque once teeth appear. Underlying both of these factors is recognition that heredity plays a fundamental role by determining the color, hardness, shape, and size of teeth, thickness of enamel, and resistance of teeth to dental caries.

A child's and an adult's teeth are only as healthy as the nutrients available during the mother's pregnancy. Prevention of dental caries really begins during pregnancy and having the expectant mother eat the proper amounts of essential nutrients. The formation of teeth begins very early

379

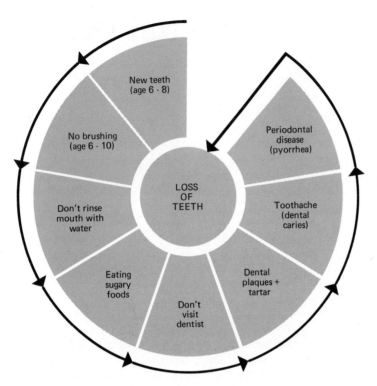

Fig. 22.1 Evolution of early stages of dental neglect that can lead to adult dental problems.

in the life history of each individual. Even the permanent teeth begin their existence five months before a child is born (Williams, 1973, p. 119). The cells responsible for tooth production during these early stages need complete nutrition—not only at that time but for many years to follow. When prospective mothers follow inferior diets, their infants grow up to have teeth that are subject to decay. The opposite is also true. Adequate nutritional (vitamins, minerals, and other micronutrients) needs remain critical throughout the period of childhood, when teeth develop and mature. Infants and children who are well nourished grow teeth resistant to dental caries. Genetic susceptibility to tooth decay

can be overcome by providing teeth with nutrition of the highest quality, i.e., plenty of calcium, phosphorus, fluoride, and ample vitamins B_6, C, and D. By contrast, refined sugar (sucrose) and foods rich in sugar, such as colas and soft drinks, candy, and pastries, should be eliminated completely from the diet.

Poor oral hygiene and bacterial plaque are the other major factors contributing to dental caries. Bacterial plaque results from the interaction of bacteria (such as *lacto bacillus*) with various sugars in the mouth. This interaction forms a sticky film along the gum lines of the teeth and in between the teeth. Such an environment provides an ideal physical and nutritional medium for the growth of bacteria—present at all times in all mouths. Brushing teeth was once considered sufficient for clearing this debris from the teeth. We now realize, however, that brushing alone removes bacterial plaque only from the exposed surfaces of teeth and is ineffective in reaching plaque between the teeth. To verify this, swish a disclosing tablet (for example, red dye obtainable from your dentist or druggist) in the mouth for one minute so that it stains the gum and tooth areas of your mouth. Dental plaque areas turn red. Complete removal of all these red markings is the ultimate goal. It is impossible to do this with just good brushing and dentifrice. It is really essential to use dental floss between the teeth, then brush and rinse your teeth and mouth with water. Brushing and the use of dental floss disturb the bacterial colonies between the teeth and stop the plaques from producing harmful acidic toxins.

One key to controlling dental caries is the continual breaking up of the fertile bacterial areas between and around the teeth and gums. At the present time, the only techniques available to assist in preventing such bacterial growth are physical in nature—brushing the teeth and using toothpicks, dental floss, and other such mechanical aids. When these aids are effectively utilized, the large bacterial colonies, or plaques, are disorganized, and the initial stages of tooth decay and gum disease are kept in check.

Most children and adults fail to take proper care of the periodontal areas where the gums meet the teeth. In addition to brushing up and down or as the teeth grow, dental hygienists suggest that the soft bristles be hand-vibrated in these areas. Such bristle action, if properly used in the way described by your dentist, at least once a day, not only disrupts the bacterial plaques, but also massages the gums. If not removed regularly, the bacteria in plaque produce acids which may dissolve tooth enamel and cause cavities. Bacterial plaque also can cause periodontal disease by producing chemicals that

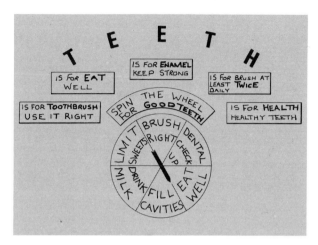

Fig. 22.2 A bulletin board suggesting that dental care is an everyday chore.

irritate the gums. In addition, when plaque accumulates over a long period of time, it may harden to become calculus or tartar. Calculus dams up the toxins produced by plaque, heightening gum irritation, causing swelling of gums and hence periodontal disease. (Topical application of fluoride or drinking fluoridated water helps prevent dental caries in children.)

These approaches to dental hygiene are new ways of conserving teeth and healthy mouths. New research suggests that brushing teeth once a day with proper and regular use of dental floss may be more effective than the often suggested approach of brushing teeth after every meal. Mouth washes have no effect on the bacteria in the mouth and are a waste of money and effort in tooth-decay prevention. Among the many new approaches, dental hygienists are most optimistic that a new kind of chewing gum and serum as immunity to dental caries can be developed as an adjutant to more effective dental care.

After all this, how should the teacher approach dental health education in the classroom? The answer is twofold. First, since most children suffer from dental caries and since children tend to receive most of their permanent teeth between six and twelve years of age, there is a need to reinforce proper brushing technique early in the primary grades. The brushing technique and the correct

technique for using dental floss should actually be introduced at the preschool age. Emphases at all levels should be on regular dental habits and sound nutrition and not on education. Teachers will do far more good by providing time each day for dental care, as after the noon meal, than offering a once-a-year instruction. Good habits need to be cultivated each day and instituted before the child has reached age 12. The lesson plans that follow are suggested ways to introduce and initiate a sound and effective school dental health program.

. . . .

TOPIC: BRUSHING TEETH

Grade Level: Primary

Outcome: The student will be able to brush his or her teeth correctly.

Concept: All surfaces of teeth should be brushed.

Content	*Learning Experiences*
1. Top inside surfaces—left, front, right 2. Bottom inside surfaces—left, front, right 3. Top outside surfaces—left, front, right 4. Bottom outside surfaces—left, front, right 5. Chewing and biting surfaces—top, left, right 6. Tongue	1. *Demonstration:* Teacher demonstrates steps in brushing teeth correctly on a large model of teeth, using a large toothbrush. Stress brushing action and organized approach so all surfaces will be brushed. (See Fig. 22.3.) 2. *Practice—simulation session:* Two students work together as "buddies." One uses popsicle stick or tongue depressor and pretends to brush his or her teeth, and the other corrects. Reverse. Teacher walks around and also corrects.

Fig. 22.3   Correct method of brushing teeth. (From "Effective Oral Hygiene," pp. 2-6, developed by the USAF School of Aerospace Medicine, Brooks Air Force Base, Texas. Reprinted courtesy of the American Academy of Periodontology.)

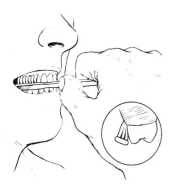

Place brush where teeth and gums meet.

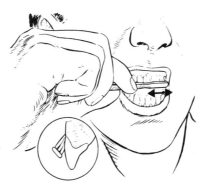

Look at the arrows on the brush. (VIBRATE, using short back-and-forth strokes, without disengaging the bristles from the edge of the gum.)

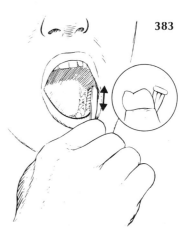

Keep brush where teeth and gums meet. VIBRATE.

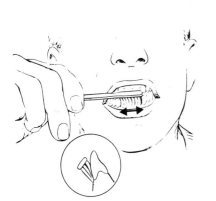

Use short *vibrating* strokes.

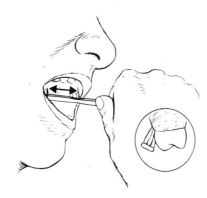

Use same method on inside surfaces.

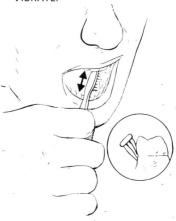

VIBRATE brush *back* and *forth.*

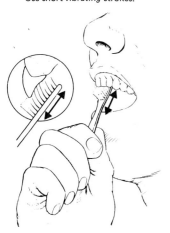

Brush (vibrate) *up* and *down.*

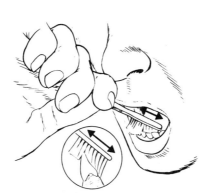

Keep strokes short and vibrate brush.

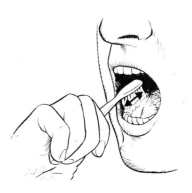

Brush back and forth on biting surfaces.

3. The techniques of brushing teeth should be repeated until children have acquired correct brushing skills and the practices become habits. To add variety to the repetition, the following alternatives are suggested:

a) Teacher and children recite the brushing-teeth rhyme while brushing teeth. (Note: This rhyme stresses areas of teeth to brush; it does not stress correct technique for plaque removal.)

The Brushing Teeth Rhyme (sing to melody of "Around the Mulberry Bush")

This is the way we brush our teeth
Brush our teeth
Brush our teeth

This is the way we brush our teeth
So early in the morning

Upper teeth, upper teeth
Brush them downward
Lower teeth, lower teeth
Brush them upward.

Brush upper teeth, Brush lower teeth
Brush also the grinders

This is the way we brush our teeth
Brush our teeth
Brush our teeth
This is the way we brush our teeth after
every meal

b) Children draw a happy face in Tommy Tooth (see Fig. 22.4).

c) Children brush to the accompaniment of "My Toothbrush Song" by Ann Lloyd and the Sandpipers, Golden Record R43R.

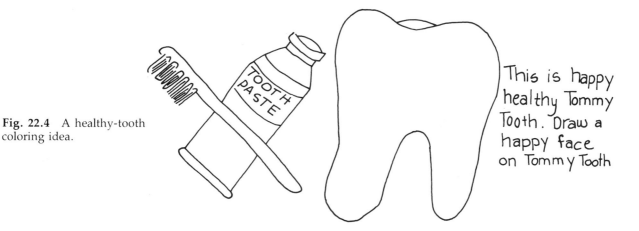

Fig. 22.4 A healthy-tooth coloring idea.

This is happy healthy Tommy Tooth. Draw a happy face on Tommy Tooth

Toothbrush Song

(Organize class into two groups—boys and girls sing own parts.)

Girls: Mr. Toothbrush and Mr. Toothpaste have very often said—

Boys: Please use us in the morning and before you go to bed.

Girls: Scrub your teeth each morn and night.

Boys: Scrub your teeth so they'll be white.

All: Put the toothpaste on your brush and rub-a-dub, scrub-a-dub, do not rush!

Girls: Mr. Toothbrush and Mr. Toothpaste have very often said—

Boys: Please use us in the morning and before you go to bed.

All: Rinse your teeth and after a while you will have a winning smile. When you're through, put toothpaste back and hang your toothbrush on the rack.

. . . .

TOPIC: USING DENTAL FLOSS

Grade Level: Primary, intermediate

Outcome: The student will be able to demonstrate proper use of dental floss.

Concept: Using dental floss once a day helps to prevent dental caries.

Content: Techniques of utilizing dental floss are:

1. Pull about 24 inches of floss from dispenser or use toothbrush that has dental flosser.
2. Wrap most of the floss around one finger.
3. Wrap the remaining floss around the same finger of the other hand. This finger can take up the floss as you use it.
4. Use thumbs as guides for flossing upper teeth.
5. Use index fingers for lower ones.
6. Hold floss tightly and work it gently between the teeth (back and forth).
7. Curve floss around tooth and work it under the gum line and scrape.
8. Repeat on adjacent teeth.
9. Follow same pattern each time.
10. Rinse vigorously with water after flossing to remove food particles and plaque that has been cut loose.

Learning Experiences

1. Teacher demonstration (see Fig. 22.5).
2. Pupils practice flossing just as they do brushing.

Key Questions

1. Why is flossing helpful?
2. How often should you use dental floss?

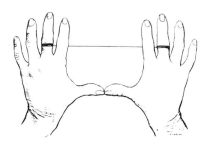

Wrap floss on middle fingers.

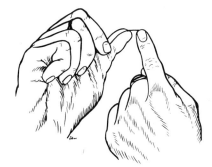

Thumb to the outside for upper teeth.

Fig. 22.5 Correct method of using dental floss. (From "Effective Oral Hygiene," pp. 8-10, developed by the USAF School of Aerospace Medicine, Brooks Air Force Base, Texas. Reprinted courtesy of the American Academy of Periodontology.)

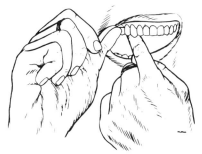

Flossing between upper back teeth.

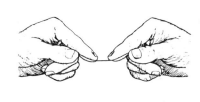

Holding floss for lower teeth.

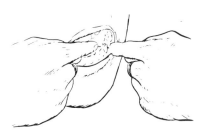

Flossing between lower back teeth.

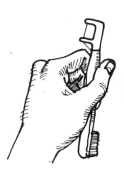

Toothbrush – Flosser

. . . .

TOPIC: VISITING THE DENTIST

Grade Level: Primary

Outcome: The student will show willingness to accept the dentist as a friend.

Concept: The dentist protects our teeth in many ways.

Content: The dentist is our friend in the following ways:

Learning Experience

1. Shows us how to clean our teeth.
2. Cleans our teeth (with special machine).
3. Protects our teeth with fluoride.
4. Checks the growth of our teeth.
5. X-rays our teeth.
6. Finds and fills cavities.
7. Corrects crooked teeth and may pull out sick teeth if necessary.
8. Shows us how to care for our teeth, gums, and mouth.

1. Skit or playette.

A Visit To The Dentist

Characters

Jerry Mahoney: a boy of from 5 to 7 who has never been to the dentist. (Instead of a pupil playing the part, a dummy, Jerry Mahoney and a dental unit, may be obtained from the local Dental Association.)
Jerry's mother
Ms Goodday: (receptionist); dressed in yellow, has a sparkling, bubbling disposition, wears hat with "HI" on it!
Ms Sparkles: (dental assistant); dressed in light blue, is neat and is a good conversationalist.
Dr. Gums: (dentist); wears a light green top jacket, has a great sense of humor, easy-going manner.
Props: The dress as described for the dental team.
Act II: *Dental chair* and *simulated drill, X-ray, spittoon,* dental *instruments,* mirror; explorer; packer; paper cups; paper towels; bib; reception desk.

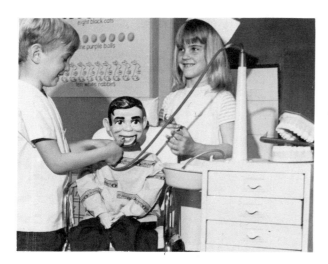

Fig. 22.6 Kindergarten children simulating a visit to the dentist, using Jerry Mahoney and the dental unit. (Photograph courtesy of the Women's Auxiliary to the San Diego County Dental Society.)

Suggested Approach: This script may be acted out or the lines ad-libbed by grades 4-6 pupils, who could put on the play for the kindergarten or grade 1 pupils. Or, the teacher could help the class ad lib and simulate the scripts.

Act I

Setting: The dentist's office—10:30 a.m. Mother and Jerry enter the office. The receptionist, with a sparkling, happy disposition, greets them. There is soft music and singing about teeth and dental hygiene. (Set props for Act I.)

Receptionist: Good morning Mrs. Mahoney, and a special good morning to you, Jerry! Won't you please sit down, and I'll tell Dr. Gums that you are here! (She goes out and comes back immediately.) You are lucky, Jerry, Dr. Gums and his assistant will be able to see you in a few minutes. How are you feeling today?

Jerry: Okay, I guess. Will this visit take long? My friends and I are going to the beach this afternoon.

Receptionist: No, just a few minutes! My, but you have a beautiful smile—and such white teeth! My goodness, you must take good care of your teeth—how do you do it?

Jerry: Naw, I brush them because Mom wants me to!
(A bell rings from the inner office.)

Receptionist: Okay, Jerry, they are ready for you now.

Act II

Setting: (Props as described in introduction.) Receptionist takes Jerry by the hand, and they enter Dr. Gums's office, where the dental assistant greets them. *Dentist's room* has dentist's chair, with simulated drill and spittoon, a small shelf, and an X-ray machine. On the table are small plastic animals, a small rag doll, several comic books, a large set of teeth, a large toothbrush.

Receptionist: Jerry, this is Dr. Gums's assistant. She will help you and Dr. Gums.

Assistant: Hi, Jerry, I am glad you could make it today. I hear you and your friends are going to the beach today—where?

Jerry: Where they swim and the waves are this high!

Assistant: You must be a good swimmer. Jerry, would you like to sit in this big chair?

Jerry: (apprehensive) Okay.

Assistant: Now, make yourself comfortable, and I'll put a bib on you. Do you build sand castles at the beach, Jerry?

Jerry: Gee, what are those?

Assistant: You have heard of castles where kings and queens lived, with large towers and high walls—(she gets a colored picture of a castle). Here is a picture of an ancient castle where the Sleeping Beauty lived.

Jerry, you hold this picture and look at it, if you want to. Meanwhile, I would like to look at your teeth. Would you open your mouth wide—yes, like that, thank you, Jerry. (She examines his teeth with the small mirror.) You have some new teeth, Jerry. And they look real healthy; they could stand a cleaning though. You know, Jerry, Dr. Gums takes his son and daughter, about your age, to the beach on weekends. And they build sand castles. Why don't you ask him how to build sand castles?

Jerry: Gee, I didn't know dentists like to build sand castles.
(Dr. Gums enters.)

Assistant: Dr. Gums, this is Jerry Mahoney.

Dr. Gums: (Smiling and thumbs Jerry's hand as a greeting.) Good morning, Jerry, I see from the way you shook hands with me that you and I have a lot in common. What's that picture you have?

Jerry: It's a picture of a Sleeping Beauty's castle.

Assistant: Jerry is going to the beach this afternoon and was thinking of building a sand castle.

Dr. Gums: Why, I build them every time I go to the beach. Building castles is one of my hobbies. Now, Jerry, show me how big and white your teeth are, open wide! Good, let me look at your back teeth. (Dr. Gums readjusts headrest and puts napkin under chin. As Dr. Gums examines Jerry's teeth, they continue to talk.) Castles are a lot of fun to make, and I'll be happy to make one with you this Sunday. Would you like that?

Jerry (nods and smiles).

Dr. Gums: Your teeth tell me you are about six years old (continues to examine the teeth). Open your mouth wider.—Oops, not too wide, (smiling), I don't want to fall in! Gee, Jerry, looks like you have a tooth missing on this side. How did you lose it? (Dr. Gums stops and lets Jerry explain.)

Jerry: It came loose last week and just fell out. I have it here in my pocket (pulls it out).

Dr. Gums: That is a very healthy tooth. Don't lose it. (He picks up the set of big teeth and brings it in front of Jerry.) See this big set of teeth—this is what your teeth will look like when you get all new teeth in a few years. This is the tooth that is missing now. (Gives the teeth to his assistant.) May I have an explorer, Ms Sparkles! Jerry, with this instrument, I can find all the secret hiding places of your food and also check to see that your teeth are healthy. Let's see, hum! Ms Sparkles, would you like to bring that large model of teeth in front of Jerry again! Great! Thank you! (Ms Sparkles, smiling, holds it.) (Dr. Gums points explorer between teeth.) Do you see the place where these two teeth meet? Food gets in between here. Yes, that's it—Ms Sparkles (she uses the toothbrush to waft the food out between the crevice). See how Ms Sparkles brushed to pull the food particles out! You do that when you brush your teeth. Let's take another look at your teeth—hm, I bet you had peanut butter and jam on your toast this morning. I just found a part of a peanut in between your teeth. And I bet you like to eat candy? Do you, Jerry?

Jerry: I like "Oh Henry Bars"—they are delicious.

Dr. Gums: What do you do right after you eat a candy bar, Jerry?

Jerry: Play, what else!

Ms Sparkles: Do you rinse your mouth with water or brush your teeth right after eating the bar?

Jerry: Naw, I don't have time.

Ms Sparkles: If I can't brush my teeth, then I always rinse my teeth after I eat a bar! Look how clean my teeth are. (She smiles and shows her teeth.)

Dr. Gums: Aren't her teeth clean and white. And she has such a pretty smile. Ms Sparkles, it's good to work with you. Now, Jerry, let me clean your teeth for you. You have no cavities as yet. You know, some of your teeth are a little dirty — let's clean and freshen them up a bit. Ms Sparkles, some cleaning compound! Jerry, this is a cleaning machine; it helps to clean your teeth. It won't hurt! (He proceeds to clean the teeth.) There, now sip some water from this paper cup and spit out!

Good! One more sip, swish the water all around—good, now spit! How does that feel, Jerry?

Jerry: That stuff smells better than it feels. It tastes like candy!

Dr. Gums: Yes, it does, it removes the tartar, or slime, that coats the teeth. Jerry, remember the candy bar you like so much?

Jerry: Oh yes, I do!

Dr. Gums: Well, what is on the outside of the bar?

Jerry: Chocolate, and it tastes good.

Dr. Gums: Yes, and if we imagine that the center of the candy bar is your tooth, we can say that the chocolate on the outside is like the slime that coats the outside of your teeth! By cleaning your teeth just now, I removed this slime. Now your teeth can feel healthy again. But, Jerry, let's cut out all these sweets, for they are not good for your teeth! Miss Sparkles, why don't you take some pictures of Jerry's teeth. He may have some decay that I am not able to see. (He turns to Jerry.) Ms Sparkles will take an X-ray of your teeth, and that will be all for today. I would like to check your teeth again in about six months. Jerry, would you like to come and see me again?

Jerry: Oh, yes, and where on the beach will we meet to build the sand castles?

Dr. Gums: I will be at Life Guard Station 3 with my son, Mark, and daughter, Wendy. I want you to meet them. Why don't you bring your mom and dad, and we can all have fun building sand castles!

Jerry: Are you coming also, Ms Sparkles?

Ms Sparkles: I'm not sure yet, but I'll try!

Dr. Gums: See you Sunday, Jerry!

Ms Sparkles: Let's have you sit up, Jerry! (She places a negative in Jerry's mouth and takes X-rays of his mouth. As she does this, she talks to Jerry.) Jerry, you're going to have fun with Dr. Gums on Sunday. Here, now bite this—good. There, that's it! (She removes the bib.) Jerry, would you like this comic book? It has pictures of many kinds of castles. Maybe you'll get an idea for your castle on Sunday!

Jerry: Gee, may I?

(Both return to the reception room.)

Jerry: (Runs to his mother exuberantly.) Hey, Mom, Dr. Gums and I are going to build sand castles on the beach Sunday! Would you and Dad like to come?

Mom: Why that's wonderful. We'll plan on it. (Turns to Ms Sparkles and Ms Goodday.) Thank you so much for helping Jerry with his teeth! Bye, bye for now.

Ms Sparkles: See you here in six months' time, Jerry, unless the X-rays show us something that needs to be fixed right away.

Jerry: Okay, Ms Sparkles, bye, bye!

Key Questions

1. Did you like the play?
2. Were the dentist and his helpers friendly?
3. What does the dentist do?
4. How was the dentist Jerry's friend?
5. Would you like to visit the dentist?
6. How often should you visit the dentist?
7. When are you going to visit the dentist?

TOPIC: CAUSE OF TOOTH DECAY

(This lesson is one of a sequence of several on this topic.)

Grade Level: Primary

Outcome: The student will be able to describe how tooth decay is caused by lacti.

Concept: Bacteria such as lacti causes tooth decay.

Content: The steps in the decay process are:

1. Sugars in the mouth
2. Lacti (germ) in the mouth
3. Lacti eats sugar.
4. Lacti produces acid.
5. Acid and saliva make more acid.
6. Acid attacks tooth.
7. Tooth decay is the result.

Learning Experience

1. *Matching bee:* Process is identified in formula fashion and conceptualized by illustrations (see Fig. 22.7).
2. *Alternative experiences*
   a) Make plaster of paris casts of teeth to show progress of tooth decay.
   b) Perform cola and tooth experiment: drop an extracted tooth in a cola bottle overnight. Observe tooth next day and compare action of lactic acid to cola.
   c) Children color pictures of lacti, tooth, and apple (see Fig. 22.8). A comic-coloring book, *Casper's Dental Health Activity Book*, is available from the American Dental Association.

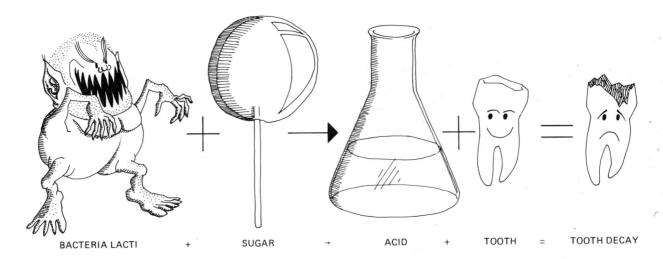

BACTERIA LACTI   +   SUGAR   →   ACID   +   TOOTH   =   TOOTH DECAY

Fig. 22.7 Pictures conceptualizing the tooth decay process.

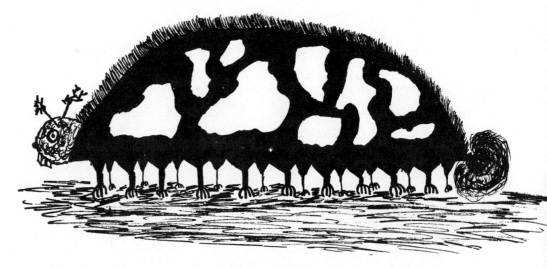

Fig. 22.8 A child's concept of "lacti."

TOPIC: TEETH TYPES AND FUNCTIONS

Grade Level: Intermediate

Outcome: The student will be able to classify teeth according to type and function.

Concept: Four kinds of teeth help us eat food.

Content: Four kinds of teeth and their locations and functions are (see Fig. 22.9):

Learning Experience

1. Incisors (central, lateral)
   a) location: front of mouth
   b) function: cutting; e.g., scissors

1. *Matching bee:* Teacher and pupil.
   a) Large diagram of mouth and large pictures of the four kinds of teeth. These are matched

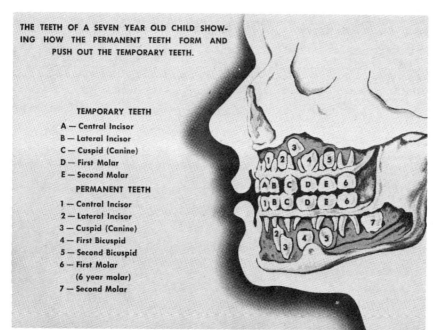

THE TEETH OF A SEVEN YEAR OLD CHILD SHOWING HOW THE PERMANENT TEETH FORM AND PUSH OUT THE TEMPORARY TEETH.

TEMPORARY TEETH
A — Central Incisor
B — Lateral Incisor
C — Cuspid (Canine)
D — First Molar
E — Second Molar
PERMANENT TEETH
1 — Central Incisor
2 — Lateral Incisor
3 — Cuspid (Canine)
4 — First Bicuspid
5 — Second Bicuspid
6 — First Molar
      (6 year molar)
7 — Second Molar

Fig. 22.9 Illustration of the teeth of a seven-year-old, showing how the permanent teeth form and push out the temporary teeth. (From "The Teeth and Their Care." Reproduced courtesy of Whitehall Laboratories.)

c) subconcept: Incisors cut food like scissors do.

2. Cuspid
   a) location: corners of mouth
   b) function: tearing; e.g., pick
   c) subconcept: Cuspids tear food like a pick does.

3. Bicuspids
   a) location: back of mouth
   b) function: crushing; e.g., nutcracker
   c) subconcept: Bicuspids crush food like a nutcracker does.

4. Molars:
   a) location: back of mouth
   b) function: grinding; e.g., masher
   c) subconcept: Molars grind teeth like a grinder does.

to proper location in mouth and jaw. Teeth are then labeled by name and their functions recorded. Household objects are also matched to conceptualize tooth function.

Key Questions

1. How many teeth do we have?
2. What four basic kinds of teeth do we have?
3. What is the function of each kind?
4. What is the purpose of teeth?

REFERENCES AND BIBLIOGRAPHY

A Dental Health Guide for the Teachers of Kentucky (Frankfort, Ky.: Department of Education, 1962).

A Guide to Dental Health Education (Martinez, Calif.: Contra Costa County Health Department, 1956).

A Guide Design for Teaching Dental Health in Florida Schools (Tallahassee, Fla.: State Department of Education, 1963).

A New Plan to Keep Your Teeth for a Lifetime (Cincinnati, Ohio: Procter and Gamble, 1971).

"Dentist Says Serum Cuts Cavities 90%," *Los Angeles Times*, November 17, 1972.

Effective Oral Hygiene (Chicago: American Academy of Periodontology).

Garn, Bernard J. *A Visit to the Dentist* (New York: Wonder Books, 1959).

Peterson, Shailer. *Clinical Dental Hygiene* (St. Louis: C. V. Mosby, 1959).

Sangnes, Gudrun, *et al.* "Effectiveness of Vertical and Horizontal Brushing Techniques in Plaque Removal," *Journal of Dentistry for Children* **39** (March-April 1972): 94-97.

Stoll, Francis A. *Dental Health Education.* (Philadelphia: Lea and Febiger, 1967).

Stoll, Francis A., and Joan H. Catherman. *Dental Health Education* (Philadelphia: Lea and Febiger, 1967).

Williams, Roger J. *Nutrition and Disease* (New York: Bantam, 1973).

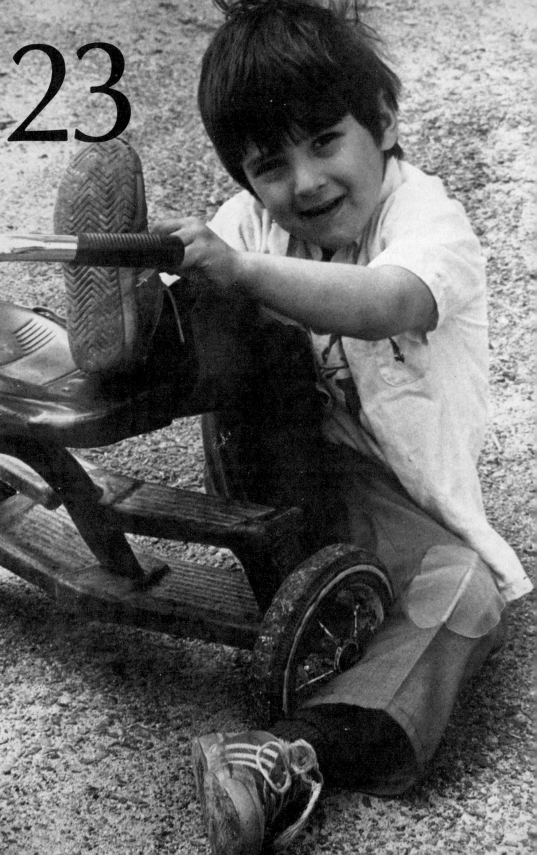

tionally and creatively solve problems that allow them to experience safe, but nonetheless exciting and challenging, adventures.

The elementary school teacher's responsibility is to instill within the pupils those atittudes that encourage them to act in the interest of their own safety, that of their families, and that of society. It is not only training in conservation of life and in the prevention of accidents, but also instruction in how to be good citizens. Another responsibility of the teacher is to create opportunities that guide the students in molding sound values, in directing their thinking and their decision making in positive ways, and in regulating their behaviors. Education for the elementary child thus becomes an ongoing process of living, and safety education, specifically, becomes a continuous process of conserving children's well-being and lifestyles.

Concern for safety in the classroom and life should not stifle initiative, adventure, and discovery. Indeed, such concern should evolve opportunities for a more abundant and richer style of living. Freedom from accidents and injuries provides opportunities for optimal well-being. It is only in this mental setting that children can mature and maximize their innate potentialities. Children can and should develop as many dimensions of their being as possible. In so doing, they acquire the capacity to function more fully as "total human beings." Safety education provides insurance for children to develop in this direction. Such a philosophy should be generated by teachers through the school environment and classroom instruction.

The lesson plans that follow suggest a few of the many learning experiences that will help the child to live safely.

. . . .

TOPIC: EMERGENCY CARE

Grade Level: Intermediate

Outcome: The student will be able to demonstrate proper emergency care procedures.

Concept: Correct emergency care may save a life.

Content: Proper emergency care includes:

1. Lay victim down.
2. Comfort victim and treat for shock.
   a) Reassure victim.
   b) Cover up victim.
   c) Disperse the crowd.
   d) Remain calm, talk slowly.

Learning Experiences

1. *Simulation role playing accidents.* Have pupils act out accidents and the provision of emergency care—both correct and incorrect!

3. Send for help—nurse, teacher, principal, parent, doctor.

Suggested Simulation Situations

Situation 1: Skinned knee on playground. Mark skins his knee while playing hopscotch. His friend, Paul, must decide immediately what to do.

Key Questions

1. How serious is the burn?
2. Is there serious bleeding?
3. Will Mark die?
4. How does Mark feel?
5. What would happen if the burn was not washed?
6. Does he need to see a doctor?

Situation 2: Deep cut in an art class. John punctures his hand with the scissors. His friend, Helda, must decide what to do.
   Follow with key questions similar to those used in first situation.

Situation 3: Broken arm. Sam breaks his arm playing football. His playmate, Ron, must decide what to do.
   Follow with key questions.

Situation 4: Fainting. Mary feels dizzy and woozy. She faints. Her friend, Sandy, comes on the scene. What should she do?
   Follow with key questions.

Situation 5: Bite by stingray. Mabel is bitten by a stingray while swimming. She is in pain and shock. Mary and Arthur are beside her. What should they do?
   Follow with key questions.

Situation 6: Heat burn in the kitchen. Mary's mother gets a serious burn on her finger from handling a hot pan and is in great pain. What should Mary do?
   Follow with key questions.

2. *Pictures* to suggest correct care.
3. *Alternative learning experience: How to Have an Accident in the Home,* a Donald Duck film cartoon depicting the many kinds of accidents that can happen in the home due to carelessness. (This film could also be used with another lesson plan.)

TOPIC: CROSSING THE STREET SAFELY

Grade Level: Primary

Outcome: The student will be able to cross the street safely.

Concept: Stop, look, and listen before crossing the street.

Content

1. Stop
   a) at crosswalk
   b) on curb
   c) for green light
2. Look—all four ways
3. Listen—for cars
4. Walk
   a) use crosswalk
   b) keep to right
   c) when crosswalk is clear

Learning Experiences

1. *Demonstration—simulation:* An intersection is laid out in the classroom, using masking tape. Pupils simulate crossing under different traffic conditions: no cars present, cars present, traffic lights, and patrol person (see Figs. 23.2 and 23.3).

   Teacher explains briefly how to cross a street safely, while a student demonstrates.

   Students take turns crossing street alone, then in twos.

   A signal light should be introduced. Children cross when the light is green.

   Have three to five students put on a large paper picture of a car and simulate car traffic. Children practice crossing street with simulated traffic.
2. *Practice crossing the street.* After practicing inside, students should try to cross a real street.
3. *Crossword puzzle*

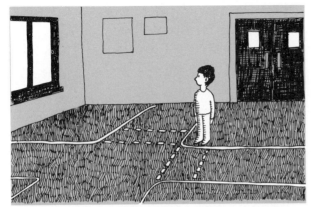

(a)   Crossing street by yourself

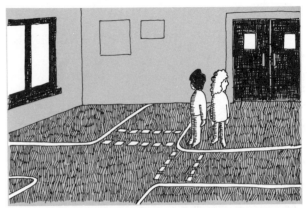

(b)   Crossing street with others

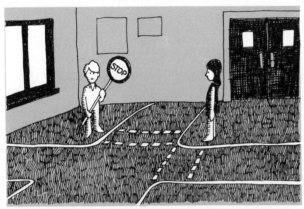

(c)   Crossing street with patrol boy

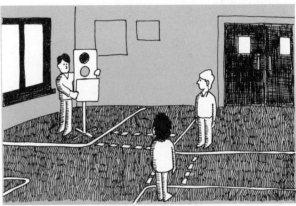

(d)   Crossing street with signal lights

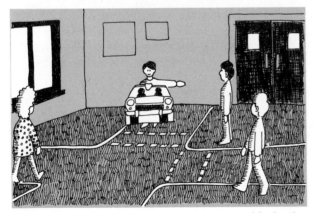

(e)   Crossing street with traffic

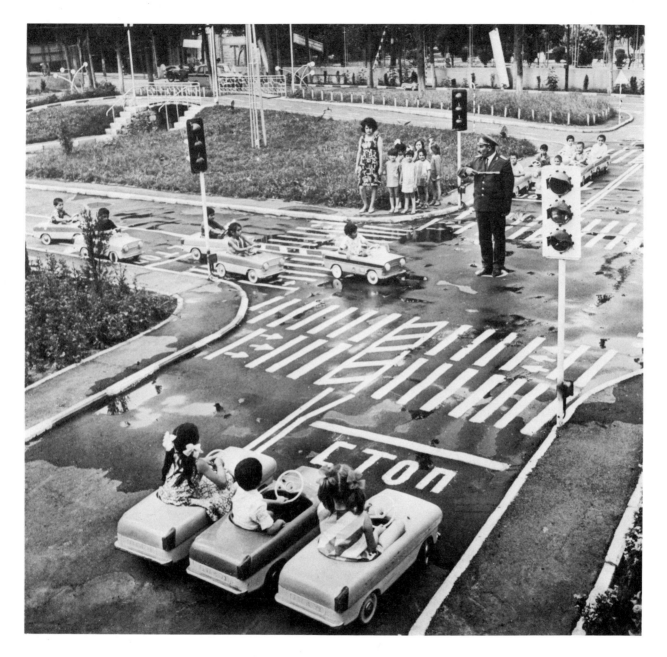

◀ **Fig. 23.2** Illustrations simulating street conditions. Pictures suggest that the teacher should provide a series of progressive learning experiences on how to cross the street safely. Children should simulate the situations above inside a classroom. Then the teacher can supervise the children in crossing a real street.

Fig. 23.3 Children in Kirovabad, Russia, study traffic rules and practice them while driving miniature cars. The "auto town" was set up after research tended to show that many traffic accidents involving children occur because they ignore traffic rules. (Novosti from Sovfoto.)

. . . .

TOPIC: MAINTAINING A SAFE BICYCLE

Grade Level: Intermediate

Outcome: The student will be able to demonstrate how to keep a bicycle in good working condition.

Concept: A bicycle in good working order is an important safety measure (see Fig. 23.4).

Content: Ways of keeping bicycle in good working order are:

1. Handlebars
   a) keep tightened
   b) adjust to appropriate level
2. Saddle
   a) tilt upward in front
   b) adjust to body height
   c) tighten all nuts
3. Wheels
   a) run freely
   b) spokes straight
   c) no wobble
   d) oil bearings
4. Reflector—visible for 300 ft
5. Brake
   a) quick
   b) even
6. Chain
   a) fits snuggly
   b) links in good condition
   c) clean and oiled frequently

Learning Experiences

1. *Demonstration:* Have several pupils bring their bicycles into class and have them identify the parts, by name, and describe how to care for each part (see Fig. 23.4).

WHAT'S YOUR BIKE MAINTENANCE RATING?

Have the cyclists draw a line from the printed description to the arrow pointing to the corresponding part on the bike drawing

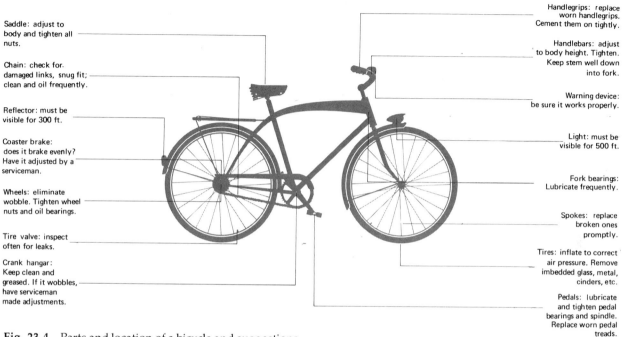

Saddle: adjust to body and tighten all nuts.

Chain: check for damaged links, snug fit; clean and oil frequently.

Reflector: must be visible for 300 ft.

Coaster brake: does it brake evenly? Have it adjusted by a serviceman.

Wheels: eliminate wobble. Tighten wheel nuts and oil bearings.

Tire valve: inspect often for leaks.

Crank hangar: Keep clean and greased. If it wobbles, have serviceman made adjustments.

Handlegrips: replace worn handlegrips. Cement them on tightly.

Handlebars: adjust to body height. Tighten. Keep stem well down into fork.

Warning device: be sure it works properly.

Light: must be visible for 500 ft.

Fork bearings: Lubricate frequently.

Spokes: replace broken ones promptly.

Tires: inflate to correct air pressure. Remove imbedded glass, metal, cinders, etc.

Pedals: lubricate and tighten pedal bearings and spindle. Replace worn pedal treads.

Fig. 23.4 Parts and location of a bicycle and suggestions for maintaining a bicycle in good working order.

7. Pedal
  a) tread in good condition
  b) lubricate and tighten pedal bearings and spindle
8. Tires
  a) inflate to correct air pressure
  b) remove foreign objects
9. Spokes—replace broken ones
10. Light—visible for 500 ft
11. Warning device—horn or bell in working order
12. Frame—clean

2. *Matching quiz:* Match parts and function with bicycle diagram (Fig. 23.5).

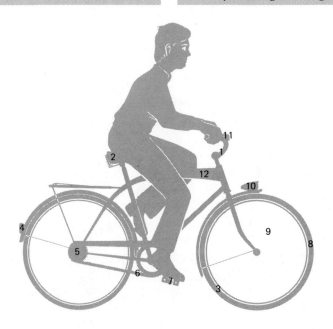

Identify the parts of a bicycle:

1. _____   7. _____

2. _____   8. _____

3. _____   9. _____

4. _____   10. _____

5. _____   11. _____

6. _____   12. _____

Fig. 23.5 Identifying parts of a bicycle. (Adapted from "Bike Quiz Guide," Bicycle Institute of America.)

3. *Inspection chart:* Each pupil uses the chart to check the condition of his or her bike (see Fig. 23.6).

INSPECTION CHART

USE THIS CHECKLIST REGULARLY TO PROTECT YOUR BIKE

PART	DATE	CONDITION	CLEANED	GREASED OR OILED	NEW PARTS	NOTES
FRONT CONES						
FRONT BEARINGS						
REAR CONES						
REAR BEARINGS						
COASTER BRAKE						
CRANK HANGER BEARINGS						
CHAIN						
PEDAL BEARINGS						
HANDLE BARS						
FRONT FORKS						
SADDLE						
FRAME						
FRONT WHEEL						
REAR WHEEL						
FRONT TIRE						
REAR TIRE						
HEAD-LIGHT						
TAIL-LIGHT						
REFLECTORS						
HORN OR BELL						
HAND BRAKE						
SPEEDOMETER						
GENERATOR						
TOOL KIT						

How to Keep Your Bicycle in Good Condition

Fig. 23.6 Bicycle inspection chart.

4. *Bicycle Safety Matching Test,* and *Bicycle Words Test.*

   a) *Bicycle Words Test:* Here is a list of 30 words commonly associated with bicycles and bicycle safety. These words can be used as a simple spelling test, definition test, sentence use, parts of speech, etc.

basket	handlebars	saddle
bearings	horn	safety
bell	hub	signals
bicycle	light	spoke
caution	pedal	tire
chain	pedestrian	traffic
crank	policeman	tube
cyclist	right	valve
fender	reflector	vehicle
fork	responsibility	wheel

   b) *Bicycle Safety Matching Test:* On the left are ten bicycle-safety words. On the right are definitions or phrases that apply to them. Have cyclists match them up.

1	spokes	A	is the safe way to ride
2	tires	B	always have right of way
3	brakes	C	replace broken ones immediately
4	chain	D	are the proper places for packages and books
5	reflector	E	should be adjusted to your height
6	bike headlight	F	clean and oil it regularly
7	Baskets	G	should be properly inflated
8	pedestrians	H	should stop smoothly and evenly
9	single file	I	must be visible for 300 ft
10	saddle	J	must be visible for 500 ft

   Correct Answers: 1—C, 2—G, 3—H, 4—F, 5—I, 6—J, 7—D, 8—B, 9—A, 10—E.

TOPIC: REACTING TO TRAFFIC SIGNALS CORRECTLY

Grade Level: Intermediate

Outcome: The student will be able to discuss the correct use of traffic signals.

Concept: Signals tell others what we are going to do.

Content: Three types of signals to know are:

1. Light signals:
   a) red—stop
   b) yellow—caution
   c) green—go
2. Arm signals:
   a) right turn
   b) left turn
   c) slowing and stopping
3. Basic traffic signs and shapes:
   a) octagonal—stop
   b) diamond—danger, caution
   c) rectagonal—traffic regulations
   d) triangular—yield

Learning Experiences

1. *Simulation game:* Teacher has regulation-size signals prepared. Students organized into four groups—each group pretends it is cars lined up in two lanes at an intersection. A student pretends to be a traffic patrol officer.

   Teacher changes signals, and pupils move forward, stop, change direction, etc. One student bumping another is considered an accident. Failure to signal correctly or react to a signal results in a traffic fine. Pupils make up additional rules.

2. *Traffic signals quiz*

Traffic Signals Quiz

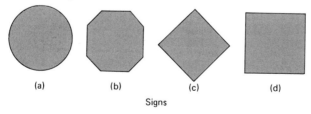

(a)   (b)   (c)   (d)

Signs

Questions:

1. What does each of the signs (a) through (d) mean?

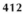

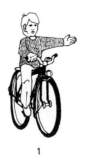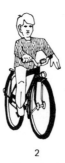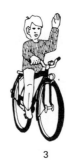

1   2   3

Turn signals

2. What does each hand signal mean?

. . . .

TOPIC: RULES FOR SAFE BICYCLE RIDING

Grade Level: Intermediate

Outcome: The student will be able to list the rules of the road.

Concept: Rules of the road help us to be safer and to live longer.

Content: Basic rules of the road are:

1. Always ride with the traffic.
2. Ride on the right side of the road.
3. Never hitch a ride.
4. Walk your bike across busy intersections.
5. Ride single file.
6. Don't carry riders.
7. Yield right of way to pedestrian.
8. Do not carry anything in your hands.
9. Keep both hands on the handlebars.
10. Give proper arm signals.

Learning Experiences

1. *Picture simulation* of traffic situations. Students pick out what the bicycle rider is doing right or wrong. *Film strip: Perception of Driving Hazards, Urban and Suburban,* by Shell Oil Company.

2. Traffic situations simulated by flannel board or magnetic board. Class reacts to various situations.

11. Look before changing direction or lane.
12. Obey all traffic signals.
13. Have bicycle inspected for safety twice a year (bike in good condition).
14. Adjust speed to road conditions, weather, traffic, and experience as a rider.
15. Select the safest route to your destination—avoid busy streets and intersections.

3. Crossword puzzle

Crossword Puzzle *

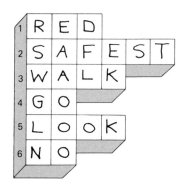 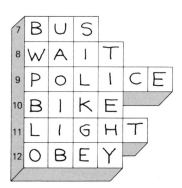

Can you fill in the blocks?

Look	Wait
Police	Bus
Safest	Go
No	Red
Obey	Walk
Bike	Light

1. A_____ light means stop.
2. Always take the_____ route to and from school.
3. Otto the Auto wants all of his little friends to _____ in the crosswalk.
4. Green means _____.
5. Stop, _____ and listen.

---

*Adapted from *Learning for Living, September/October, 1972,* a publication produced by the Automobile Club of Southern California. All rights reserved.

6. Opposite of "yes."

7. Many children ride to school on a big yellow _____ .

8. _____ your turn at the drinking fountain.

9. The _____ are your friends.

10. Walk your _____ across the street.

11. Always wear _____ or bright clothing at night.

12. Bike riders should _____ traffic rules too.

4. Traffic-Bicycle Riding Quiz or Bicycle Riding Quiz

Traffic—Bicycle Riding Quiz

Directions: Circle the letter of the answer that you think *best* answers the statement.

1. When riding a bike at night
   a) a light in front and back is necessary.
   b) a front light and a back reflector are necessary.
   c) only a front light is necessary.
   d) only a back reflector is necessary.

2. When making a right turn on your bike, you should
   a) make the turn from the left lane.
   b) make the turn from the right lane.
   c) ignore the lanes because you are on a bike.

3. While riding your bike, you may
   a) carry a rider if he or she is not too heavy.
   b) carry a rider only when you have a luggage rack.
   c) never carry a rider.
   d) carry a rider on the handlebars.

4. If you come to intersection marked "NO LEFT TURN," the sign
   a) applies to cars only and not to bikes.
   b) applies to bikes as well as cars.
   c) can be ignored if there are no cars coming.

5. A bike rider in heavy traffic should
    a) make a hand signal, then turn left.
    b) make a hand signal and make turn at same time.
    c) force the traffic to stop so that you can make the left turn.

6. Signaling to stop is
    a) helpful but is not always necessary for bike riders.
    b) necessary to let other drivers know what you are going to do.
    c) not necessary because cars pay little attention to bikers.

7. When passing a slow-moving car, you should
    a) go on the sidewalk to pass car.
    b) pass car on the left side.
    c) pass car on the right side.
    d) never pass a car.

8. A bike rider should
    a) always keep both hands on the handlebars.
    b) keep both hands on the handlebars except when carrying things.
    c) keep both hands on the handlebars except when signaling.

9. You should
    a) hitch a ride on a car or truck only if it is going slow.
    b) never hitch a ride on a car or truck.
    c) hitch a ride if you have a strong rope or chain.

10. When riding in the street, a group of riders should
    a) ride double file.
    b) ride single file.
    c) weave across the lanes.

Bike Riding Quiz

The correct answers to these 50 true or false questions are circled.

1. A bicycle is considered a vehicle and should be ridden on the right-hand side of the street.	Ⓣ	F
2. Bicycle riders should observe and obey all traffic signs, stop signs, and signals and other traffic control devices.	Ⓣ	F
3. Bike riders should try to crowd ahead between cars at a stop sign so they can be in front when the light changes.	T	Ⓕ
4. Pedestrians do not have the right of way on sidewalks or crosswalks.	T	Ⓕ
5. The signal for a right turn is extending the right arm straight out.	T	Ⓕ
6. Night riding without a white headlight and red taillight or reflector is unsafe.	Ⓣ	F
7. Bicycle riders hitching a ride on another vehicle can easily have an accident.	Ⓣ	F
8. It is safe and proper for a bike rider to carry a passenger.	T	Ⓕ
9. A bike in poor mechanical condition is safe if the rider is skilled.	T	Ⓕ
10. It is safe to ride bikes three abreast when riding in a group.	T	Ⓕ
11. The roadway is a safe place to park your bike.	T	Ⓕ
12. Bikes should be inspected twice a year by a reliable service person.	Ⓣ	F
13. The headlights of a bicycle should be seen from at least 500 ft.	Ⓣ	F
14. Riding single file is the sensible thing to do.	Ⓣ	F
15. The proper way to make a left turn is to cut the corner.	T	Ⓕ
16. It is safe to enter the street from the sidewalk without first seeing whether a car is coming.	T	Ⓕ
17. When passing a slow-moving car going in the same direction, you should pass to the left.	Ⓣ	F
18. Bicyclists should keep to the right while riding in the street.	Ⓣ	F
19. Bike riders should give hand signals when stopping or turning.	Ⓣ	F
20. Hitching a ride on another vehicle is safe if the rider is careful.	T	Ⓕ
21. Icy or slippery streets are dangerous places to ride a bike.	Ⓣ	F
22. A bike rider should look only straight ahead when crossing an intersection.	T	Ⓕ
23. It is safe for two people to be on a bike if one is on the handlebars.	T	Ⓕ

24. Cyclists should ride at least three feet away from parked cars. (T) F

25. On country roads cyclists should keep to the left, same as pedestrians. T (F)

26. Broken or loose spokes should be replaced immediately. (T) F

27. Pedals should not be worn or broken. (T) F

28. A broken coaster brake can be easily fixed at home. T (F)

29. Handlebars should be loose so you can change riding positions. T (F)

30. Your chain should be loose enough to slip off easily. T (F)

31. The whole bicycle should be cleaned and oiled occasionally. (T) F

32. Saddle and handlebars should be adjusted to your height. (T) F

33. Riding bikes off curbs doesn't damage the bikes. T (F)

34. It is permissible to ride small children in baskets. T (F)

35. Persons riding bikes are subject to the same traffic laws that govern automobile drivers. (T) F

36. Blue is a good color to wear when biking after dark. T (F)

37. It is not necessary to stop at intersections if there is no traffic. T (F)

38. You can drive a bike, but not a car, in either direction on a one-way street. T (F)

39. There is danger of skidding on curves even if the road is not wet. (T) F

40. If you live in the country, you can ride on either side of the road. T (F)

41. Even a skilled bike rider should walk his or her bike through heavy traffic. (T) F

42. If you don't ride on busy streets, you don't need a horn or bell. T (F)

43. Cyclists have the right of way over pedestrians. T (F)

44. The faster you ride, the safer it is. T (F)

45. A warped wheel rim can cause an accident. (T) F

46. When riding at night, ride to the left so you can see approaching headlights. T (F)

47. A good bicycle really never needs greasing and oiling. T (F)

48. A loose saddle is a potential danger to the cyclist. (T) F

49. It is a bad idea to wax the metal finish of your bike. T (F)

50. When cycling, you should pay strict attention to what you're doing. (T) F

5. *Picture Quiz:* Students pick out what rider is doing wrong in various riding situations. (See Pictures Quizzes 1-5.)

Picture Quiz (perceptivity) 1 *

What are the riders doing wrong in each picture situation (a) through (d)?

Picture Quiz 2

The rider in each picture situation (e) through (h) is doing something right or wrong. Which situations are safe? Which are dangerous?

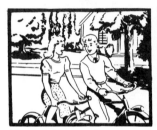

(a) Not paying attention to road ahead.

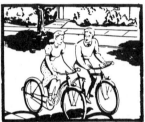

(b) Riding two abreast.

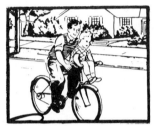

(e)

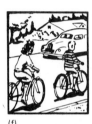

(f)

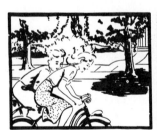

(c) Excessive speeding.

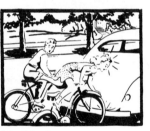

(d) Tailgating

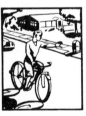

(g)

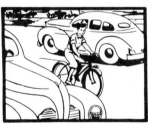

(h)

---

* The illustrations for Picture Quizzes 1 through 5 are taken from *Bicycle Safety Manual,* a publication of the Berea Police Department, Berea, Kentucky.

Picture Quiz 3

Two pictures make a complete situation. What did the rider do wrong?

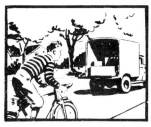 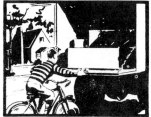

Picture Quiz 4

Two pictures make a complete situation. What did the rider do wrong?

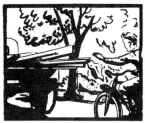 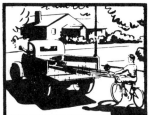

Picture Quiz 5

Three pictures make a complete situation. What did the rider do wrong?

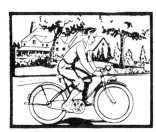 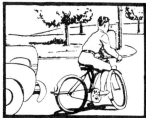 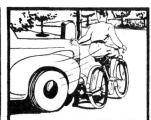

REFERENCES AND BIBLIOGRAPHY

Bicycle Safety in Action (Washington, D.C.: National Commission on Safety Education, 1964).

Bicycle Safety Pamphlet (Washington, D.C.: National Automobile Club, 1963).

Bike Safety Pamphlet (San Diego, Calif.: Fire Department).

California Driver's Handbook (Sacramento, Calif., 1972.).

Evans, William. *Everyday Safety* (Chicago: Lyons and Carnahan, 1962).

Florio, A. E., and G. T. Stafford. *Safety Education* (New York: McGraw-Hill, 1969).

Leaf, Munro. *Safety Can Be Fun* (New York: Lippincott, 1961).

CHAPTER 24

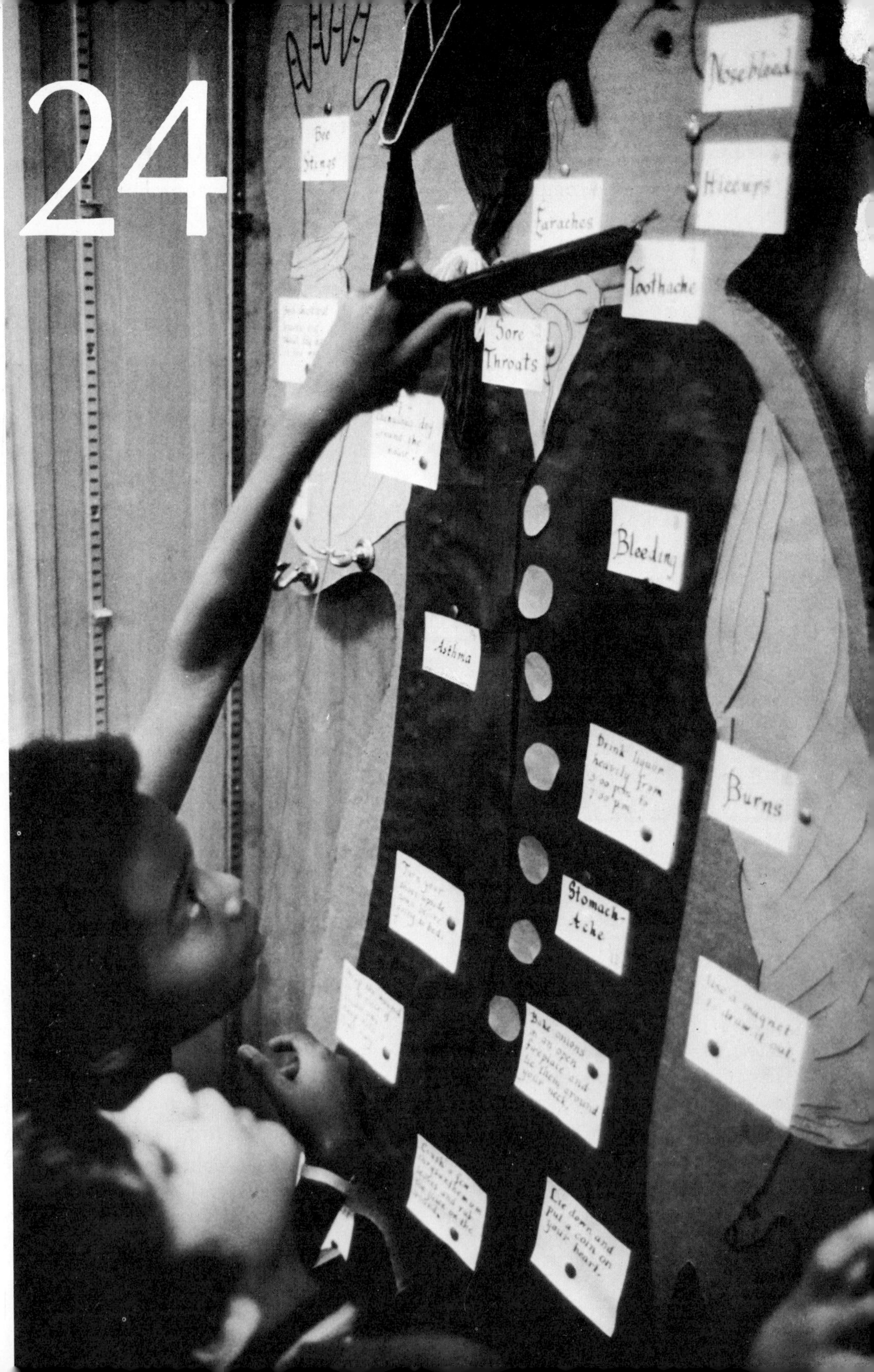
Nosebleed
Bee Stings
Hiccups
Earaches
Toothache
Sore Throats
Bleeding
Asthma
Burns
Stomach-Ache
Use a magnet to draw it out.
Bake onions in an open fireplace and tie them around your neck.
Lie down and put a coin on your heart.

teaching about diseases

INTRODUCTION

Today complete freedom from disease and illness is a mirage. However great the benefits of medical progress, improved sanitation, having regular medical care, and enjoying a high standard of living, they do not ensure complete freedom from disease. Children are especially susceptible to numerous infections and ailments.

Almost 50 percent of all childhood diseases are respiratory. The common cold, influenza, measles, mumps, diphtheria, and strep throat are just a few of the common infections from which children suffer. Obviously, children will react emotionally to such infections. They become disabled physiologically, their social life is disrupted, and they react emotionally with fear and anxiety. Such reactions disrupt learning, as well as overall development. Children need help in allaying such emotional stresses. Hence teachers need to be aware that children need not only guidance in immunizations as protection against diseases, but also general information about illnesses and diseases, how to care for oneself during illness, and how to keep from getting sick.

Not even doctors dare mention well-being without considering disease and illness in the total health spectrum. Illness and disease, like well-being, are interpreted through the use of society's value system and, as such, are cultural concepts. For example, whether one becomes bedridden with a cold or disregards the cold symptoms in his or her daily routine is directed by one's cultural perception of illness. Our interpretation of "mental illness" provides another such example. Cultural evaluation varies, and as a result, we find that there is a great deal of confusion over what disease, infection, and disorder are. The quandary can be resolved only by taking into account that information which falls within the province of medical fact.

Disease is an abnormal process in which there is alteration of anatomy or physiology of an individual for a long period of time. Such alterations give rise to physiological symptoms or signs which may be mild, severe, acute, or chronic and may end in recovery or death. There are many causes of diseases: (1) microorganismic invasion of the body, (2) general stress, (3) malnutrition, (4) genetic disorder

421

of body processes, and (5) aging. Any one of these causes can wear down body defenses, overcome its tolerance, and upset the constancy of the body's internal environment, thereby causing a disease.

Infection is part of the disease process. It occurs when bacteria or viruses multiply in or on human tissues in an unusual place or in unusually large numbers. Most infections do not cause diseases. A viral infection, causing one to have the usual cold and respiratory symptoms, is temporary and usually does not last longer than two or three weeks. Thus a cold and influenza are not diseases, but infections. The viruses multiply to an unusually large number in the respiratory tract and temporarily overwhelm the body's defense mechanisms. Infections subside when the body's antibody resistance is elevated, the infectious host runs short of food, its growth conditions become unfavorable, or it chokes from its own waste products. Most of the illnesses of early and middle childhood are of an infectious respiratory nature.

A disorder is a dysfunction of an organ or body system, and readjustment takes place. A prolonged disorder may lead to prolonged disability or disease. For example, lack of insulin secretion by the pancreas could occur in most individuals; however, such imbalance generally reverts to normalcy. If it does not, this condition becomes a chronic disorder, diabetes. When such a disorder persists for three months or longer, we refer to it as a disease.

We have been brainwashed into thinking that there is a single cause of disease or disorder. This thinking has prevailed since the turn of the century, when a single bacteria was identified as the direct cause of an infection. It is possible that many infections and diseases are initiated by more than one factor. This possibility has given rise to the multicausation theory of diseases. Viruses, for example, have been identified as a causative agent of colds, but other etiological factors such as poor nutrition, fatigue, low body resistance, and a poor mental outlook on life are also predisposing factors.

Most acute or short-term infections, e.g., colds and influenza, probably have several causes.

The human body has numerous defense mechanisms to resist infections and diseases. Three lines of body defense that must be overcome by a pathogen before it can establish an infection are: (1) the mechanical-chemical barrier, such as the skin, sweat cells, the mucous membranes, secretions of the nose and respiratory tract, hairs and cilia acting as air filters, saliva in the mouth, and tears; (2) the cellular barriers, such as white blood cells and the process of phagocytosis, or white blood cells engulfing and destroying bacteria; and (3) the antibodies, or chemical substances in the blood serum that destroy foreign bodies and toxins or waste products. As part of these three lines of defense, the body has a special system for clearing undesirable particles, such as bacteria, dust, and antigens, from the blood and lymph. This reticuloendothelial system consists of fixed phagocytic cells in the lymphoid tissues, liver, spleen, bone marrow, lungs, and other vital tissues. These organs have tissues that remove particulate matter from the lymphatic and blood streams.

Teachers should make children aware that the body gives off symptomatic warnings whenever something is wrong with the body—whenever homeostasis has been disrupted. Among the usual symptoms of illness are: inflammation (swelling, pain), watery eyes, running nose, headache, and fever. These are nature's ways of letting us know that something is wrong with our bodies.

Living in the world today presents many challenges and problems. Diseases are part of the scene. Anthropologists have interpreted disease as a byproduct of a civilized way of life. Each civilization evolves a lifestyle that incubates its own peculiar diseases. This concept helps us to understand why disease or infection may be very virulent at one time of history or in one country, but not very virulent at another time or in another country. We should also be aware that infectious diseases replace one another, and when one is rooted out, it is likely to be replaced by others. Thus the epidemic diseases, such as typhoid, cholera, and tuberculosis, have been replaced in the Western world by viral and chronic diseases. As always, the environment in which the individual lives and his or her manner of living are of great importance in determining susceptibility to the diseases of modern times.

It should be apparent by now that well-being and disease cannot be defined or distinguished merely in terms of anatomical, physiological, or mental attributes. Their real measure is in the ability of the individual to function in a manner acceptable to self and to the group of which she or he is a part. The interpretation of whether a person is able or unable to function varies with age, the conditions of living, and one's cultural value system. How a young child perceives illness or disease may be very different from how an adolescent or teacher perceives these. Perhaps it may be of help for teachers to perceive illnesses and diseases as at the opposite end of the wellness spectrum (see Fig. 1.3). Illnesses and diseases may be a consequence of irresponsible behaviors and poor ways of coping with life. On the other hand, optimal well-being may be interpreted as a consequence of responsible behavior and good ways of coping with life problems. Teachers should impress this "consequence" concept on children, for it ties in harmoniously with the current ecological and risk-taking behavior themes.

Finally, as our technological lifestyle changes, we can expect new habits to emerge which may be deleterious to our well-being. Although such habits are initiated early in life, their consequences remain latent. It is not until the child has become a middle-aged adult that the symptoms become acute and the person becomes prematurely disabled. Heart disease is a good example of this process. A child's deleterious habits of living, as reflected by overeating; not exercising regularly; academic, social, and emotional stresses; and cigarette smoking form a syndrome of behaviors predisposing him or her to heart disease at a later age. Many other diseases have similar latent and chronic overtones. Children need to be made aware that they will continuously evolve new health problems in an effort to adapt to technological progress and social change. They need to be made aware that such problems may start as acute disrupting illnesses or diseases and emerge into chronic disabling diseases for which there are as yet no general cures. As such, chronic diseases need to be anticipated during the formative years. Prevention against social and chronic diseases of progress must begin with the elementary children, even though chronic diseases are a health problem of later life.

Obviously, the suggested lesson plans that follow are interrelated with other lesson-plan chapters. These lessons could have been included with their appropriate topical lessons. But we chose to put these into a special chapter, for at the elementary school level, childhood illnesses occur often and thus become a significant part of growing up for the child. Teachers should study the lesson plans presented in this chapter and adapt them to their teaching situations.

. . . .

TOPIC: COLDS—AND HOW TO AVOID THEM

Grade Level: Primary

Outcome I: The student will be able to describe the symptoms of a cold.

Concept: Cold symptoms tell us that something is wrong.

Content: Symptoms of a cold are:

1. Throat irritation
2. Fever
3. Coughing
4. Sneezing
5. Running nose
6. Watery eyes
7. Loss of appetite
8. Feeling tired.

Learning Experiences

1. *Matching bee:* Pictures of sick and well person are matched with symptoms by pupils (simulate with comic characters—Snoopy, etc.)
2. *Alternative experience:* Pupils take turns simulating symptoms; e.g., "How Cathy feels when she has a cold," and class tries to identify symptom.

Outcome II: The student will be able to state ways to avoid catching a cold.

Concept: Right style of living helps us avoid colds (good habits help prevent colds).

Content: Good habits helping us to avoid a cold are:

1. Using paper tissue when coughing or sneezing
2. Eating balanced diet regularly
3. Getting proper amount of sleep
4. Drinking plenty of fluids
5. Wearing warm clothes
6. Washing hands before eating

Learning Experiences

1. *Flannel board—Snoopy Fights a Cold:* Snoopy and various pictorial situations depicting good and bad health habits. Children place Snoopy in situations preventing cold: "Give Snoopy right style of living!" Let class react to pupil choices.
2. *Demonstration:* Proper way to blow nose and to use paper tissue.

7. Keeping feet dry
8. Getting regular exercise
9. Getting plenty of rest
10. Being cheerful
11. Not playing with someone who has a cold
12. Not using same drinking glass
13. Disposing of paper tissue properly.

3. *Alternative suggestions*
   a) *Picture Quiz* on how to avoid a cold.

Picture Quiz

Which picture in each pair shows how to prevent colds? Which picture is incorrect (has something wrong with it)? Circle the correct face.

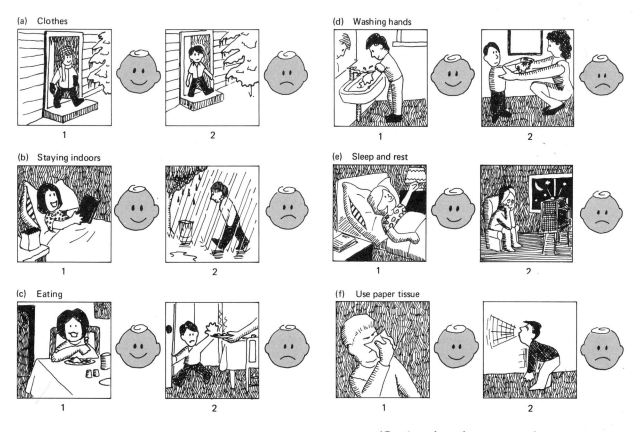

(a) Clothes

(b) Staying indoors

(c) Eating

(d) Washing hands

(e) Sleep and rest

(f) Use paper tissue

(Continued on the next page.)

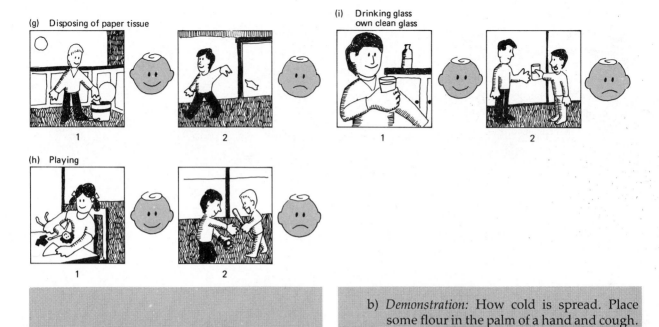

(g)   Disposing of paper tissue

(h)   Playing

(i)   Drinking glass
own clean glass

b) *Demonstration:* How cold is spread. Place some flour in the palm of a hand and cough. Observe flour dispersing. Flour conceptualized to germs.

Key Questions

1. When should you wash your hands?
2. How do you feel when you have a cold?
3. What should you do when you want to cough?
4. What should you do when you get tired?
5. What should you do with paper tissue which you have used?
6. How can you prevent catching a cold?

TOPIC: IMMUNIZATION

Grade Level: Primary

Outcome I: The student will be able to describe how immunization gives us a protection (medicine) against disease.

Concept: Immunization protects us from diseases.

Content: Immunization:	*Learning Experiences*
1. Is a medicine that enters our body. 2. Helps our body to make fighters (in blood) against disease. 3. Is helpful in fighting germs.	1. *Storytelling:* Silly, Sassy, and Smarty

Silly, Sassy, and Smarty

by Nancy Rice

Once upon a time there were three friends who always played together. Their names were Silly, Sassy, and Smarty. One bright summer day, they were running and skipping when all of a sudden Silly, who was silly for not wearing shoes, felt something sharp going into her foot. This sharp thing was a nail, and it hurt Silly very badly. Sassy told Silly not to be a baby, to pull it out, and that it would be just fine. Silly and Sassy were anxious to start playing hopscotch, but Smarty told them to wait, that they would have to take Silly to the hospital or to the doctor's office or to that clinic to get a shot. Silly said that she didn't need a shot, that she never gets any of those diseases with the big words. Sassy told Silly that Smarty just thinks she's a doctor or something like that. Besides, Sassy asked Silly if she has one of those funny-looking scars on her arm from when she was a baby. Silly quickly rolled up her sleeve and found that sure enough—she did have one. Well, Sassy said she had nothing to worry about, because that's all the shot you need. So the three friends kept on playing until it was time to go home for dinner.

The next day, Sassy and Smarty met at their favorite place, but Silly never showed up. The friends told themselves that she must have had something else to do. So the two of them just played hopscotch and jumped rope for the rest of the day. Well, the next day something even more strange happened. Smarty was to meet Silly and Sassy at their favorite spot, but neither one of them showed up this time. This made Smarty sad; she thought her friends didn't like her anymore. She tried playing by herself, but it was just no fun. She went home to tell her mommy about her two friends.

Her mother suggested that they call up her two friends and find out why they didn't come to play. First, Smarty's mother helped her dial Silly's number. Silly's mother answered the phone and told Smarty that Silly was a sick little girl because she had stepped on a nail two days ago and had not told her. Silly's mother explained that she needed a tetanus shot because she hadn't had one in over three years. Silly's foot got swollen, she had a fever, and she started to hurt all over. Her mother told Smarty that she took Silly to Dr. Welby for a tetanus shot, so Silly would feel better in a few days. Smarty was glad to find that Silly was still her friend, even if she was a sick friend. Smarty then called Sassy and her mother answered the phone. She said that Sassy was sick with flu and couldn't speak to Smarty. Her mother also told Smarty that Sassy wouldn't have caught the flu or would have had a much milder case if she had had a flu shot, but Sassy had thrown such a fit at the clinic about how much it was going to hurt that her mother had decided not to make her have one after all. Smarty hung up the phone, telling Sassy's mother she hoped Sassy would be able to play soon.

Smarty then went and told her own mother why Silly and Sassy couldn't play. Her mother told her that she didn't miss very many school or play days because her daddy and mommy take her regularly to get the different shots she needs. Her mommy and daddy know that a shot might sting for a minute, but that Smarty will be well, happy, and able to play more all year long. I'll bet Smarty was named after her mommy and daddy, don't you?!

Key Questions

1. Did you like the story?
2. Why did Silly get sick?
3. Why did Sassy get sick?
4. Why didn't Smarty get sick?
5. Who would you like to be?
6. What should you do to stay healthy?

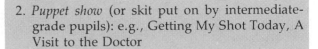

2. *Puppet show* (or skit put on by intermediate-grade pupils): e.g., Getting My Shot Today, A Visit to the Doctor

Outcome II: The student will be able to state how immunizations are given.

Concept: Immunizations or shots are given by a doctor or nurse.

Content: Shots are given:

1. When you are healthy.
2. Mom or Dad makes appointment at doctor's office.
3. Nurse rolls up sleeve.
4. Nurse cleans arm by rubbing alcohol over it.
5. Nurse gives shot.
6. Nurse wipes arm with alcohol.

Learning Experiences

1. Puppet show (or skit)
2. *Demonstration:* A mock immunization with a medicine dropper (filled with water), rubbing alcohol, and cotton ball.
3. *Alternative experiences*
   a) *Film: Magic Touch,* to be presented by teacher and pupils who will take part in the skit or play.
   b) Permission slips and immunization history slips to be taken home and filled out by parents.

TOPIC: BODY DEFENSES AGAINST DISEASES

Grade Level: Intermediate

Outcome: The student will be able to describe the three lines of body defense.

Concept: Our body has three lines of defense against diseases.

Subconcept 1: Skin and mucus membranes are our first line of defense.

Content: Physical barriers include:

1. Skin is tough and acts like an armor.
2. Mucous membranes in nose, lungs, and stomach trap germs.

Learning Experiences

1. Picture simulation in sequences and matching bee. Visual aid in different colors.

3. Tears in eyes and nose wash out and kill germs.

2. Compare body to castle. Castle wall is equivalent to skin, doors and windows to nose and mouth (see Fig. 24.1).

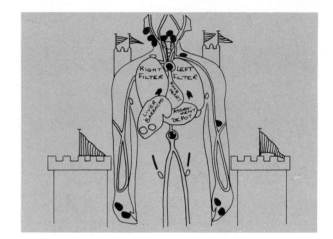

Fig. 24.1 Conceptualization of body defenses against diseases.

Subconcept 2: Phagocytes and lymph are our second line of defense.

Content: Second line of defense includes:

1. Phagocytes, or white blood cells—engulf and immobilize germs and cause pus and inflammation.
2. Lymph carries bacteria to lymph nodes.
3. Macrophages (scavenger cells) kill germs.
4. Thymus gland helps lymphatic system.
5. Liver and spleen lined with phagocytes which destroy bacteria in blood.

Learning Experiences

1. Same as for first subconcept.
2. Conceptualize phagocytes and macrophages as soldiers, and lymphatic system as roadway for soldiers.

Subconcept 3: Antibodies are the third line of defense.

Content: Third line of defense includes:

1. Many chemical antibodies.
2. Each antibody is specific for each foreign substance.
3. Antibodies and germs create a neutral condition.

Learning Experiences

1. Same as for first subconcept. Conceptualize antibodies as king's special guard.
2. *Alternative learning experiences*
   a) *Chart* displaying the three body defenses.
   b) *Film: How Our Bodies Fight Disease.*

Key Questions

1. How does the skin protect you against bacteria?
2. What are phagocytes?
3. What are macrophages?
4. What happens once bacteria gets inside your body?
5. What is an antibody?
6. How does an antibody fight a disease?
7. How do the hairs in the nose act as barriers to infection?
8. Are tears a first, second, or third line of defense?

. . . .

TOPIC: HOW DISEASES ARE SPREAD

Grade Level: Primary, Intermediate

Outcome: The student will be able to identify ways in which diseases (bacteria and viruses) may be spread in many ways.

Concept: Diseases are spread in many ways.

Content: Diseases are spread in following ways:

1. *Through the air:* by coughing and sneezing.
2. *Personal contact:* directly by touching another person or indirectly by touching objects (glass, towel, washcloth, etc.) handled by another.

Learning Experiences

1. *Simulate ways* of spreading microbes.
   a) *Demonstration:* Place cocoa or flour in palm of hand and cough. Action of flour can be compared to that of microbes.

3. *By insects:* flies, mosquitoes, ticks, etc.
4. *In food:* touched by insects and humans.
5. *In water:* drinking infected water.
6. *By animals and pets:* cats, dogs, and birds; ringworm, ticks, fleas.

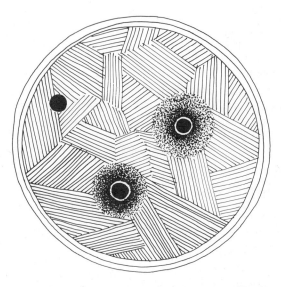

Fig. 24.2 Determination of sensitivity of bacteria to different antibiotics (single-paper disk-diffusion method). A Petri dish of agar was heavily inoculated with the test organisms. Disks of filter paper impregnated with different antibiotics were dropped on the freshly inoculated surface. Note the white bacterial growth with a zone of no growth around two of the disks. There is no inhibition of growth around the third. A zone of inhibition indicates that the growth of the organism would probably be limited in a patient receiving an antibiotic.

b) *Demonstration:* Place red lipstick on palm of hand of student or clean glass. Have another student touch palm or infected glass. Observe for tracings of lipstick on hand of second student.

c) *Demonstration:* Attach transparent sticky tape to feet of a large model fly. Have fly land on flour, and dust, then on some flat white paper. Observe color tape tracings on white paper.

d) *Demonstration:* Cultivate culture plates of several foods and observe for bacteria growth.

e) *Demonstration:* Cultivate culture plates of different samples of water (pond, river, tap) and observe for bacterial growth and contamination.

f) Refer to demonstration of drinking glass and lipstick.

2. *Alternative learning experience*

a) *Demonstration:* Plant antibiotic paper disks on jar media inoculated with infectious bacteria. Incubate for 36-48 hours. Observe. (See Fig. 24.2.)

b) *Simulate* bacterial growth needs with several plants. All living things need oxygen, water, food, and warmth.

c) *Demonstration:* After conceptualizing, by use of flour or lipstick, how germs are spread, have infected student wash hands with soap and water. Do same with use of paper tissue and coughing. Likewise wash dirty glass with soap and water.

d) *Pictures simulating* ways of spreading diseases. Add to this a pupil matching bee technique.

e) *Demonstration:* With oral disclosing pill. Red coloring of teeth and germs identifies bacterial plaques.

Key Questions

1. Can you think of other ways that diseases are spread?
2. How can pets spread diseases?
3. How do humans spread diseases?
4. Where do we find germs?
5. How can we stop the spread of germs and diseases?
6. How can you get a cold?
7. How can you get a skin infection?
8. How does washing hands prevent infection?
9. How many ways can we spread disease?

. . . .

TOPIC: PERSONAL CLEANLINESS

Grade Level: Primary

Outcome: The student will be able to exhibit personal cleanliness and tidiness.

Concept: Cleanliness keeps us healthy and helps us have friends.

Content: Ways of keeping clean are:

1. Hands and fingernails—water, soap, and file
2. Face and ears—soap and water
3. Hair—brush and washing
4. Body—shower and soap
5. Teeth—toothbrush, toothpaste, dental floss
6. Clothes—washing machine, iron, hangers
7. Shoes—shine, brush, and polish

Learning Experiences

1. *Matching bee:* The part of body with article used to keep it clean.
2. *Puppet shows:* e.g., Stinky

Stinky

by Barbara Burch

Characters: Stinky the Skunk, Ollie the Alligator, Dopey the Dog, Ms Smarty the Teacher

Act I

Scene: The Classroom. Stinky is sitting by himself. Ollie goes up to the teacher and says:

Ollie: Ms Smarty, nobody wants to sit by Stinky because he smells bad.

Ms Smarty: Now, Ollie, that's not a nice thing to say! He's a skunk and he can't help it.

Ollie: But Ms Smarty, his hair is dirty and messy too, and he didn't brush his teeth.

Ms Smarty: Go back to your seat, Ollie. I'll talk to Stinky.

Act II

Scene: On the playground. Ms Smarty asks the children to pick a partner to play with. Nobody picks Stinky. He goes to Ms Smarty and says:

Stinky: Ms Smarty, nobody wants to be my partner. What's wrong with me?

Ms Smarty (laughing): Stinky, when was the last time you had a bath?

Stinky: A bath? I don't like to take baths, Ms Smarty. My mother doesn't make me.

Ms Smarty: Well, Stinky, do you ever wash your hair, or brush your teeth? And your fingernails—they're a mess!

Stinky (defensively): But Ms Smarty, only girls and sissies do that stuff!

Ms Smarty: But Stinky, everyone should keep clean and smelling nice, because if we don't, other people won't like to be around us.

Stinky: Oh, is that why nobody wanted to be my partner, Ms Smarty? Because I smell bad?

Ms Smarty: That's right Stinky. Ollie said that you smell bad. That's why you should take a bath, and wash your hair, and brush your teeth. Then people will think you look nice and smell nice, and they will want to be around you.

Act III

Scene: Next day, on the playground. Ms Smarty asks the children to pick partners to play with. Dopey the dog says to Stinky:

Dopey: I'll be your partner Stinky. You smell nice today.

Stinky: O.K., Dopey, but maybe I should change my name. I'm not stinky anymore because I take baths now.

And they all shout:

ALL: HOORAY FOR STINKY!!!

Key Questions

1. Did you like our puppet show?
2. Why did the children not want to play with Stinky?
3. What did Stinky do in order to be able to play?
4. What should we do to make us look and smell nice?
5. Why do we want to look and smell nice?
6. How often should you wash your hands and face?
7. How often should you take a shower?

3. *Alternative suggestions*
   a) *Health clock:* Opposite the hours of the day, there are objects for caring for our bodies. Children dial the hands of the clock and discuss/demonstrate the use of each item.
   b) *Films: How Billy Keeps Clean—Cleanliness and Health*. Order from: Coronet Instructional Films.

. . . .

TOPIC: HOW SOAP CLEANSES THE BODY

Grade Level: Primary

Outcome I: The student will be able to describe how soap cleanses the body.

Concept: Soap removes dirt and bacteria from the skin.

Content: Soap removes dirt and bacteria from skin as follows:

1. Dirt and bacteria stick to oily skin.
2. Soap and water form a soapy film around dirt.
3. Bacteria and dirt inside soapy film.
4. Shower water rinses soapy film.
5. Skin is now clean.

Learning Experiences

1. *Demonstration:* Cultivate bacteria from various parts of body in Petri dishes for 48 hours at room temperature. Display dishes to class. Observe bacterial growth.
2. *Demonstration:* Blow up a small colored balloon to simulate a bacteria. Put the balloon in a clear plastic bag. Plastic bag conceptualizes soapy film.
3. *Alternative suggestions*
   a) *Film: Soapy the Germ Fighter.*
   b) *Demonstration:* Washing dirty hands with and without soap. Observe the difference in cleanliness.
   c) *Demonstrate:* Inoculate Petri dish agar growth media with various soaps. Have a control dish (no soap). Observe how soap inhibits bacterial growth.

Key Questions

1. Does skin always have oil?
2. Why does dirt stick to the skin?
3. Why should one have a clean body?
4. How do bacteria cause body odors?

TOPIC: IMMEDIATE SYMPTOMS OF GONORRHEA

Grade level: Junior High

Outcome I: The student will be able to identify the immediate symptoms of gonorrhea.

Concept I: Immediate symptoms of gonorrhea in a man are easily recognized.

Content: Male symptoms of infection are:	*Learning Experiences*
1. Inflammation of urethra 2. Swelling of urethra 3. Burning-itchy sensation during urination 4. Thick, creamy, greenish yellow discharge	1. Case history

A Case History

by Charles Peveler

William S., a slight, brown-haired 18-year-old boy, was invited to a party. At the party he met a pretty 17-year-old girl, Carol. William and Carol became good friends at the party. Two hours after the party had started, things become boring, so William and Carol decided to take a ride. After driving around for about 30 minutes they decided to park. While parked, William and Carol had sexual intercourse.

Seven days later William began to feel a burning-itchy sensation during urination. He also noticed a thick, creamy, greenish yellow discharge during urination. William had heard that these were the signs of gonorrhea, so he went to his family doctor. William explained his situation to the doctor. The doctor took a sample of the discharge and analyzed it. William found out that he was infected with gonorrhea. William was treated with penicillin. The doctor explained to William the dangers of untreated gonorrhea and emphasized that the person or persons with whom he had had sexual intercourse should also be treated. Carol was brought in for testing, and it was found out that she was infected with gonorrhea. Carol did not realize that she had gonorrhea because she did not feel anything wrong with her. In the course of ten days before Carol was treated, she had infected two other boys. All were brought in for testing.

Key Questions

1. How did William become infected with gonorrhea?
2. What were his symptoms?
3. Was it smart for William to see a doctor immediately? Why?
4. Why didn't Carol know she had gonorrhea?
5. How were all the victims with gonorrhea treated?

2. *Alternative learning experiences*
   a) *Film: Attack Plan-VD*. Order from Walt Disney Productions.
   b) Lecture/discussion
   c) Diagram of body. Pupils identify reproductive structures affected by infection.

Concept II: Immediate symptoms of gonorrhea in a woman are often difficult to recognize.

Content: Female symptoms of infection are:

1. Similar to males if urethra is infected.
2. Different in that they are not recognizable if vagina or uterus is infected.

Learning Experiences

1. Same as for concept 1.

REFERENCES AND BIBLIOGRAPHY

Bender, Stephen J. *Venereal Disease* (Dubuque, Iowa: Wm. C. Brown, 1971).

California State Department of Education. *Suggestions for Instruction About Gonorrhea and Syphilis in Junior and Senior High Schools* (Sacramento: State Department of Education, 1972).

Hellman, Hal. *Defense Mechanisms* (New York: Holt, Rinehart and Winston, 1969).

Pelezar, Michael J., and Roger D. Reid. *Microbiology* (New York: McGraw-Hill, 1965).

Slaton, William. *Bacteria and Viruses: Friends or Foes* (Englewood Cliffs, N.J.: Prentice-Hall, 1965).

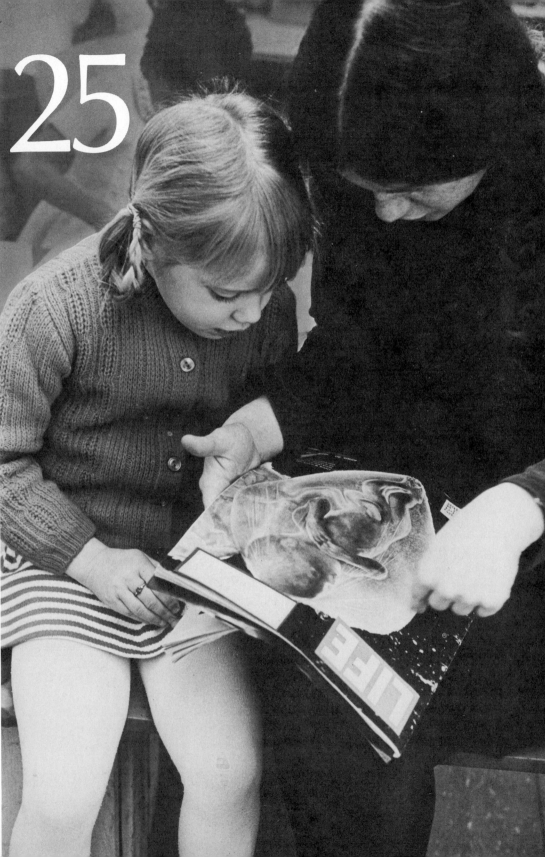

teaching about family living

INTRODUCTION

Family life education is perhaps the most controversial content area of the elementary health education curriculum. The mere mention of sex education is bound to create conflict in most communities. This is indeed unfortunate.

All of us are potentially capable of performing and of experiencing the impulses associated with performing sexual activity, mating, and reproduction. Closely related to the performance of those basic functions are the keen passions, satisfactions, and devotions that we feel. These feelings range from the primarily physical to the essentially psychic. Our entire psychophysical sexual development is an extremely complicated, demanding, and important developmental task. It involves emotions, societal influences, parental guidance, cognitive information, experience, etc. Ideally, the end-product is a fully functioning person who has achieved a sensible, humane, and healthy attitude toward all aspects of sex, marriage, and life.

Within this context, it can be stated that sex and reproduction are natural and fundamental. However, the range of behavior within this spectrum is most diverse. Sexual behavior can be approached for immediate, selfish, and totally physical gratification. On the other hand, it can also be experienced as a harmonious blending of both physical and psychological forces. In the long run, it is the latter approach that will contribute the most to positive and healthy sexual adjustment.

Today's society does little to provide support for the premise above. We still continue to operate under a double standard that implies sexual freedom for males and chastity for females.

Our culture continues to encourage the young male to sexually exploit his female counterpart. And yet sexual encounters that are based solely on physical attraction lack the tenderness and total satisfaction that can be derived only from a meaningful relationship. When sex is approached from the purely physical standpoint, it is only a matter of time before the participants lose their ability to give of themselves and find true happiness and peace of mind with their partners. The attitudinal connotations of sexual behavior are extremely important when you consider the vast number of people who are presently afflicted with sex-related emotional problems.

Sexual information and the impulses connected with such behavior are far too complex and important to the child's personality development to be ignored or left to instinct. As with all other matters of the child, the parents have the prime responsibility for the sexual education of the youngster. However, it is generally agreed that most children receive very little, if any, sexual education at home. Therefore, the school in its supplementary role becomes a logical choice to assist the home in the development of the child's sexual knowledge. Obviously other agencies, such as the church, can be helpful in contributing to the child's family living education.

The elementary level is the only time in our educational process when everyone attends school and may receive the benefits of such education. And the subject is far less likely to encounter conflict at the elementary level than at other levels. The elementary school child accepts sexual education readily and naturally. Thus it does not represent the emotional hurdle at the early elementary level that occurs during puberty. More important, most elementary school children are likely to become the victims of inaccurate street information and unwholesome lavatory-wall-type attitudes. Children want answers about reproduction, birth, sex, and family living. They need to be given straightforward, honest information at appropriate times during their lives. The teacher should provide enough information to satisfy the child's immediate curiosity and leave the door open for the child to come back for more imformation when he or she needs it.

The emphasis at the elementary level should help children to evolve healthy attitudes toward family living. Such attitudes have been referred to as a "healthy sexuality" and are reflected in the degree to which one feels comfortable with (and toward): sexual roles (father, mother, sister, brother); relationships with the same and with the opposite sex; and fulfilling personal, family, and social responsibilities (as a worker, student, family member, housewife, etc.). A healthy sexuality needs to be compatible with a healthy attitude toward life. Children need to structure their identity with sexual roles early. They need to appreciate the role of the body in reproduction and to understand the part that emotions play in sexual behavior. They need to learn the social mechanics of how to relate to others in positive ways. And they need to learn to assume responsibilities in general. Obviously, such an educational approach is interrelated with emotional and social well-being.

Numerous school systems have initiated, or are initiating, family life and sex education programs. It can be safely hypothesized that family life and sex education will be an integral part of most elementary health education curriculums throughout the United States in the foreseeable future. Implementation of such instruction requires a great deal of forethought about what, when, and how it should be taught, as well as about who should teach it.

Often, there are groups in the community opposed to family life and sex education programs being offered in the schools. Some states have even legislated guidelines for or against offering such education. The logical question all teachers, administrators, and parents need to answer is: How can we avoid triggering the social machinery in the community and still evolve and offer good, sound, and socially acceptable family health education programs? One way to do this is to avoid bootlegging sex education into the schools.

We bootleg family life education into the schools when: *

1. We label the course as "sex education." This immediately focuses attention on the course and causes a sensation.

---

* Reprinted by permission from Walter Sorochan, "Don't Bootleg Sex Education into the Schools," *Kentucky Association for Health, Physical Education, and Recreation Journal,* April 1969, pp. 12-14.

2. *We offer a "one-shot" type of program. Examples of this would be a one-unit, a one-semester, or a one-year type of program. Such programs tend to be ineffective because the value structures of the pupils do not have time to become established. Only continuous and progressive programs of a comprehensive nature can help to structure the "maturational preparedness" of the pupils necessary to receiving further instruction.*

3. *Family health education is inserted or integrated into a subject other than health education, with the exception of the primary grades. Science teachers tend to place emphasis on physiological processes and to skimp over the psychosocial and value aspects of family health education. Teachers in other subjects may likewise stress their area more than the desirable eclectic balance of physiology, psychosociology, and values. An imbalance may be countered by offering health instruction in the schools on a continuous, progressive, and comprehensive basis, from grades "K'" through 12. In this steadily evolving plan, family health education unfolds quite naturally and assumes a definite and an accepted place in the total school curriculum.*

4. *We offer such instruction with a special emphasis in either physiology, psychology, or morals. Instead, there needs to be a blending of physiology, psychosociology, and values. We need to teach both conduct and knowledge, and to make this education a part of personality-character development.*

5. *We plan syllabae or units directed specifically toward adolescent needs and interests alone. Content selected should also reflect heavily upon the developmental tasks of children and adolescents. By structuring the content solely on the basis of needs and interests, educators make a false assumption that children have a mature concept of values.*

6. *Teachers with little or no background in family living and sex education are assigned the responsibility of offering instruction and guidance in this area. Teachers need exposure to group-projection techniques, sensitivity training, psychology, sociology, health education, physiology, and family living courses. Above all, teachers need*

to have a good sense of humor, a healthy and mature outlook on life, and also be able to relate and communicate effectively with youngsters.

7. *The study guide for teachers is used alone. Instead, before teaching a topic, the teacher should specify in writing exactly what will be taught and how it will be taught. Such lesson plans should be approved by the school administration and a copy kept on file in the principal's office for reference.*

8. *We borrow or copy another school's successful family health education program. The content may be similar, but subcultural groups in the two communities may be different. Instead of borrowing, schools should adapt and evolve a program to suit the needs, interests, and developmental tasks of their particular students.*

9. *A part of the school's program is not directed toward adult education in family life. Such programs would help to keep the parents continuously informed about the ongoing units in family health education. Then, too, many parents need sex education and such classes should be offered to make the parents feel more adequate and at ease with their children. It would also give them a sense of belonging and of having a hand in the program.*

10. *We initiate such programs without properly preparing the pupils, the parents, the school administrators, the churches, and the community as a whole. Since education is a shared responsibility, all segments of the community must be oriented to the program. One of the best ways of doing this would be to form a school health education council. The family health education committee would be part of this council. Such a council and committee would provide the school with the social machinery that is needed to get acceptance for the program.*

The best advice for those involved or about to be involved with such programs is to avoid bootlegging family health education into the schools. Second, the effort should be undertaken with the development of a comprehensive health education program. By so doing, numerous opportunities will be opened up for much-needed instruction about personal, family, and community well-being. Such an approach would provide numerous opportunities to crystallize and reinforce the value system of youngsters and to make life in school, the home, and community more meaningful and worthwhile.

In light of the discussion above, peruse the following lesson plans, keeping in mind that they are indicative of the type of lessons that you would be expected to implement in this content area. Remember that they are only exemplary in nature and by no means encompass a complete unit. They are simply provided as a guide or basis for the formation of a complete unit dealing with family life and sexual education.

. . . .

TOPIC: FAMILY RESPONSIBILITIES

Grade Level: Primary

Outcome: The student will be able to define the various responsibilities of each member of the family.

Concept: Every person has family responsibilities.

Content: Responsibilities of family members are:

1. Mother and/or Father
   a) keeps house clean
   b) washes/irons clothes
   c) mends clothes
   d) buys groceries
   e) cooks meals
   f) takes care of all of us
   g) has a job sometimes
2. Father and/or Mother
   a) works at a job
   b) earns money
   c) helps around the house
   d) takes care of garden/lawn
   e) fixes things

Learning Experience

1. *Puppet show:* Pupils put on a puppet show. The written dialogues for "The Rabbit Family" are included merely as a guide for teachers, and teachers should structure the situation for their pupils and encourage children to make own puppets, evolve, and ad-lib the dialogue.

3. Me
   a) help with dishes
   b) help prepare meals
   c) make my bed
   d) clean up room
   e) pick up toys
   f) polish own shoes
   g) feed pet
   h) take care of younger brother or sister
   i) hang up clothes
   j) take out trash
   k) help with garden/lawn

The Rabbit Family

by Christine West

Characters:	Father, Mother, Brother Peter, Sister Susie, Narrator
Narrator:	Once again in the household of the Rabbit family, they see how important it is for each member to assume responsibility, to perform certain duties, and to cooperate. Sharing in the responsibility makes work easier for everybody and makes a happier family.
Mother:	Good morning, Father Rabbit.
Father:	Good morning, Mother Rabbit, and good morning, my children. Isn't this a beautiful Saturday morning? Perhaps we should use this fine day for a family picnic, since I don't have to work in the carrot factory today.
Susie/Peter:	Oh yes, Daddy. Let's go to the big meadow for a picnic. (Jump.)
Mother:	Yes, that sounds like fun. But before we leave for the day, we all have some responsibilities to take care of. Each one of us has a few duties to help the family to run smoothly.
Father:	That's right. We must all cooperate and help one another. If we all do our duties quickly and help one another, we will have more time for fun and play.
Susie:	I think that is nice to help other people because when you need help, they will help you back. That makes life a little easier for everybody.
Peter:	Susie and I will clean our rooms like we always do, then I can take out the trash and help Dad in the yard.

Susie:	And when I'm done cleaning my room, I will dust the furniture and help Mommy. If I feed the baby his carrot juice, Mommy can mend Daddy's shirts so that he will have some clothes to wear. Then together we can pack a picnic lunch.
Father:	I will fix Peter's bicycle and mow the lawn.
Mother:	Fine. Let's all do our duties so that we can have a fun afternoon. (Everybody down.)
Narrator:	Two hours have passed.
Father:	Well, my rabbit family, are we ready to go and enjoy the rest of this beautiful day?
Mother:	Yes, dear, I think that we are.
Susie & Peter:	Yes. Let's go.
Mother:	I feel so good now. If we didn't all cooperate together, I would have to do everything! Thank you, children.
Susie & Peter:	It was fun to do the chores with you!
All:	We are all happy helping each other!
(Curtain goes down!)	
Narrator:	That's all folks!

Key Questions

1. Did you like the puppet show?
2. Weren't all of our actors and puppets great?
3. Which puppet did you like the most? Why?
4. Would you like to help mother rabbit or father rabbit?
5. Do you help mom and dad with chores at home?
6. What chores do you have each day?

2. *Alternative learning experiences*
   a) *Posters* illustrating chores.
   b) *Inventory:* "Do you help?" (See p. 447.) Have children react to it at end of puppet show.
   c) *Film: Beaver Valley.* Animal film of how beaver families live.
   d) *Film: Families,* for primary grades, 10 min. Order from: Perennial Education Inc., 1825 Willow Road, Northfield, Ill., 60093.

b) *Filmstrip: How Shall I Tell My Child About Sex?* (for teacher)

c) *Demonstration:* Raise gerbils

Purpose: To explain reproduction in mammals to make children aware of the animal family unit.

Procedure: Purchase a pair of gerbils 9-12 weeks prior to the beginning of unit. Sexual maturity occurs between 11 and 12 weeks. This gives the gerbils time to get used to each other. Gerbils will mate by 14 weeks. The gestation period is 24-30 days. Since the pregnant gerbil gains very little weight, it is often difficult to tell whether a gerbil is pregnant.

Both mother and father are affectionate toward the babies, and there is no reason to separate the parents. A hamster cage may be used. Use hamster litter or cedar shavings as a floor cover for the cage. Gerbils are odorless rodents and hence very clean. The cage needs to be cleaned about every two weeks. They nibble on sunflower seeds and corn. Carrots, celery, and lettuce may also be included in the diet. Keep the diet high in protein and low in fat. Add a little evaporated milk to the diet during pregnancy and nursing. Gerbils drink very little water, but water should be provided in a trough so that they can drink in a standing, upright manner.

Do not handle gerbils after a litter is born or attempt to clean the cage, as they are very sensitive at this time.

For more insight on raising gerbils in the classroom, refer to: D. G. Robinson, *How to Raise and Train Gerbils*, T.F.H. Publications Inc., New Jersey City, 1967.

. . . .

TOPIC: FEMALE REPRODUCTIVE SYSTEM

Grade Level: Intermediate

Major Outcome: The student will be able to summarize how the female reproductive system helps a woman to have babies.

Major Concept: The reproductive system helps a woman to have babies.

Outcome I: The student will be able to describe how many forms of life start as tiny eggs.

Concept I: Chickens come from eggs.

Content	Learning Experiences
1. The egg is made inside the mother. 2. The egg grows in the nest. 3. The egg contains all the nourishment the baby needs.	1. Picture illustrations (fish, birds, reptiles, humans) and descriptions by teacher. 3M-SHES overhead projection

Concept II: Humans come from eggs.

Content	Learning Experiences
1. The egg is made inside the mother. 2. The egg grows inside the mother. 3. The egg gets its nourishment from the mother.	1. Description by teacher 2. Illustrate size of human egg and compare to common objects of similar size.

Outcome II: The student will be able to identify the four basic parts in the female reproductive system.

Concept I: Four basic parts make up the female reproductive system.

Content

1. There are two ovaries (size of almond nuts).
2. There are two fallopian tubes.
3. The uterus is a muscle.
4. The vagina is a canal.

Learning Experience

1. *Matching bee:* teacher using the flannel board; shows the basic parts. Use a green or blue background for flannel board and have all parts white in color.

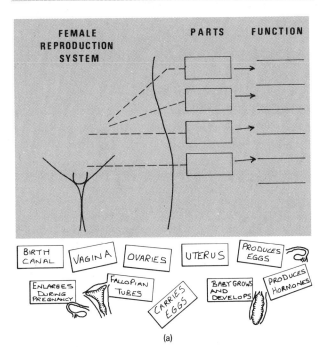

(a)

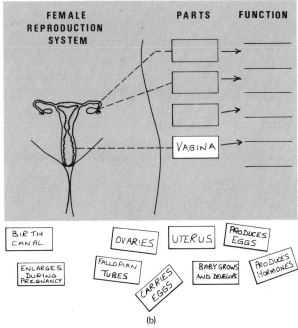

(b)

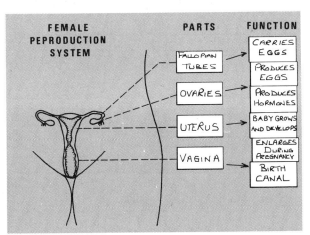

(c)

Fig. 25.2 Using a matching bee to teach about the female reproductive system. In (a) the parts, their names, and their functions are mobile. The parts and their names have been matched on the outline of the body in part (b). The matching bee has been completed in part (c).

Concept II: The sex organs are located in the lower part of the abdomen.

Content	*Learning Experience*
1. There is one ovary on each side of the body.	1. *Matching bee:* Teacher using the flannel board; shows the location of the basic parts.
2. The fallopian tube goes from the ovaries to the uterus.	
3. The uterus is between the two ovaries.	
4. The vagina is below the uterus.	

Concept III: Each part of the female reproduction system has a different function in helping a woman to have a baby.

Content	*Learning Experiences*
1. The ovaries produce the egg and sex hormones.	1. *Matching bee:* Teacher using flannel board; shows the function of each part.
2. The fallopian tubes fertilize the egg and carry the egg to the uterus.	2. *Alternative learning experiences:*
3. The uterus stores the egg.	a) *Matching bee:* Teacher and pupil. Use flannel board with mobile parts and functions. Match all three on a cardboard silhouette outline of lower abdominal area (see Figs. 25.2 and 25.3).
4. The vagina is the birth canal.	

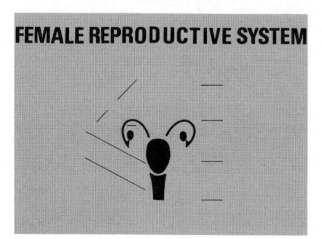

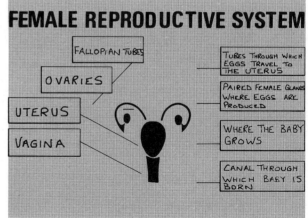

b) *Film: The Story of Menstruation* by Walt Disney.

c) *Film: Human and Animal Beginning*, 1966, 13 min. Order from: Perennial Education Inc., 1825 Willow Road, Northfield, Ill., 60093.

Key Questions

1. Where does the ovary come from?
2. What is the function of the ovary?
3. How do the eggs get from the ovary to the uterus?
4. What are the four main parts of the female reproductive system?

. . . .

TOPIC: MALE REPRODUCTIVE SYSTEM

Grade Level: Intermediate

Outcome: The student will be able to describe the structure and function of the male reproductive system.

Concept: The male reproductive system is an integral aspect of the process of conception.

Content: Key components of male reproductive system are:

1. Testes
2. Epididymis
3. Vas deferens

Learning Experience

1. *Matching Bee:* Teacher uses the flannel board to show the location of the basic parts. (See female reproductive system lesson plan as an example.)

◀ **Fig. 25.3** An alternative suggestion for a matching bee on the reproductive system. The parts are all of the same color, and the outline of the pelvic area has been omitted.

4. Seminal vesicles
5. Prostate gland
6. Cowper's glands
7. Penis
8. Urethra

Key Questions

1. Where are sperm produced?
2. What route do sperm take out of the male reproductive system?
3. What contribution do the seminal vesicles, prostate gland, and Cowper's glands make to the male aspect of the reproductive process?
4. What is the key structural difference between the male and the female urethra?

. . . .

TOPIC: MENSTRUATION

Grade Level: Intermediate

Outcome I: The student will be able to describe the process of menstruation.

Concept: Menstruation is the shedding of the inner lining of the uterus.

Content	*Learning Experiences*
1. Thick inner lining does not receive a fertilized egg. 2. Thick lining is made up of endometrial cells and rich supply of blood vessels. 3. Cells and blood vessels discarded as flow. 4. Menstrual flow occurs for a period of several days, hence menstrual period.	1. *Film: The Story of Menstruation,* by Walt Disney. Order from Association Films (10 min, color). Teacher should first introduce film by suggesting what pupils should look for in the film. This may be done by listing key words on the blackboard: pituitary gland ovaries

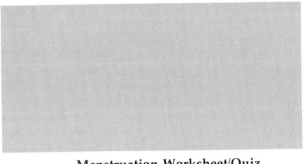

fallopian tubes
uterus
ovulation
menstruation

2. *Worksheet:* To accompany film showing. Work sheet may be used by pupils during the showing of the film or as a quiz or review after the showing of the film.

Menstruation Worksheet/Quiz

Directions: Select the best answer.

1. The pituitary gland:
   a) sends out growth hormones
   b) is located in the upper arm
   c) affects the ovaries
   *d) a and c

2. Ovulation:
   a) occurs every other week
   b) is when the uterus lining is discarded
   *c) is the process in which a ripe egg leaves the ovary
   d) involves the liver and the small intestine

3. Menstruation occurs:
   a) every 14 days
   b) every other week
   *c) about every 28 days
   d) every three months

4. What is the correct sequence of passage for the egg?
   a) ovary, uterus, fallopian tubes, vagina
   *b) ovary, fallopian tubes, uterus, vagina
   c) uterus, ovary, vagina, fallopian tubes

5. A special lining of blood and tissue builds up in the:
   *a) uterus
   b) ovaries
   c) fallopian tubes

* Correct answer is marked with the asterisk.

6. The menstrual period usually lasts:
   a) 3-10 days
   *b) 4-5 days
   c) 10-15 days
   d) 28 days
7. Menstruation is:
   a) a basic part of growing up for a girl
   b) one long, natural, continuous cycle of life
   c) should be regular within each girl
   *d) all of above
8. Suggest five ways a girl can take care of herself during the menstrual days.

Suggestion: teacher should stop the film whenever she or he wishes to emphasize or clarify a point or to direct student's attention to an answer on the work sheet.

Key Questions

1. What is menstruation?
2. Where does it occur?
3. What is the purpose of menstruation?
4. Is menstruation a normal process?
5. Do all girls and women experience it?
6. Does menstruation continue into old age?
7. How long may the menstrual cycle be?
8. What is the normal length for a girl?
9. Should a girl avoid bathing and swimming during her menstrual period?
10. Is exercise harmful or helpful during the menstrual period?
11. What kind of attitude should a girl have during menstruation?

3. *Alternative suggestion:* Should film not be available, the process of menstruation should be explained by use of:
   a) Picture illustrations

b) The Story of the Four Seasons (compare the process of menstruation to nature's cycle of the seasons).

The four seasons compared to menstruation

Seasons	Tree (one-year cycle)	Process of menstruation in young girl (28-day cycle)
Winter	During the winter the tree is dormant, but while it is dormant it prepares for spring internally.	It is during this time of the month that the ovaries receive a hormone which triggers the production and maturation of an egg.
Spring	During the spring the tree begins to grow, and new leaves begin to appear.	It is at this stage that the egg is really beginning to mature and at the same time nature prepares the uterus for its arrival by lining the walls of the uterus with a soft lining called endometrium.
Summer	In the summer the tree continues to grow, but it now also begins to prepare for fall and the eventual onset of winter.	The egg continues to grow and is now mature and released from the ovaries into the fallopian tubes. If the egg is not fertilized, it is then passed to the uterus and disintegrates.
Fall	During the fall the tree begins to shed its leaves and prepare for winter.	Since the egg has disintegrated, the endometrium lining is no longer needed so the uterus releases the lining to the vagina where it is then passed to the outside. The cycle is now ended and the body begins the entire process again.

Outcome II: The student will demonstrate understanding of the process of menstruation.

Concept: The process of menstruation prepares the woman's body to have a baby.

Content: The process of menstruation involves:

1. Pituitary gland secretes growth hormones.
2. Growth hormones activate ovaries to secrete mature sex hormones and eggs.
3. Sex hormones activate inner lining of uterus to thicken.
4. One egg released about every 28 days.
5. If egg is not fertilized, menstruation begins.
6. Inner lining (endometrium) of uterus is shed.
7. Shedding called menstrual flow.

Learning Experiences

1. Film
2. Worksheet
3. Key questions

Outcome III: The student will be able to accept menstruation as a natural process of living.

Concept: Menstruation is a natural cyclic process.

Content: Ways in which menstruation is a natural process are:

1. A continuous cycle
2. Occurs once a month (28 days)
3. Happens to all girls
4. Starts between ages 9 and 17
5. A part of growing up
6. Process of preparing a girl's body to have children
7. Lasts three to seven days
8. A part of becoming a woman

Learning Experiences

1. Film
2. Worksheet
3. Key questions

Outcome IV: Girls will be able to practice good menstrual hygiene.

Concept: There are ways of caring for the body during the menstrual period.

Content: Ways of caring for the body during menstruation are:

1. Shower daily.
2. Exercise moderately.
3. Eat a balanced diet every day.
4. Sleep eight or more hours.
5. Drink plenty of liquids.
6. Maintain good, correct posture.
7. Keep yourself well groomed.
8. Keep a calendar record of your periods.
9. Go to doctor if your periods are very irregular or if you have other problems.

Learning Experiences

1. Film
2. Worksheet
3. Key questions

REFERENCES AND BIBLIOGRAPHY

Duvall, Evelyn Millis. *About Sex and Growing Up* (New York: Association Press, 1968).

Growing Up and Liking It (Milltown, N.J.: Personal Products Co., 1969).

Guyton, Arthur. *Function of the Human Body* (Philadelphia: Saunders, 1960).

Kirkpatrick, Clifford. *The Family, As Process and Institution.* (New York: Ronald Press, 1955).

Lerrigo, Marion, and Michael Cassidy. *A Doctor Talks to 9-to-12-Year-Olds* (Chicago: Budlong Press, 1964).

Lerrigo, Marion, and Helen Southard. *A Story About You* (Washington, D.C.: NEA and AMA, 1966).

The Miracle of You, What it Means to Be A Girl (Neenah, Wisc.: Kotex Products, Kimberly-Clark Corporation, 1968).

Robinson, D. G. *How to Raise and Train Gerbils* (Jersey City: T.F.H. Publications, 1967).

Sorochan, Walter. "Don't Bootleg Sex Education Into the Schools," *Kentucky Association for Health, Physical Education, and Recreation Journal* (April 1969): 12-14.

Very Personally Yours (Neenah, Wisc.: Kimberly-Clark Corporation).

Winch, Robert. *The Modern Family* (New York: Holt, Rinehart and Winston, 1963).

index